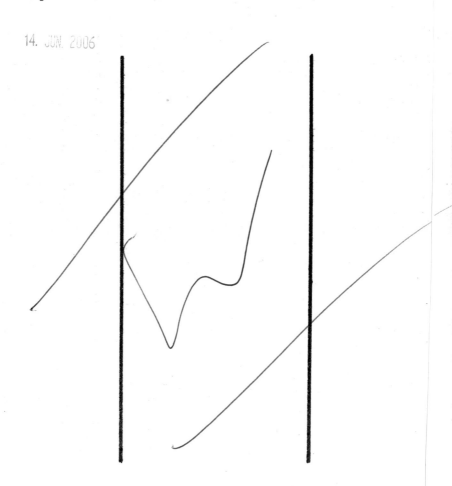

Telepsychiatry and e-mental health

Edited by

Richard Wootton

Centre for Online Health, University of Queensland, Brisbane, Australia

Peter Yellowlees

Centre for Online Health, University of Queensland, Brisbane, Australia

Paul McLaren

South London and Maudsley NHS Trust London, UK

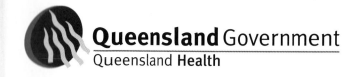

Queensland Government
Queensland **Health**

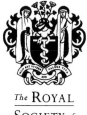

South London and Maudsley
NHS Trust

The ROYAL
SOCIETY *of*
MEDICINE
PRESS *Limited*

British Library Cataloguing in Publication Data
A catalogue record for this book is available from the British Library

ISBN: 1-85315459-7

Typeset by Phoenix Photosetting, Chatham, Kent

Printed by Bell and Bain, Glasgow

▶ Contents

Telepsychiatry and e-mental health

Edited by

Richard Wootton

Centre for Online Health, University of Queensland, Brisbane, Australia

Peter Yellowlees

Centre for Online Health, University of Queensland, Brisbane, Australia

Paul McLaren

South London and Maudsley NHS Trust London, UK

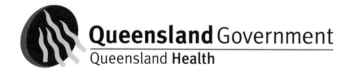

Queensland Government
Queensland **Health**

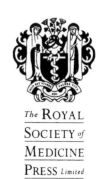

The ROYAL
SOCIETY *of*
MEDICINE
PRESS *Limited*

South London and Maudsley
NHS Trust

British Library Cataloguing in Publication Data
A catalogue record for this book is available from the British Library

ISBN: 1-85315459-7

Typeset by Phoenix Photosetting, Chatham, Kent

Printed by Bell and Bain, Glasgow

► Contents

► List of Contributors

Paul Baker Mental Health Foundation, London, UK

Chris Ball South London and Maudsley NHS Trust, London, UK

Svein Bergvik Telenor Research and Development, Norway

Luke Birmingham University of Southampton, Southampton, UK

Ilse Blignault Centre for Online Health, University of Queensland, Brisbane, Australia

Anne Buist Department of Psychiatry, University of Melbourne, Austin Repatriation Medical Centre, West Heidelberg, Australia

Robbie Campbell St Joseph's Health Centre, London, UK

Kate Cavanagh Ultrasis plc, London, UK

William J. Chimiak Center for Health Sciences Communication, Brody School of Medicine at East Carolina University, Greenville, North Carolina, USA

Helen Christensen Centre for Mental Health Research, Australian National University, Canberra, Australia

David Cook University of Kansas Medical Center, Kansas City, USA

Catherine Ebenezer South London and Maudsley NHS Trust, London, UK

Deede Gammon Norwegian Centre for Telemedicine, Tromsø, Norway

Harry Gelber Royal Children's Hospital, Melbourne, Australia

Kathleen M. Griffiths Centre for Mental Health Research, Australian National University, Canberra, Australia

John M. Grohol Cape Cod Institute, Greenwich CT, USA

Chloe Groves Centre for Mental Health Research, Australian National University, Canberra, Australia

Esther Gwinnell Department of Psychiatry, Oregon Health Sciences University, Portland, Oregon, USA

Donald Hilty University of California Davis, Sacramento, USA

Robert C. Hsiung Department of Psychiatry, University of Chicago, Illinois, USA

Martin A. Jenssen Norwegian Centre for Telemedicine, Tromsø, Norway

Barbara Johnston Kaiser Permanente, Oakland, California, USA

Robert King Department of Psychiatry, University of Queensland, Brisbane, Australia

Sarah Leonard School of Nursing and Midwifery, University of Southampton, Southampton, UK

Paul McCrone Centre for the Economics of Mental Health, Health Services Research Department, Institute of Psychiatry, Kings College London, UK

Paul McLaren South London and Maudsley NHS Trust, London, UK

Edward Alan Miller Department of Health Management and Policy, University of Michigan, Ann Arbor, USA

Wendy Reid Kids Help Line, Brisbane, Australia

David Shapiro Universities of Leeds and Sheffield, UK

Scott C. Simmons Center for Health Sciences Communications, Brody School of Medicine at East Carolina University, Greenville, North Carolina, USA

Susan Simpson Department of Clinical and Counselling Psychology, Royal Cornhill Hospital, Aberdeen, UK

Warner V. Slack Departments of Medicine and Psychiatry, Harvard Medical School, Massachusetts, USA

Ashley Spaulding University of Kansas Medical Center, Kansas City, USA

Darren Spooner Norfolk Mental Health Care NHS Trust, UK

Jean Starling Department of Psychological Medicine, The Children's Hospital at Westmead, Sydney, Australia

Gunnvald B. Svendsen Telenor Research and Development, Tromsø, Norway

Doug Urness Alberta Mental Health Board, Ponoka, Canada

Lydia Weisser Medical College of Georgia, Augusta, USA

Vivian L. West Center for Health Sciences Communication, Brody School of Medicine at East Carolina University, Greenville, North Carolina, USA

Richard Wootton Centre for Online Health, University of Queensland, Brisbane, Australia

Peter Yellowlees Centre for Online Health, University of Queensland, Brisbane, Australia

Jason Zack JSZ Behavioral Science Inc., USA

Charles Zaylor University of Kansas Medical Center, Kansas City, USA

► Foreword

Mental Health is often described as the 'Cinderella of health services' despite the huge burden which mental illness places on the public health. Even in the industrialized world, it is a challenge for services to meet demand. In much of the developing world, suffering from mental illness goes without recognition. Most treatment-delivery episodes involve a service user meeting with a professional. Thus mental health services are expensive in terms of human resources and vulnerable to geographical inequalities in service delivery.

The title of this book is *Telepsychiatry and E-mental Health*. Telepsychiatry is that area of telemedicine, which has explored the use of communications technology in mental health service delivery. The technology most often used has been videoconferencing, connected by analogue or digital communications links. E-mental health incorporates information technology and the development of computerized therapies.

The notion that communications technology can enhance mental health service is not new. The earliest reports in the literature date from the late 1950s when an interactive television link was used in Nebraska to connect a teaching hospital department of psychiatry with a state institution. This work raised issues, which have recurred in subsequent telepsychiatry research. These are how best to use communications technology to:

1. improve the quality of care for service users in institutions
2. address geographical inequalities in access to mental health care
3. improve clinical communications between mental health service professionals
4. deliver psychotherapy
5. deliver new educational opportunities to staff working in remote institutions.

Although these issues are not entirely resolved, the practice of telepsychiatry is becoming well established in many health systems around the world and is also being translated into the Internet era, where it is becoming known as 'e-mental health'.

This book is the first substantial academic review of the fields of telepsychiatry and e-mental health, and it covers over 20 years of experience from all around the world. The book has a significant Australian flavour, which is appropriate since, for example, organizations like Queensland Health have used telemedicine for health service provision for many years. Indeed, the partnership of a major health service with the Centre for Online Health at the University of Queensland has resulted in a substantial number of research papers demonstrating that telepsychiatry and e-mental health techniques do indeed offer promising solutions to the problems of delivering mental health care. This is particularly important in a state like Queensland, which is larger than Texas, but has a population of only 3.8 million people. Not surprisingly, many Queenslanders find access to health services very difficult for geographical reasons.

Telepsychiatry and E-mental Health covers both clinical and educational work and describes three major types of technologies: videoconferencing, the Internet and the conventional telephone. The editors have selected highly experienced practitioners from a wide range of clinical and academic centres on three continents. All of the major mental health disciplines, including medicine, psychology, nursing and social work, are represented. This gives the book an unusually broad perspective. Patients with mental health problems are increasingly being treated by multidisciplinary teams of clinicians, and in future will receive improved access to care using the sorts of techniques and technologies described in this book. Whilst electronic mental health services will never replace face-to-face care – nor should they – they will increasingly be integrated into face-to-face programmes. Just as patients now quite commonly email their psychiatrists, so in future they will increasingly receive assessment and therapy electronically if they so choose. Mental disorders such as depression, anxiety and substance abuse are increasingly recognized around the world as being very substantial public health burdens with enduring economic and social costs. It is vital that the sorts of approaches described in this book are further explored, and that the challenges, particularly to prove that these techniques can improve health outcomes, are taken up.

This book will be of great service to clinicians, and to patients, around the world. It will help to guide the development of twenty first century mental health services and should help to ensure that health care becomes more accessible and affordable for those who are at present out of reach of such services. The overwhelming message of the book is that 'no one size fits all' and that there are now many different approaches that can be used to deliver mental health care electronically. As such the chapters can be read independently, depending on the reader's specific interest, and as a whole they provide an extensive review of the latest global literature, ideas, thoughts, technologies and approaches in this exciting field. Queensland Health is pleased to have been able to assist in its publication.

Dr Robert Stable
Director General
Queensland Health

▶ Preface

This is the fourth book in the Royal Society of Medicine's telemedicine series. Its predecessors are:

- *The Legal and Ethical Aspects of Telemedicine*, B.A. Stanberry, 1998
- *Introduction to Telemedicine*, R. Wootton and J. Craig (eds), 1999
- *Teledermatology*, R. Wootton and A.M.M. Oakley (eds), 2002

The present volume describes how telemedicine applies to psychiatry and mental health generally. The book represents the collective experience of practitioners in different parts of the world, practising a wide range of telepsychiatry and related applications. Both the South London and Maudsley NHS Trust in the UK, and Queensland Health in Australia, have extensive experience of these techniques. It is a pleasure to acknowledge the support of these major health service organizations in the production of the book. We think that anyone involved in telemedicine will find the material interesting because much of it is relevant to other fields than simply mental health.

The aim of the book is principally to permit those who are involved in mental health to begin to assess how telemedicine might be applied to their working practice. Clinicians should find it particularly useful, of course, but many chapters are also of relevance to health service managers, planners and information technology staff. Parts of the book may also be useful to patients themselves.

The book is an eclectic collection of essays. Contributors have come from Europe, North America and Australasia, and work in a variety of medical, technical and administrative specialties. The majority are practising clinicians with substantial practical experience of telemedicine and health informatics.

The book is divided into four sections:

1. An introductory section dealing with background information about telemedicine and online health in relation to psychiatry, including technical matters.
2. A section describing the global experience of diagnosis and patient management using real-time video techniques.
3. A section concerning e-mental health and the Internet, especially distance education, for the patient, the doctor and the student.
4. A final section about techniques which look promising for the future, but which are currently experimental. This includes the development of standards, a topic, which is still in its infancy in telemedicine generally.

We hope you enjoy reading it.

Richard Wootton and Peter Yellowlees
Brisbane, Australia
Paul McLaren
London, UK
November 2002

Section 1: Background and Technical Matters

1. **Introduction**
   Peter Yellowlees, Edward Alan Miller, Paul McLaren and Richard Wootton

2. **Telecommunications and Videoconferencing for Psychiatry**
   Scott C. Simmons, Vivian L. West and William J. Chimiak

3. **Health Economics of Telepsychiatry**
   Paul McCrone

4. **Telepsychiatry and Doctor–Patient Communication – an analysis of the empirical literature**
   Edward Alan Miller

5. **E-therapy: Opportunities, Dangers and Ethics to Guide Practice**
   Robert C. Hsiung

6. **Cybermedicine in Psychiatry and Psychology – a personal recollection**
   Warner V. Slack

▶ 1

Introduction

Peter Yellowlees, Edward Alan Miller, Paul McLaren and Richard Wootton

Introduction

Telepsychiatry has generally been thought of as being the delivery of health care and the exchange of health care information for purposes of providing psychiatric services across distances. This is essentially a reworking of the generic definition of telemedicine which was used in the introductory book in this series.[1] The relatively recent term 'e-mental health', however, is increasingly being applied, and is widely used by authors in the present book. E-mental health typically relates to mental health services provided through any form of electronic medium, most commonly via the Internet or telephony. This is in contrast to the more traditional term, telepsychiatry, which is still primarily used in reference to videoconferencing. Although their technological emphasis differs somewhat, e-mental health and telepsychiatry both relate to the providers' and patients' ability to access specialist knowledge through the use of telecommunications and information technologies. While teleconsultations between a patient and/or their primary care provider, and a psychiatrist or mental health specialist are generally performed for either diagnostic or management reasons, they are frequently used for educational purposes, particularly among providers, as well as for administration. Not only has there been a convergence of technologies, but there has increasingly been a convergence in terminologies as much of e-mental health now incorporates what has traditionally been called health informatics or telematics.

Equipment for telepsychiatry and e-mental health

As noted in previous books in this series,[1,2] the fundamental components of a telemedicine system required to bring about an interaction between a therapist and a patient are a means of information capture, a means of information transport and a means of information display. This interaction is almost always a two-way process and can be done either in real time or in a pre-recorded fashion, often called 'store and forward'.

Real-time telepsychiatry primarily uses videoconferencing or telephony for real-time clinical interactions, while store and forward systems transfer pre-recorded information in a fashion that allows it to be dealt with at a convenient time. E-mental health on the Internet raises the interesting possibility of both styles of care being provided with the same equipment.

Telepsychiatry and e-mental health can be practised almost anywhere if the appropriate equipment is available and there is access to adequate communications bandwidth. Telemedicine patients in general have been seen in clinics and hospitals, in their own homes, in nursing homes, in remote locations around the globe and even in space. Increasingly satellite systems are being used to reach remote locations, while DSL (digital subscriber line) connections allow faster downloads via ordinary telephone networks. In this book, for example, e-mental health systems are described that use a wide array of telecommunications including ordinary telephone lines, digital lines such as ISDN, T1 leased lines, microwave links, mobile phones, ATM (asynchronous transfer mode) systems and fibreoptic cables. The networks include local area networks, wide area networks and of course the Internet. E-health, a term that is increasingly being used in place of telemedicine, is now possible in ways that were not even conceivable a decade ago. In this book some sophisticated futuristic e-mental health systems, proposals and possibilities are described, but they represent only one end of a spectrum that also includes simple telephony-based systems for transmission of ordinary voice or low resolution videoconferencing.

Background

Mental health care seems especially well suited for telemedicine since most diagnostic and treatment information is gathered audio-visually.[3,4] There is also little need for laboratory tests for consultation or diagnosis. Not surprisingly, therefore, most early telemedicine applications were psychiatric in nature. The first reported use of telemedicine, for example, took place during the 1950s and 1960s at the Nebraska Psychiatric Institute, which initially used closed circuit television for medical education purposes,[5] followed by group psychotherapy,[6] consultation, assessment, collaboration and teaching.[7,8] The phrase telepsychiatry was subsequently coined in the early 1970s with Dwyer's[9] description of the Massachusetts General Hospital project, in which psychiatrists at the hospital consulted via closed circuit television with patients at a medical station located at the airport. Other early projects involved consultation between psychiatric consultants, family physicians and patients in rural New Hampshire[10] and child psychiatrists, nurses, inner city children and parents in New York City.[11]

Although early telepsychiatry projects such as these often closed or experienced usage reductions after the initial funding ran out,[12,13] government support and lower equipment and transmission costs has increased utilization over the last few years. The number of US-based telepsychiatry programmes, for example, grew from 9 to 29 between 1994 and 1998.[14] The total number of consultations also grew, increasing from 948 in 1994 to more than 8640 in 1998. At an average of 48 consultations per month, however, individual programme activity is still comparatively low. Relatively few rural facilities, moreover, use telemedicine, and even among those that do, the number of teleconsultations is typically small.[15]

A variety of factors have contributed to the slow adoption of telepsychiatry and telemedicine, including a general lack of third party reimbursement, state licensing requirements, inadequate telecommunication networks, and insufficient privacy and security standards. Another often cited barrier is the dearth of evaluation data about the effects of telemedicine.[16–19] While much of the literature supports the feasibility of telepsychiatry and other applications,[4,20] data concerning its effect on cost, quality and access has been somewhat limited. This is a point highlighted by Baer et al[4] who argued that 'additional studies are needed to determine when and for what age groups and conditions telepsychiatry is an effective way to deliver psychiatric services'. It is also an issue emphasized by Capner[21] who suggested that 'there is a dearth of evidence regarding the reliability of psychological services provided using videoconferencing', and by Liss et al[22] who concluded that 'there is currently a substantial gap between the widespread demand for [telehealth] and the scientific evidence supporting its efficacy and cost effectiveness'. Ball and McLaren[23] added that 'psychiatric assessment by videoconferencing remains at an early stage of development with much work to be done before it can be routinely employed as a clinical tool'.

To facilitate more research, numerous telemedicine evaluation frameworks have been proposed.[16,18,24,25] To varying degrees all emphasize the careful specification of evaluation methods, including the application of experimental and quasi-experimental designs. Most also suggest a comparison of costs and benefits, or costs and effects and, not surprisingly, that investigators ascertain the effect of telemedicine on cost, quality and access. The effect of telemedicine on quality is a particular concern given the novelty of the video medium in health and mental health care.

In thinking about the relationship between quality and telemedicine, it is helpful to consider Donabedian's[26] distinction between medicine's technical and interpersonal components.[27] While the technical dimension refers to the clinical processes of care (e.g. diagnosis, treatment and follow-up) and its outcomes (e.g. health status, quality of life), the interpersonal dimension refers to the social and psychological aspects of treatment, including user acceptance and satisfaction, and the doctor–patient relationship. Many researchers have emphasized the technical dimensions of quality; that is, whether telepsychiatry adversely affects clinical diagnosis and outcomes. Others, however, have explored user acceptance and satisfaction, finding that while patients appear willing to accept telepsychiatry after they have had some experience with it, providers exhibit considerably more resistance.[3,21] This is particularly true of general practitioners and psychiatry consultants who may be concerned about abdicating control of patient care, interrupting existing referral patterns, experiencing equipment failures and scheduling delays, not to mention the inconvenience of travelling to the telemedicine studio when desk-top systems are not available.[28–30] Non-physician providers appear to be more accepting.[20]

Essential components for telepsychiatry and e-mental health

Psychiatrists and other mental health clinicians were early adopters of telemedicine. This is because mental health consultations primarily involve taking a careful history, which is entirely possible via videoconferencing. Furthermore, history-taking has long occurred via the telephone, and more recently with the aid of computerized interviews.

Psychiatrists have always been particularly interested in communication, and more specifically in communication across a variety of media. The process of psychiatric diagnosis, moreover, is essentially one of observation, reasoning and deduction, without the need for frequent recourse to medical or pathological investigations. It is hardly surprising, therefore, that psychiatrists, such as Warner Slack as described in this book (see Chapter 6), have had longstanding interests in the application of technology to the diagnostic process.

Requirements for examination

In order to make a diagnosis a number of demographic details are required including the patient's age, sex, ethnicity and geographical residence. Of particular importance is the biological and cultural family history as well as the individual's personal history and experiences, or otherwise, of trauma and difficulty in their past. It is important to determine if patients have major medical problems and to examine their level of ingestion of medications as well as other substances such as alcohol, cigarettes, illegal drugs and caffeine. A history typically includes examination of each patient's relationships, assessments of their personality style and character, and most crucially, careful examination and documentation of their mental state at the time of the assessment.

The mental state assessment of the patient is the psychiatrist's core clinical objective and includes assessment of the patient's appearance, their behaviour, their conversation, for both its content and style and whether the patient suffers from any abnormalities of perception, such as hallucinations. It also includes an assessment of the patient's cognitive state – incorporating their memory, attention, orientation and thought processes, and a review of their capacity for insight and judgement into their situation. Finally, the mental state focuses on both the clinician's and patient's own perceptions regarding the danger that they pose to themselves and to others.

On a number of occasions it is crucial that physical examinations be performed, in addition to a variety of other medical investigations, including blood and urine screens, X-rays and EEGs.

Whilst the history and mental state assessment can be performed in real time on most e-mental health systems which allow good quality visual contact, it is of course not possible to perform physical examinations or diagnostic testing. These are normally arranged at the request of the psychiatrist by the patient's local medical providers, or, in the case of a physical examination, can be done by the patient's general practitioner if there are particular aspects of the physical examination, such as a tremor, which might be difficult to pick up over video. There have been a number of studies which confirm that videoconferencing allows a similar range of diagnostic accuracy to face-to-face psychiatric assessments, although such studies have not been performed when only email or telephone-based systems are used.

The advent of web-based systems of care, such as that described by Johnston in this book (see Chapter 19), will allow mental health therapists and patients to interact on the Internet in a therapeutic relationship using chat rooms, email and telephony. They will also allow patients to undergo structured cognitive behavioural programmes and receive mental health education individualized to their needs.

Psychotherapy

Mental health clinicians are increasingly providing their patients with health information. A relevant example is cognitive behavioural therapy, which requires that patients receive substantial amounts of education about their disorders. This is an area where e-mental health is particularly strong and where clinicians will increasingly be able to teach both patients and other providers through simultaneous video transactions, as well as through downloadable material available at Internet sites.

In respect of the delivery of psychotherapy, the potential of information technology for the delivery of talking treatments has long been recognized. Warner Slack in his chapter (see Chapter 6) gives a personal account of the development of his ideas in this area, while Kavanagh reviews the research on the computerization of cognitive behavioural therapies, a field with huge potential (see Chapter 20). Pychotherapy research has matured from the generation of models to a more evidence-based discipline, which allows for the dissection of effective treatment components. Developing computerized treatments continues the search for key elements, while challenging existing dogma. Telepsychiatry projects have also challenged the assumption that therapists and patients need to be in the same room to develop effective therapeutic relationships. Evidence supporting this statement is found in Miller's chapter in this volume (see Chapter 4).

Requirements for consultation

Security and privacy are the two core requirements for any telepsychiatry or e-mental health consultation. All systems must keep patient data secure, no matter whether consultation has taken place via video, email, telephony or in the form of electronic information. Privacy is crucial for both real-time and store and forward approaches. There are now a number of documented clinical guidelines (see Chapter 21) and ethical guidelines (see Chapter 5) available which have been published by groups in the USA, the UK and Australia. Some countries require certification for telepsychiatry practitioners to be able to claim government payments for their consultations. In Australia, this certification process is focused on ensuring that clinicians have a good understanding of prevailing clinical, technological and ethical practices.

During a video session there are now certain well-documented, clinically sensible ways of preparing the patient, of running the session itself, and of terminating the session. Patients need to understand the process fully before any consultation, and ideally should have a friend or colleague, or perhaps another provider sitting with them during the encounter. In telepsychiatry these consultation facilitators are often clinical case managers who are in effect acting as the specialist's hands and the patient's ears. This is an important role and it is one that will increasingly develop in the future, particularly in a discipline such as mental health where multidisciplinary-team-based treatment programmes are common.

No one has ever argued that videoconferenced psychiatric consultations are as good as in-person consultations. Consequently, telepsychiatry sessions should be interspersed with face-to-face meetings to allow a deeper doctor–patient relationship to develop over time. This may not always be possible for patients in very remote regions. Nonetheless, health systems should back up telepsychiatry programmes with face-to-face consultations, even if they are not necessarily by the same psychiatrist or mental health clinician.

Suitable cases for e-mental health

Patients with a remarkable range of diagnostic categories have been seen using telepsychiatry and e-mental health. At present there is no evidence that any particular group of patients is more or less likely to benefit from these techniques. Most studies show that a small proportion of patients find the technology difficult to manage, and would strongly prefer to be seen face to face. But such studies have also identified others, probably about 5% of those patients seen, who actually prefer to meet with their therapists electronically in some form or the other. This group of patients is often characterized by people who have phobic disorders or who are paranoid. They feel more in control using such consultations, and find it much less distressing to have consultations close to their homes, rather than having to travel long distances where the journey itself may be extremely anxiety provoking. As Slack notes in his chapter (see Chapter 6), there is also a group of patients who are much more open about their problems whilst using computers, and the ability within e-mental health to combine computer-based assessments with human assessments is likely to be particularly popular with these individuals.

All major diagnostic groupings of patients have been successfully assessed using telepsychiatry, including patients who are actively psychotic and hallucinating from the television screen through which they are consulting with a telepsychiatrist.[31] The bulk of psychiatric treatments have been performed electronically including most forms of assessment, cognitive and behavioural psychotherapy and insight-oriented psycho-therapies. The people who have more difficulty in the interaction are providers, rather than patients, and it is crucial to devote substantial effort to train providers in the best techniques and approaches to providing care over these systems. Such training needs to be continuing and to be based on adult learning processes; some of the better training programmes have provided this training via the videoconferencing equipment itself, literally training on the job.

Telepsychiatry for education

The provision of health information via telepsychiatry and the Internet is an area that is expanding rapidly. There are now a number of books (e.g. *The Patient's Internet*

Handbook[32] by Kiley and Graham) dealing specifically with health information provision by electronic means, particularly the Internet, and several of the chapters in this book have this as a major focus. Mental health, in particular, is a clinical area where the provision of good quality health information to patients is vital. Much of the cognitive behavioural therapies depend on the ability of patients to access high-quality information, and the whole area of 'bibliotherapy', the use of information for treatment, is by definition core to e-health and telepsychiatry. Large numbers of professional training programmes in mental health use telepsychiatry techniques, and medical students are increasingly being trained in an environment where the majority of their learning resources are captured and displayed electronically via the Internet. E-health has broadened the ability that teachers have to conduct sessions with their students, both locally and globally, an issue raised by Yellowlees in his chapter (see Chapter 22). As doctors and other health professionals are increasingly trained in programmes using adult learning principles, it is likely that e-health approaches will underpin a very high proportion of professional undergraduate and postgraduate education in the years to come.

Patient self-help

While some videoconferencing programmes are aimed at patients, and are used by support groups, it is mainly the Internet that will be the focus of self-help groups, programmes and educational initiatives in the future. Large numbers of patients are already using the Internet for accessing health information[33] and mental health professionals are frequently confronted by patients who have downloaded volumes of health information from the Internet. Of course the problem with much of the information so discovered is that it is unreliable at best, and mischievous at worst. The chapter by Christensen explores many of the issues surrounding patient information on the Internet (see Chapter 15), and provides examples of good quality websites that are available for patients, and which can be recommended by clinicians. There are some indications that patients with mental health disorders, who often feel isolated and stigmatized, use the Internet to a greater extent than patients with other disorders. The Internet has been described as a level playing field, and it is hardly surprising that people who may be anxious in real life find it easier to communicate and learn through such a medium. Certainly there has been a proliferation of self-help sites in the last few years and a number of excellent patient-focused portals also exist.

Legal aspects of telepsychiatry

The legal and ethical issues in telepsychiatry are generally the same as in any other branch of e-health or telemedicine. These have been extensively described in a number of books and documents, and of course vary between countries.[34] Whilst a number of psychiatrists have expressed very reasonable concerns about the legal implications of telepsychiatry, there is growing acceptance that these can be overcome. The area in which telepsychiatry is different from other specialties, of course, relates to the potential capacity of psychiatrists to write legal orders restricting or confining patients under relevant mental health act legislations. There is so far only one report in the literature[35] describing such a legal certification as having taken place using telepsychiatry. In this case, the psychiatrist interviewed a patient using videoconferencing and wrote a formal recommendation to a magistrate who accepted the telepsychiatry recommendation and implemented the Mental Health Act Order. There are other examples, in Australia, of videoconferencing being used by mental health guardianship boards who are empowered to make orders under the Act. In Victoria and in Queensland, for example, the Mental Health Act of 2002 mentions the use of videoconferencing as a medium by which psychiatrists may perform legal assessments.

Cross-boundary consultations continue to give rise to difficulties. Most state systems around the world, particularly in America and Australia, insist that practitioners are licensed to practice in the state in which the patient is situated. This potentially restricts the practice of telepsychiatry as it means that most practitioners, who are only registered in one state, can only practice within those state boundaries. In Australia, however, state medical boards are starting to look at mutual recognition issues, although in the USA this seems to be less the case.

The final medicolegal issue relates to standards and accountability. Large numbers of ethical and clinical standards are being developed for various e-mental health technologies, and these are reviewed in Chapters 5 and 21, by Hsiung, and Wootton and Blignault, respectively.

The current scene

A number of recent reviews have concluded[36-38] that videoconferencing is clinically effective. Whilst there are still relatively few trials with large numbers of patients, there does seem to be a growing body of evidence that supports the use of videoconferencing as an effective means of providing psychiatric services, mainly for diagnosis but also for treatment. As Internet-based videoconferencing becomes available we can expect that telepsychiatry processes will be transferred to the World Wide Web. This should be an effective medium for providing mental health services, and at least in theory, should be considerably cheaper. When combined with some of the technologies and processes discussed in the fourth section of this book, this should make mental health services much more accessible to patients around the world.

International collaborations

Telepsychiatry is regarded as being the most common form of real-time teleconsultation (i.e. excluding teleradiology). The most recent survey from the Association of Telehealth Service Providers, for example, suggested that mental health represented 40% of all teleconsultations in the USA in 2001.[39] Unlike some other areas in telemedicine, however, no international telepsychiatry or e-mental health organizations have evolved. This is despite the fact that there are now a number of case reports of international consultations occurring, and some email telemedicine programmes, such as that run by the Swinfen Charitable Trust (http://www.coh.uq.edu.au/swinfen [last checked 6 September 2002]) include psychiatric consultations that occur around the world. Major conferences, however, frequently feature substantial numbers of papers on telepsychiatry and e-mental health. The development of fast open communications on the Internet will facilitate such linkages, and will certainly improve educational initiatives in this area.

Conclusion

The two major trends in mental health care in the last quarter of the twentieth century have been the de-institutionalization of psychiatric services with a shift to community care and the resurgence in talking treatments including a rise in cognitive behavioural models. Community mental health services and the new psychotherapies are heavily dependent on human resources. Standards of delivery of community care have moved up the political agenda in many countries and models of case management have been developed to improve the coordination of care delivery. Information and communications technology has received little attention in the development of case management models and we believe this book is timely in highlighting its potential. In the UK tragic failures of community care in which mentally ill service users have committed homicide or suicide have stimulated wide public debate. They have been attributed at least in part to failures of communication and led to major revisions in service organization. While this has led to major revisions in service organization in order to improve communication, little attention has been paid to the role of information and communications technology. Email and electronic patient records (EPR) have not developed as rapidly in mental health care as in other specialities. Zaylor (see Chapter 10) highlights the importance of records following patients in the US penal system. The EPR in mental health will arise from a generic EPR, but it is essential that mental health services are not left behind.

A common finding in telepsychiatry outcome research has been the wariness of professionals to use mediated communication for therapeutic tasks, in contrast to the enthusiasm of service users. This user enthusiasm is apparent at all ages and across ethnic groups. The reasons for professional wariness are complex and range from ethical concerns about harming vulnerable users with an unknown treatment model to challenges to fundamental views on professional roles through to outright protectionism. These themes are explored in this book and their understanding will be critical to the further development of e-mental health.

Telepsychiatry and e-mental health are certainly here to stay. The authors who have contributed to this book have demonstrated, through the breadth and depth of their experiences, just how mature this discipline has become. The days of psychiatric treatment being delivered by Freud-like figures in an analytical style are gone and the future for e-mental health is bright, with mental health services being delivered widely around the world, in many different ways, but with an increasing emphasis on providing good access to care for patients any time, anywhere.

E-mental health has tremendous potential to improve the care of patients, and is now being practised in most western countries, with access to some programmes from underdeveloped nations. With illnesses such as depression, anxiety and substance disorders all rising rapidly in prevalence, telepsychiatry and e-mental health seem likely to be important approaches to providing effective mental health care on a global basis.

References

1   Wootton R, Craig J. *Introduction to Telemedicine*. London: Royal Society of Medicine Press, 1999.
2   Wootton R, Oakley A. *Teledermatology*. London: Royal Society of Medicine Press, 2002.
3   Maheu MM, Whitten P, Allen A. *E-Health Telehealth, and Telemedicine: a guide to start-up and success*. San Francisco: Jossey-Bass, 2001.
4   Baer L, Elford R, Cukor P. Telepsychiatry at forty: What have we learned? *Harvard Review of Psychiatry* 1997;**5**:7–17.
5   Wittson C, Dutton R. A new tool in psychiatric education. *Mental Hospitals* 1956;**7**:11–14.
6   Wittson CL, Afflect DC, Johnson V. Two-way television in group therapy. *Mental Hospitals* 1961;**12**:22–23.
7   Benschoter RA, Wittson CL, Ingham CG. Teaching and consultation by television. 1. Closed circuit collaboration. *Mental Hospitals* 1965;**16**:99–100.
8   Menolascino FJ, Osborne RG. Psychiatric television consultation for the mentally retarded. *American Journal of Psychiatry* 1970;**127**:515–520.
9   Dwyer TF. Telepsychiatry: psychiatric consultations by interactive television. *American Journal of Psychiatry* 1973;**130**:865–869.
10 Solow C, Weiss RJ, Bergen BJ, Sanborn CJ. 24-hour psychiatric consultation via TV. *American Journal of Psychiatry* 1971;**127**:1684–1687.
11 Straker N, Mostyn P, Marshall C. The use of two-way TV in bringing mental health services to the inner city. *American Journal of Psychiatry* 1976;**133**:1202–1205.
12 Maxmen JS. Telecommunications in psychiatry. *American Journal of Psychotherapy* 1978;**32**:450–456.
13 Baer L, Cukor P, Coyle JT. Telepsychiatry: application of telemedicine to psychiatry. In: Bashshur RL, Sanders JH, Shannon GW, eds. *Telemedicine: theory and practice*. Springfield, IL: CC Thomas, 1997:265–288.
14 Wheeler T, Allen A. Current telepsychiatry activity in the U.S., Australia, Canada, and Norway. Available at http://www.isft.org/interarticles/telemed.htm [last checked 12 September 2002].
15 Hassol A, Irvin C, Gaumer G, Puskin D, Mintzer C, Grigsby J. Rural applications of telemedicine. *Telemedicine Journal* 1997;**3**:215–225.
16 Joint Working Group on Telemedicine, Department of Commerce. Telemedicine Report to Congress, January 31, 1997. Available at http://www.ntia.doc.gov/reports/telemed/ [last checked 17 September 2002].
17 Bashshur RL. Rethinking the evaluation and priorities in telemedicine. *Telemedicine Journal* 1998;**4**:1–4.
18 Field MJ, ed. *Telemedicine: a guide to assessing telecommunications in health care*. Washington, DC: National Academy Press, 1996.
19 Grigsby J, Kaehny MM, Sandberg EJ, Schlenker RE, Shaughnessy PW. Effects and effectiveness of telemedicine. *Health Care Financing Review* 1995;**17**:115–131.
20 Grigsby J. Telemedicine in the United States. In: Bashshur RL, Sanders JH, Shannon GW, eds. *Telemedicine: theory and practice*. Springfield, IL: CC Thomas, 1997:291–325.
21 Capner M. Videoconferencing in the provision of psychological services at a distance. *Journal of Telemedicine and Telecare* 2000;**6**:311–319.
22 Liss HJ, Glueckauf RL. Ecklund-Johnson EP. Research in telehealth and chronic medical conditions: critical review, key issues, and future directions. *Rehabilitation Psychology* 2002;**47**:8–30.
23 Ball C, McLaren P. The tele-assessment of cognitive state: a review. *Journal of Telemedicine and Telecare* 1997;**3**:126–131.
24 Grigsby J, Schlenker RE, Kaehny MM, Shaughnessy PW, Sandberg EJ. Analytic framework for evaluation of telemedicine. *Telemedicine Journal* 1995;**1**:31–39.

25   Sisk JE, Sanders JH. A proposed framework for economic evaluation of telemedicine. *Telemedicine Journal* 1998;**4**:31–37.

26   Donabedian A. *Explorations in Quality Assessment and Monitoring: Vol 1 The Definition of Quality and Approaches to its Assessment.* Ann Arbor, MI: Health Administration Press, 1980.

27   Miller EA. Telemedicine's technical and interpersonal aspects: effects on doctor–patient communication. *Journal of Telemedicine and Telecare* 2003;**9**:1–7.

28   Reid J. *A Telemedicine Primer: understanding the issues.* Billings, MT: Innovative Medical Communications, 1996.

29   Shannon GW. Telemedicine and the health care system. In: Bashshur RL, Sanders JH, Shannon GW, eds. *Telemedicine: theory and practice.* Springfield, Illinois: CC Thomas, 1997:37–51.

30   Kavanagh S, Hawker F. The fall and rise of the South Australian telepsychiatry network. *Journal of Telemedicine and Telecare* 2001;**7**(suppl. 1):41–43.

31   Kavanagh SJ, Yellowlees PM. Telemedicine – clinical applications in mental health. *Australian Family Physician* 1995;**24**:1242–1247.

32   Kiley R, Graham E. *The Patient's Internet Handbook.* London: Royal Society of Medicine Press, 2002.

33   Yellowlees P. *Your Guide to eHealth – third millennium medicine on the Internet.* Brisbane: University of Queensland Press, 2001.

34   Stanbury B. *The Legal and Ethical Aspects of Telemedicine.* London: Royal Society of Medicine Press, 1998.

35   Yellowlees P. The use of telemedicine to perform psychiatric assessments under the Mental Health Act. *Journal of Telemedicine and Telecare* 1997;**3**:224–226.

36   Hilty DM, Luo JS, Morache C, Marcelo DA, Nesbitt TS. Telepsychiatry: an overview for psychiatrists. *CNS Drugs* 2002;**16**:527–548.

37   Roine R, Ohinmaa A, Hailey D. Assessing telemedicine: a systematic review of the literature. *Canadian Medical Association Journal* 2001;**165**:765–771.

38   Baer L, Elford DR, Cukor P. Telepsychiatry at forty: what have we learned? *Harvard Review of Psychiatry* 1997;**5**:7–17.

39   Dahlin MP, Watcher G, Engle WM, Henderson J. *2001 Report on US Telemedicine Activity.* Portland, OR: ATSP, 2001.

2

Telecommunications and Videoconferencing for Psychiatry

Scott C. Simmons, Vivian L. West and William J. Chimiak

Introduction

The practice of telemedicine involves numerous technologies, including telecommunications, computer networking, digital signal processing and audio/video production. The technology required for telepsychiatry is fairly straightforward – the primary technical need is interactive videoconferencing to allow clinical sessions to be conducted with the highest quality possible within constraints such as cost.

There are several variables important to the quality of any videoconferencing system used for interactive telemedicine consultations. The variables include colour, illumination, sound, movement, depth and image quality. Several interdependent technology-related factors influence these variables, including:

- networking and communications
- audio and video compression
- videoconferencing standards
- audiovisual peripherals.

Recent research at East Carolina University has explored the effect of components that affect interactive telemedicine sessions. These include the network load and the audiovisual coder/decoders (CODECs), which change audiovisual information from its original source into a digital format and convert it back into audiovisual content when it arrives at its destination. The variables varied in importance based on physician specialty. In psychiatric consultations, movement and sound were found to have the most effect on the comfort level of the physician participating in an interactive consultation (unpublished work).

Networking and communications

Bandwidth

Bandwidth represents the theoretical maximum rate that data can travel through a network and is often expressed in units of bits per second (bit/s) with the usual *Systeme*

Internationale prefixes of kilo (k or 10^3), Mega (M or 10^6) or Giga (G or 10^9). The fundamental building block of the telecommunication system is the 64 kbit/s digital data circuit. Some parts of the telephone network (PSTN) still use analogue connections, but the main trunk circuits are all digital nowadays.

In Japan and the USA, data services are provided by aggregating or *multiplexing* 64 kbit/s channels to achieve higher bandwidth. A T-1 connection (more properly known as DS-1) represents 24 multiplexed channels and provides a bandwidth of 1.54 Mbit/s. Often, fractional T-1 services are used for telemedicine applications, e.g. ¼ T-1 (384 kbit/s) or ½ T-1 (768 kbit/s). An aggregate of 28 multiplexed T-1's is called a T-3 (DS-3). In Europe, the Conference of European Post and Telecommunications (CEPT) system is used, which is also based on 64 kbit/s building blocks. A CEPT-1 (or E-1) connection represents 32 multiplexed channels and provides 2.048 Mbit/s.

Another class of telecommunication services is the Integrated Services Digital Network (ISDN). ISDN is widely available. A fundamental unit of the ISDN is the so-called Basic Rate Interface (BRI), which provides the user with a bandwidth of 128 kbit/s. Aggregates of BRI ISDN, called the Primary Rate Interface (PRI), are 1.47 Mbit/s in the USA and 1.92 Mbit/s in Europe.

The conventions and terminology described were developed when the telecommunications infrastructure was based on transmitting electrical signals through copper wires. Today, many of the high-speed links are optical, based on converting electrical signals to light waves which are transmitted over optical fibres. Optical fibres have a much greater transmission capacity than copper wires of similar diameter. Therefore, optical networking is used in much of the current backbone infrastructure. The capacity of fibreoptic networks can be increased with the use of wavelength division multiplexing, which involves the use of different wavelengths (i.e. colours) simultaneously over the same optical fibre. Each wavelength carries a separate signal.

In much of the world, digital transmission from homes and rural sites uses a modem connected via an analogue telephone line. The maximum bandwidth that can be achieved in this way is limited to 56 kbit/s. Two new technologies have recently made higher bandwidth services available and affordable. *Asymmetric Digital Subscriber Line* (ADSL) technology uses existing copper telephone wiring but permits much faster transmission. It is asymmetric, so that the incoming data flow to the home is faster (usually 1.5–9 Mbit/s) than the outgoing data (usually 16–640 kbit/s). This technology allows both voice (telephone) and data connections simultaneously. *Cable modem* technology uses existing cable television infrastructure for high-speed connectivity. Cable modem connections are also asymmetric, with a typical incoming bandwidth of 1.5 Mbit/s and an outgoing bandwidth of 500 kbit/s.

Packet vs. circuit-switching

One concept central to understanding networks is the way networks route traffic from originating source to destination and back. Most telephone services use *circuit-switching* to route voice calls through their networks. In a circuit-switched network, a request for a connection, for example a telephone number dialled with a telephone handset, results in a dedicated link being established from switch to switch right through to the destination. That point-to-point link, called a *circuit*, is dedicated to the call until it is terminated. Traffic can flow in both directions via the circuit, which acts like a long cable that connects the two points together. PSTN, ISDN and T-1 (E-1) services are all circuit-switched.

Other services, such as data transmission, use *packet-switching* to route traffic from source to destination. In packet-switched networks, traffic is divided into smaller chunks, or packets, and each packet is transmitted individually through the links joining the nodes in the network. The route that each packet takes through the network is independent of the routes of the other packets, as the network equipment determines the path for each individual packet, which can depend on the conditions at the time. The packets are put back in order and reassembled when they reach their intended destination. Each packet may traverse a different path to reach its destination. This means that the return paths may also be independent from the send paths. In packet-switched networks, data competes for network bandwidth.

The differences between circuit and packet-switching are essential to understanding the way that different videoconferencing systems operate and perform. Circuit-switched networks are designed for real-time (synchronous) applications such as videoconferencing. A circuit established for the videoconference is dedicated to that session, and is not at risk for competing for bandwidth with other network traffic.

Standards approved by the International Telecommunication Union (ITU) define how videoconferencing data travels over networks. H.320 and H.324 videoconferencing standards, which are discussed below, are designed for circuit-switched networks. Internet Protocol (IP) videoconferencing (H.323 and MPEG standard) systems are designed for packet-switched networks. IP videoconferencing systems require more bandwidth than their H.320 counterparts to achieve the same quality, because networking information is contained in each packet. In an H.320 system, this is not necessary, as a point-to-point circuit connection negates the need for networking information. Packet-switched services are usually less expensive than circuit-switched, however, and can be used for many other applications, for example email and text file transfers. In practice, most networks use a combination of circuit and packet-switching. The pros and cons of each must be considered to select the right solution for specific telemedicine applications.

Packet-based networks

IP communications are packet-based and are becoming an increasingly common form of telecommunication. Rapid growth in the use of personal computers (PCs) and corporate and academic computer networking, and the subsequent popularity of the Internet and World Wide Web, have resulted in the widespread adoption of IP communications. Most telemedicine systems still rely largely on circuit-switched networks for videoconferencing, but as more videoconferencing systems are designed to work with packet-based networks this will change.

Packet-based network communications involve a set of rules, or protocols, that define how data will be transferred from one device to another. The upper 'layer' protocol defines services using the services provided by the layer below it. This keeps the layers distinct and simplifies the design of the hardware and software. The protocols that specify how computers communicate, networks connect, and how traffic is routed over packet-based networks are collectively called the Internet protocol suite. They are also sometimes referred to as the TCP/IP protocol suite. Of these protocols, the Transmission Control Protocol (TCP) and the Internet Protocol (IP) are the best known. TCP is concerned primarily with partitioning data into packets, while IP is used to address and route the packets to ensure that they arrive in the right place at the right time.[1] The Internet model is shown in Figure 2.1.

TCP is the major transport protocol used by applications in the Internet suite of protocols. It provides reliable, full-duplex streams (data can move in both directions), and relies on IP for directing the delivery of the packet. It also adapts to network congestion, which occurs when there is more traffic on the network than it can handle. With heavy congestion, most implementations respond by reducing the amount of traffic offered and then build up the data rate to the maximum that the network can handle (data rates may also be affected by time of day, and environmental factors such as storms).[2]

One of the features of TCP is that it delivers data packets using a checksum for verification. The TCP information to be sent is processed to create a numerical value that is placed in the header of the packet. When the packet is received, the checksum is again performed and compared with the header checksum for integrity. If the numerical value is the same, the packet is deemed good, delivered and acknowledged. If it does not pass the checksum, it is discarded and not acknowledged. If there is no acknowledgement at the sending site after a timeout period then the packet is resent with a new checksum. This continues until an acknowledgement is received or until the limit in the number of retransmissions occurs, in which case a failure is reported to the application.

Another transport protocol is the User Datagram Protocol (UDP), the protocol used for most teleconferencing and Internet streaming. Streaming is a technique where voice or video data are temporarily saved in reserve memory storage (i.e. buffered). When packets of the incoming stream are delayed, the data in the buffer is played. Generally the receiver of the stream does not notice this. UDP is a very simple transport protocol, which also depends on IP for delivery. Because there is insufficient time for voice or video packet re-transmission in a live voice or video transmission,

Application	
Transport	TCP, UDP, RTP: partitions data into packets
IP	Contains address
Data link	Provides access to network
Equipment	

Fig. 2.1. Layers of the Internet model.

UDP does not provide for exchange of packets with acknowledgement or guaranteed delivery like TCP.

Real Time Protocol (RTP) is the protocol for the transport of real-time audio and video data. In real-time videoconferencing, video and audio data are broken down into packets. The time relationships between packets is maintained by using a timestamp to place audio and video packets in the correct timing order. RTP also sequentially numbers each packet, providing a means to detect packet loss. Packets are delivered as fast as they can be sent. The time relationships are critical. Most systems introduce some delay (referred to as latency), ranging from a tenth of a second to about 2 seconds. A delay of more than 3 seconds is very obvious and is generally unacceptable for videoconferencing.[2]

All data on the Internet depend on the IP. This is a very flexible network layer protocol, which controls how data-traffic is sent through network devices such as routers or switches. IP is a best-effort protocol, handling data much like an ordinary letter would be handled in the postal system. All packets are mixed on a best-effort network. Each packet is sent to its destinations using every effort to ensure that it is received at the correct destination as quickly as possible. To ensure that each packet reaches its destination reliably, the upper protocol layers must detect and correct problems such as network congestion, packet loss or delay.

Some features have been implemented to differentiate how data are treated through the network. The latest networks allow for placing a class of service, or Quality of Service (QoS), request in the packet. QoS requests are designed as mechanisms to guarantee throughput levels for particular priority traffic. This allows for an increase in the urgency of transmission as data are transmitted through network switches and routers.

Routers and switches

Two or more networks are connected using routers and other networking equipment (Fig. 2.2). For data to move from one network to another, a router transfers packets sent from the site of origin to the intended receiver. Although this sounds like a simple job, when many networks are interconnected, it becomes a complex task. Improvements in protocols have simplified routing to the point that a router is not as necessary as before, except perhaps on an Internet connection operating at 45 Mbit/s or more. Although PCs can be configured as routers, commercial routers, which contain powerful processors, are used in larger networking systems.

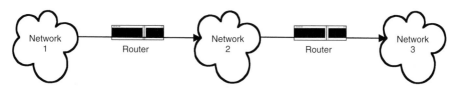

Fig. 2.2. Routers used to connect three networks.

A switch is a device that is used to move packets in a network. They are designed to work at various levels of the Internet model discussed earlier. They are not only much faster than routers, they are also much cheaper. Switches work by 'sneaking a peek' at the higher layer, allowing the switch to know the address of a packet. This allows for switching data from one place to another very rapidly.

Audio and video compression

One of the fundamental challenges of videoconferencing is that it is a bandwidth-intensive application. A video signal is composed of multiple still images, or *frames*. Each second of broadcast-quality video in the USA has 30 frames, so a single second of video can contain 30 separate images. Each image typically contains 2.5 million bits. This would require a bandwidth of approximately 74 Mbit/s. Therefore, to reduce the bandwidth requirements, compression is used.

There are many different strategies for compressing video and audio signals, but several elements are common to each. *Intraframe* compression involves the compression of individual frames (image). *Interframe* compression relies on the fact that there is often little difference between consecutive frames and redundant data can be removed between frames. Compression can be either *lossless* or *lossy*.[3,4] Lossless compression allows exact reconstruction of the image, i.e. no data are lost. A compression ratio of 3 : 1, or possibly 4 : 1, is currently the best lossless video compression that can be achieved. There is some data loss (lossy compression) in most compression schemes in videoconferencing, but much of this lost data is imperceptible to the human eye, i.e. it is *visually lossless*.

Less bandwidth is required for audio than for video, but both are compressed in videoconferencing systems. Compression is accomplished by the coder/decoder, or *codec*. This is a device used to compress audio and video signals at the origination site and decompress the signals at the receiving site. Codecs can use special electronics (hardware codec) or software for compression, and commercial videoconferencing systems often use both. A hardware codec can be either a standalone appliance, or 'black box' or a card (or set of cards) installed in a PC. A software-only codec, such as is used in commercial products like NetMeeting (Microsoft), relies on software instructions executed on the PC microprocessor to perform compression. Satisfactory performance of software-only codecs depends on the host PC's specification as well as what other tasks the computer is performing at the same time the videoconference is occurring.

Videoconferencing standards

There are three worldwide standards for colour television, or analogue video:

1. the National Television Standards Committee (NTSC standard), used in the USA, Canada, South America and Japan

2. Phase Alternating Lines (PAL), used throughout Europe (except France) and Australia

3. Sequential Colour avec Memoire (SECAM), used in France, most of eastern Europe and the Middle East.

These standards define the number of frames per second, and the number of lines and colours that can be within each frame. The NTSC standard, for example, uses video signals that allow for 30 (29.97) frames/s, 512 lines scanned (usually 484 are displayed), up to 16 million different colours, and a 4:3 aspect ratio (horizontal:vertical), i.e. the display is wider than it is tall. PAL and SECAM standards allow for 625 lines and 25 frames/s.

The International Telecommunication Union (ITU) has defined the standards for videoconferencing systems. The ITU standards are actually interrelated families of standards. For example, the 'H Series' addresses videoconferencing, but videoconferencing systems also use 'G Series' standards for audio compression and 'T Series' standards for conference control, file transfer and whiteboards.

Currently, the most widely used video compression standard in videoconferencing is H.261, which supports up to 30 frames/s in NTSC format, and 25 frames/s in the PAL and SECAM formats, and a resolution of 352 × 288 pixels. H.261 is an *interframe* compression standard, and it uses a technique called discrete cosine transformation (DCT). Commonly used audio compression standards in videoconferencing are ITU G.711 (medium quality – same as telephone), G.722 (highest quality) and G.728 (lowest quality).

Most T-1-based videoconferencing systems are H.320-based, while ISDN systems use H.321, which is H.320 adapted for ISDN. IP-based systems use the H.323 standard, and PSTN systems are based on H.324. Table 2.1 summarizes the three series of ITU standards of particular relevance to telepsychiatry.

Table 2.1. The ITU standards[5] used in telemedicine applications

Series	Application	Standards
G: 'Transmission systems and media, digital systems and networks'	Voice coding	G.711: pulse code modulation – same as standard telephone G.722: highest quality G.728: low bit rate
H: 'Audiovisual and multimedia systems'	Videoconferencing	H.320: videoconferencing over PSTN (includes T-1 and fractional T-1 networks) H.321: ISDN videoconferencing (adapted from H.320) H.323: packet-based network (IP) videoconferencing H.324: low bandwidth (PSTN) videoconferencing Note: H.261 and H.263 (low bit rate) are video compression standards used by above
T: 'Terminals for telemedicine services'	Multimedia conferencing	T.120: whiteboards, file transfer, session management

The Moving Pictures Expert Group (MPEG) standards used in digital video applications have been recently adopted in videoconferencing systems. MPEG-1 was developed to compress video for playback on CD-ROM drives at 30 frames/second, with 352×240 pixel resolution and CD-quality audio. MPEG-2 was optimized for digital versatile disk (DVD) and cable and satellite television at 30 frames/second, with 720×480 pixel resolution and high-quality audio. The new MPEG-4 standard has been designed for streaming video applications using the Internet, and is not likely to be applied to videoconferencing systems.

Audiovisual peripherals

Networks can significantly affect the quality of a videoconference. The components of the videoconferencing system or the audiovisual peripheral equipment attached to it, may also affect the quality of the videoconference. These components include cameras, monitors/displays, microphones and loudspeakers.

Audiovisual equipment must allow the patient and clinician to be seen and heard. These components all affect key technical elements that determine videoconferencing quality. These technical elements are:

- image definition, or sharpness and focus of the image
- resolution: video is usually described in terms of the number of horizontal lines on a monitor expressed as a ratio (aspect ratio); audio refers to the pickup pattern
- colour, hue and saturation, or tonal quality and purity of colour
- lip synchronization, or the relationship between the video and audio streams.

Cameras

In videoconferencing for psychiatry, the ability to see the patient both close up (e.g. to observe facial expressions[6]) and from afar (perhaps to observe for leg jitters), or to see several people during a family conference is very important. The type of camera used in the video system is particularly important. The standard for most video equipment is the pan/tilt/zoom camera (Fig. 2.3). Automatic focus is an important feature for any telepsychiatry system, so that concentration on the consultation is not shifted to the mechanics of focusing the camera when images are changed. These cameras usually provide excellent images, but tend to be expensive.

TV monitors and computer displays

The size of a TV monitor is a factor in telepresence, or the perceived presence from a physically remote location.[7,8] Television monitors typically use a 69–91 cm (diagonal) screen. The size of the screen needs to be appropriate for the distance between the monitor and the clinician. Although the resolution is not affected by the monitor size, the apparent image quality may decrease as the monitor size increases.

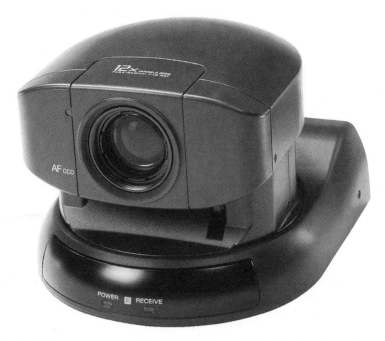

Fig. 2.3. Pan/tilt/zoom camera used during patient consultation. (Photograph courtesy of Sony Electronics Inc.)

Computer monitors, which are typically between 38 and 53 cm (diagonally), use video cards for converting analogue signals to video signals for a VGA image. VGA monitors have a higher resolution, so that the image definition is of higher quality. Monitors affect resolution by the number of pixels on the rows and columns. The greater the number of pixels, the better the resolution. For example, a resolution of 1024×768 will provide a sharper or clearer image than a resolution of 640×480.

Microphones and loudspeakers

Microphones convert sound waves into electrical signals. The quality of the signal depends on its pickup pattern, or the directions from which it picks up sounds. In telepsychiatry, it is important that microphones are omnidirectional, picking up sound anywhere in the room. If a patient moves about in the room during a consultation, an omnidirectional microphone will pick up the patient's conversation equally well from any direction. By contrast, a directional microphone picks up sound only from the front, and a unidirectional microphone from one direction only. When a unidirectional microphone is used, systems often employ extra microphones in the patient examination room to ensure that sounds are picked up in all parts of the room.[9]

Audio signals are compressed for transmission, just like video signals. When resolution is reduced, noise (artifacts of sound) and distortion of the sound increase.

This is less critical in telepsychiatry than in other specialties, for example cardiology and pulmonary medicine, but may become distracting during any videoconference.

Loudspeakers that provide sufficient tone and volume are used with most videoconferencing systems.

Lip synchronization

The visual perception that speech is coordinated with the visual movement of the speaker's mouth is called lip synchronization. Bandwidth is probably the most important factor affecting lip synchronization. The lower the bandwidth, the less there appears to be lip synchronization, creating a lag between what is said and when it is heard. This can be a distraction during telepsychiatry.[6,10]

Security

Security is a concern for telepsychiatry, or any health application that uses videoconferencing. Not only is the integrity of the data a concern, but confidentiality of that data and availability of the network are important elements in security. There are numerous technologies for security, for example firewalls, access controls, security protocols (encryption), virtual private networks (VPNs) and management controls. Security is discussed in detail in several excellent references.[1,11–13]

Future trends

Home networking

Increasingly, homes are connected to the Internet, using either a modem connected via the PSTN or higher-bandwidth ADSL or cable modem services. A recent report[14] stated that 51% of households in the USA had access to the Internet in 2001. As telemedicine becomes more commonplace and moves out of the traditional hospital settings to clinicians' offices and patient homes,[15] home networking technology will become an important vehicle for telepsychiatry.

Several companies now manufacture home (residential) gateways. These devices allow multiple personal computers to share an Internet connection and enable the creation of a local-area network (LAN) within the home (i.e. a home-area network). Home gateways have other important features, such as firewalls, and some also act as wireless access points. Perhaps more significantly, such resources permit other Internet-ready devices with embedded computers to use the same network and share Internet access.

The use of broadband connectivity to the home will enable more advanced interactive services such as IP videoconferencing. Currently, home broadband services are limited to cable and DSL and are primarily focused around population centres, i.e. 'within the city limits'. In the USA, it has been estimated that approximately 78–85% of households with Internet access have 'narrowband' or PSTN service (the proportion varies by region).[14] However, there is a steady rise in the use of broadband.

Wireless networking

Developments in wireless communications technologies are likely to have a significant effect on the future of telemedicine. Current wireless technologies can provide connectivity throughout an organization, and different technologies are best suited to particular segments of the network. There are several different categories of wireless networking applications.

Wireless backbone, or *wireless wide-area networking* (WWAN), involves the use of wireless technologies for networking across long distances, such as fixed-point microwave or satellite systems.[15] Current fixed-point WWAN systems can provide high bandwidth data transmission up to 1 Gbit/s. These WWAN systems could be used to interconnect distant hospitals or other remote clinical facilities, or to provide 'last-mile' connections from facilities to high-speed optical backbone networks.

Wireless local-area networking (WLAN) systems are becoming increasingly common, especially those based on the Institute of Electrical and Electronics Engineers (IEEE) 802.11 wireless Ethernet standard. WLAN systems are used for networking within smaller areas, such as in a clinic or on a single floor of a hospital. The current 802.11b standard supports up to 11 Mbit/s connections and the new 802.11a standard up to 54 Mbit/s.[17]

Personal-area networks (PAN) are a relatively new concept, and are intended to cover short ranges of less than 10 m, such as within one room. PAN applications include communications between personal electronics devices, and between devices and computers. The principal PAN standards are Bluetooth and Infrared Data Association (IrDA). The IrDA standard is designed for point-to-point infrared communications within a 1 m range, with a bandwidth of up to 4 Mbit/s.[18,19] Bluetooth can be used for point-to-point or point-to-multipoint connections; each device is provided with three voice channels (64 kbit/s) or 1 data channel (up to 721 kbit/s).[20]

Mobile networks comprise the final category of wireless applications, and include cellular telephone and satellite technologies. Currently, most cellular networks provide limited data connections, typically 9.6–28.8 kbit/s maximum. New technologies are being tested that may provide sufficient bandwidth to support videoconferencing.

Table 2.2 summarizes the various categories of wireless technologies, and the standards and applications relevant to each.

Internet 2

When the Internet became a viable service for commercial use, there was a need to develop and improve it. In the USA, an Internet testbed was developed for use by the federal government and universities called the Next Generation Internet (NGI). A commercial initiative called Internet 2 was also launched. Although there is a common misconception that these networks are faster, or that they provide better QoS, that is not their intent. In the USA, NGI and Internet 2 sites are not pursuing QoS initiatives, citing low utilization of the network as the reason. It is our belief that when the features of the Internet 2 and the NGI work as intended in university settings, their use will become universal.

Table 2.2. Categories of wireless capabilities, technologies and applications used to describe types of wireless network

Category	Distance	Bandwidth	Applications	Technology/Standards
Wireless wide-area network (WWAN)	Long range (> 1–2 km)	Up to 1 Gbit/s	Inter-facility, inter-campus or regional data communications	Narrow-beam, fixed-point, line-of-sight, wireless (microwave) or satellite links. Licensed or unlicensed spectrum
Wireless local-area network (WLAN)	Medium range (100–1000 m)	11–54 Mbit/s	Intra-facility or inter-computer networking	Omni-directional. Unlicensed spectrum IEEE 802.11
Wireless personal-area network (WPAN)	Short range (1–10 m)	700–1000 kbit/s	Device-to-device or device-to-computer communications	Infrared Data Association (IrDA): infrared, line-of-sight Bluetooth: RF, omnidirectional. Unlicensed spectrum
Mobile networking	Long range (depending on coverage)	Up to 64 kbit/s	Voice and data for mobile workforce or emergency response	Cellular (GSM, CDPD, PCS, GPRS) Satellite (Iridium, Echostar, etc.). Licensed spectrum

Several technologies are being investigated, such as a different version of IP (Ipv6), which provides a much larger address space. To date, however, there are no useful applications using Ipv6. A security protocol, IPSec, has also been developed. Numerous applications are being explored using the NGI and Internet 2, which will undoubtedly provide the foundation for future innovations in telecommunications and videoconferencing.

Conclusions

This chapter has described only briefly the major telecommunications and technologies used in telepsychiatry. An increasing number of clinicians are interested in or are already using telemedicine as a method of providing care. Although there remains a lack of research in telepsychiatry,[21] the number of empirical studies is increasing. With innovation in telecommunications technologies and some evidence to support its value and encourage its implementation in mental health care, the future for telepsychiatry is bright.

References

1   Minoli D, ed. *Internet and Intranet Engineering*. New York: McGraw-Hill, 1997.
2   Lemaire ED, Boudrias Y, Greene G. Technical evaluation of a low-bandwidth, Internet-based system for teleconsultations. *Journal of Telemedicine and Telecare* 2000;**6**:163–167.

3   Wang L, DeBrunner V, DeBrunner L, Radhakrishnan S. Introduction to still image compression. 1999, August. Available at http://coecs.ou.edu/vdebrunn/www/VED%20pages/pubpdf/vision%20systems.pdf [last checked 11 September 2002].

4   Wong S, Zaremba L, Gooden D, Huang HK. Radiologic image compression. *Proceedings of the IEEE* 1995;**83**:194–219.

5   International Telecommunication Union (ITU). Available at http://www.itu.org [last checked 9 September 2002].

6   May C, Gask L, Ellis N, et al. Telepsychiatry evaluation in the north-west of England: preliminary results of a qualitative study. *Journal of Telemedicine and Telecare* 2000;**6**(suppl 1):20–22.

7   Draper JV, Kaber DB, Usher JM. Telepresence. *Human Factors* 1998;**40**:354–375.

8   Tachakra S, Newson R, Wootton R, Stinson A. Avoiding artificiality in teleconsultations. *Journal of Telemedicine and Telecare* 2001;**7**(suppl 1):39–42.

9   Elford R, White H, Bowering R, et al. A randomized, controlled trial of child psychiatric assessments conducted using videoconferencing. *Journal of Telemedicine and Telecare* 2000;**6**:73–82.

10 Deitsch SE, Frueh BC, Santos AB. Telepsychiatry for post-traumatic stress disorder. *Journal of Telemedicine and Telecare* 2000;**6**:184–186.

11 National Research Council, Computer Science and Telecommunications Board. *Networking Health: prescriptions for the Internet.* Washington, DC: National Academy Press, 2000.

12 National Research Council of the National Academy of Sciences. *For the Record: protecting electronic health information.* Washington, DC: National Academy Press, 1997.

13 National Institute of Standards and Technology. *An Introduction to Computer Security: the NIST handbook.* Special Publication 800-12. Available at http://www.securiteinfo.com/ebooks/palm/nist-compsec-handbook.pdf [last checked 9 September 2002].

14 US Department of Commerce. *A Nation Online: how Americans are expanding their use of the Internet.* Washington, DC: National Telecommunications and Information Administration, 2002. Available at http://www.ntia.doc.gov/ntiahome/dn/nationonline_020502.htm [last checked 11 September 2002].

15 Chae YM, Park HJ, Hong GD, Cheon KA. The reliability and acceptability of telemedicine for patients with schizophrenia in Korea. *Journal of Telemedicine and Telecare* 2000;**6**:83–90.

16 Biesecker K. The promise of broadband wireless. *IT Professional* 2000;**2**:31–39.

17 Paulson LD. Exploring the wireless LANscape. *Computer* 2000;**33**:12–16.

18 Infrared Data Association (IrDA). Available at http://www.irda.org [last checked 9 September 2002].

19 Pfeifer T. Internet-Intranet-Infranet: a modular integrating architecture. In: IEEE Computing Society. *Proceedings 7th IEEE Workshop on Future Trends of Distributed Computing Systems.* Los Alamos, CA: IEEE, 1999:81–87.

20 Bhagwat P. Bluetooth: technology for short-range wireless apps. *IEEE Internet Computing* 2001;**5**:96–103.

21 Frueh BC, Deitsch SE, Santos AB, et al. Procedural and methodological issues in telepsychiatry research and program development. *Psychiatric Services* 2000;**51**:1522–1527.

3

Health Economics of Telepsychiatry

Paul McCrone

Introduction

Economics has been described as the 'science of scarcity' because it is concerned with the allocation of resources which are inherently limited in their supply. Clearly any society has a finite ability to produce goods and services at any point in time and yet the demand for those goods and services is likely to be high. Health care has to compete with other worthy causes such as education, social care and law and order for public expenditure, and spending money on private health care can only be accomplished at the expense of spending it on other activities. Within health care there are also competing demands placed upon resources. For instance if increased funds are made available, what proportion should be spent on services for children with leukaemia and what proportion on older people with Alzheimer's disease? If it is decided to allocate more funds to treat leukaemia then what particular treatment should be funded? Health economics provides methods by which such decisions can be informed. Telepsychiatry lends itself ideally to health economic evaluation. One of the main reasons for the existence of telepsychiatry is the perception that staff and patient time is being saved by holding case conferences and consultations remotely.

Cost measurement

The appropriate measurement and analysis of costs is fundamental to any economic evaluation.[1] At the outset a number of questions need to be asked. First, whose perspective is being considered? Second, what costs should be included? Third, over what time period should costs be measured? Fourth, who will provide the resource use data in order to generate costs? Finally, what is the source of the unit cost information?

Perspective

It is important that the perspective which is driving an economic evaluation is established when determining which costs (and indeed which outcomes) to include. Clinical and economic evaluations are frequently funded from within the health care sector and are generally conducted by researchers working in the health services or in associated academic departments. Therefore, there is likely to be a focus on costs pertaining to the health service. However, it is likely (and in mental health care it is probable) that any change in the way that a service is delivered will have an effect on non-health care services, families, patients and society in general. Economists tend to stress the need to take a societal perspective whereby the broadest range of costs is included. This is important, since health care expenditure (which is primarily funded from general taxation) could equally be used for other areas such as education, defence or aid to developing countries. In addition, the effect on families and patients can be profound. In the case of telepsychiatry this will certainly be the case since reduced travel times allow other activities to be undertaken. However, it is probably true that health care decision-makers will primarily be interested in the costs that affect their particular sector and therefore a pragmatic approach is to take a societal perspective but to report costs arising to different sectors as well as overall costs.

Costs to include

Once the relevant perspective is established the next step is to decide which costs to include. Economic evaluations usually compare at least two treatments or modes of service delivery, or alternatively focus on a single treatment or mode of delivery and compare the situation before and after its inception. With either of these designs all costs that may be affected should be included. In mental health care this may not be clear and therefore costs should generally be measured comprehensively.[2] However, if it is known that any particular component of the care package delivered to patients will not be affected then there is no need to include it if the ultimate aim is to compare relative costs.

It may not be immediately obvious what are costs. For example, if a patient's retired spouse accompanies them to psychiatry appointments and, if after the introduction of a telepsychiatry service, the time required to do this is reduced, then is there a cost saving? The spouse is unlikely to be receiving any income for caring for the patient but it is possible that they could use the time in other ways and therefore there are opportunities gained by freeing up of time. This time therefore has a value and should be included in any economic evaluation. This is the notion of 'opportunity cost' – costs incurred when opportunities are forgone by engaging in a particular activity. It should be apparent that opportunity costs and financial or accounting costs may well be different, although the latter are frequently used.

Time period over which costs should be measured

The introduction of telepsychiatry services will inevitably incur substantial start-up costs. Although there is a downward movement in the price of the necessary hardware, it still constitutes a major investment for any mental health care provider. In an economic evaluation such costs should be apportioned over the expected lifespan of the equipment. Investment in equipment has an opportunity cost – these funds could equally be spent in other ways or even invested so as to earn interest. Therefore the opportunity cost of capital investment can be estimated by combining the expected interest payments that would be accrued were the funds to be invested elsewhere over a period equivalent to the expected lifespan of the equipment. Furthermore, the initial period during which a telepsychiatry service is introduced, staff are trained and the equipment is used will be operationally different from the situation say 6 months later. Therefore, to make valid comparisons between telepsychiatry and existing services it may be necessary to wait until a 'steady-state' has been achieved.

With regard to other services that may be affected by the introduction of telepsychiatry a sufficient period of time should be used for detecting any changes in resource use. Some services (e.g. contacts with general practitioners and, community mental health nurses) may be used fairly frequently and therefore a relatively short measurement period could be used for these. A service such as psychiatry inpatient care though is going to be used relatively seldom, but it could still be affected by the introduction of telepsychiatry and if so there would be important economic consequences. Therefore, any cost period should be of sufficient length to capture all relevant effects. In mental health care evaluations, a cost period of between 3 and 12 months is generally used. Clearly longer periods of time would provide decision-makers with more definitive information, but such long-term studies are not always feasible. Standardized instruments are not particularly appropriate for measuring costs as the relevant cost items will differ between studies. However, interview schedules have been developed which can be adapted according to the particular study requirements.[1]

Sources of resource use information

Data on service use can come from a number of sources but these will differ in terms of their accuracy and comprehensiveness. It has already been stressed that a societal perspective is the ideal, in which costs are measured comprehensively. The best source of such broad information will usually be the patient or their family. However, patient recall of service use may lack accuracy and, therefore, hospital administration systems should be used to supplement and validate data reported by patients. This will be especially crucial with high cost services such as inpatient care and day care.

The evaluation of telepsychiatry is different from that of other service innovations in that many of the effects may not be realized by the patient, and in such situations data provided directly by staff may be warranted. For example, case conferences in which the patient may or may not be present could be facilitated via video links, and the main cost impact of this could be travel-time savings for professionals who would otherwise have to travel to one central location.

Unit costs

The purposes of conducting an economic evaluation of a telepsychiatry service may be to justify its existence to local managers and policy-makers, and as such the unit costs attached to the measures of resource use need to reflect local circumstances. However, evaluation findings in one area could be used to inform planning in other settings. If this potential is to be fully exploited then generic unit costs should also be considered. In the UK, for example, generic unit costs for a number of mental health care services have been published by Netten et al.[3]

Methods of economic evaluation

The aim of an economic evaluation is to determine the relationship between costs and outcomes for alternative treatments or modes of service delivery. Essentially, an economic evaluation seeks to identify which interventions produce the greatest level of 'outcome' for a given level of inputs or cost or, alternatively, which intervention incurs the lowest cost when achieving a specific level of 'outcome'. From this it should be evident that economic evaluation is not simply about identifying least-cost options – after all, one of the least costly options is usually to do nothing and this can rarely be appropriate.

Cost-minimization analysis

Discussion of this form of analysis might seem to contradict the above paragraph. However, there are some situations where the outcomes of different services are known *a priori*, and therefore only costs need to be measured. If outcomes are identical then the least cost option is the preferred one. In practice, outcomes will rarely be known beforehand and therefore cost-minimization analysis is rarely appropriate – even though it is commonly used. It is used fairly frequently in telepsychiatry studies and this implies that the process of care delivery is unlikely to affect patient outcome.

Cost-effectiveness analysis

Although the terms 'cost-effectiveness analysis' and 'cost-benefit analysis' are frequently used to describe all forms of economic evaluation, they are in fact specific forms of analysis. Cost-effectiveness analysis combines cost information with data on a single condition-specific outcome measure, for example symptomatology or social functioning. A formal synthesis of differences in costs and outcomes can enable the most efficient intervention to be identified.

Cost-consequences analysis

This is a more general case of cost-effectiveness analysis. Rather than one single outcome measure being used a number of different ones are considered. This seems appropriate for mental health care research where interventions rarely affect only one domain and where different problems for different individuals may be dominant. However, it can prove difficult if the link between costs and one outcome measure is very different between costs and other outcome measures. In such a situation which finding should be given most weight?

Cost-utility analysis

This is similar to cost-effectiveness analysis since only a single outcome measure is used, but it is different because this outcome measure is a generic measure that can in theory be used in any health care evaluation. This enables interventions in diverse areas (e.g. cancer and stroke) to be compared in terms of cost-utility. Utility is a rather abstract concept and, in order to make this form of analysis practical, health-related quality of life based on quality adjusted life years (QALYs) is usually used in its place.

Cost-benefit analysis

Perhaps the most powerful technique, and yet most difficult to conduct, cost-benefit analysis compares the costs of a particular service with the outcomes achieved, the latter also being measured in monetary terms. If the monetary outcomes exceed the costs then the service is considered to be efficient. Unfortunately it is very difficult to value outcomes in monetary terms and therefore this form of analysis is rarely used.

Sensitivity analysis

The appropriate interpretation of economic evaluations can be hindered in three ways. First, they are frequently conducted in closely controlled experimental conditions, often within the confines of a randomized trial. This can be important for determining the relative efficacy of one form of treatment or service delivery over another, but it can lead to results not being representative of those that would apply in real-life settings. Second, there may be pressures to evaluate a service as soon as it is introduced and this may mean that a 'steady-state' of activity has not been attained. This is likely to be particularly relevant to telemedicine services. Third, there will be uncertainty regarding the values of some parameters in most evaluations. A good example is patient time, for which there is no standard method of valuation. Conducting a 'sensitivity analysis' is a recognized way of determining how robust a study's findings are to changes in the parameters.

Economic evaluations in a 'systems' context

As has already been indicated, the particular aim of an economic evaluation is to determine which of two or more services or modes of service delivery is most technically efficient. This in itself is informative. However, the findings from economic evaluations need to be assessed in the light of the wider mental health care system. A service such as telepsychiatry may well produce similar patient outcomes at a lower cost than face-to-face consultations, but will cost savings necessarily arise? The reality is that psychiatrists will be able to process more 'cases' and the system will become less constrained. Savings would ultimately only occur if the number of staff were reduced because of the telepsychiatry service. One exception though is the savings in travel expenses other than time. Similarly community care, which may be less expensive than traditional inpatient care, may only produce savings if beds (and maybe whole wards) are closed. This is not to say that costs are not saved, but they are in terms of time and not money. A system that is less constrained will enable patients to be seen more quickly and will also increase access to patients who otherwise may not have received the service. This though is based on the premise that time savings are being used to provide more patient care.

Review of economic evaluations in telepsychiatry

Few economic studies of telepsychiatry have been conducted. This is ironic since one of the main aims of telepsychiatry is to reduce costs and increase access.[4] However, good quality studies have been conducted in other areas of telemedicine (see Box 3.1 for an example).

Werner and Anderson[5] conducted a feasibility study of telepsychiatry in a rural county in Michigan. They recognized the need to include a wide range of cost elements in their analysis including: equipment, clinic personnel, installation,

---

Box 3.1.   Cost-benefit analysis of teledermatology[16]

Background
15% of general practice consultations in the UK are for dermatological problems. Referral to a specialist though is problematical, as the number of dermatologists is limited. The use of telemedicine may speed up the whole process, and also save patient time.

Study methods
Two rural- and two urban-based general practices were included in the study, along with two hospital-based dermatology departments. Patients ($n = 204$) consulting their general practitioner for dermatological problems were randomized to either a face-to-face appointment with a specialist or an appointment via a video link from the general practice, with the general practitioner in attendance.

Costs
Patients recorded details of the time spent in attending the initial appointment and the subsequent consultation (if one took place). Hourly rates of dermatologists and general practitioners were £150 and £114 respectively. Patient time was based on the average annual income for those in work and travel costs were based on a standard cost per mile or the relevant public transport fares.

The average cost of professional time for the conventional consultation was £34.75. However, the average cost for the teledermatology consultation was greater at £69.08, due to the attendance of the general practitioner. Patient time and travel costs were, as would be expected, greater for the conventional appointments (£13.98 compared to £7.88). The equipment costs for the teledermatology service amounted to £124.92 per patient. Therefore, the total costs per person were £201.88 for the teledermatology patients and £48.73 for the patients receiving the conventional service.

Benefits
By being present during the teledermatology consultations general practitioners were able to learn new skills. It was estimated that this would enable them to refer 20% fewer patients to specialists, thus saving patient time and travel costs and consultant costs. These savings worked out at £9.74 per patient. To achieve these savings in the absence of teledermatology, the general practitioners would have had to attend a training course, which would amount to £60.04 when averaged across the patients seen. Therefore, the total monetary benefits were estimated to be £69.78 for the teledermatology patients, resulting in a net cost (cost minus benefits) of £132.10 for the teledermatology patients and £48.73 for the conventionally seen group.

Conclusions
The teledermatology service was more expensive than the conventional service even after subtracting the benefits that would arise from its use. However, it was noted that if the video-link equipment was purchased at current prices (and these are still decreasing), the number of sessions were increased and if the service were aimed at those having to travel further distances, then the service could become more efficient (Fig. 3.1).

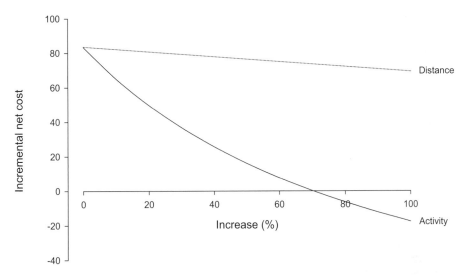

Fig. 3.1. Difference in net costs between teledermatology and conventional consultations given (i) increases in the activity rate caused by other specialities using the equipment, and (ii) an increase in the distance travelled by those having conventional consultations as a result of targeting more rural areas.[16] With the activity rates and travel time saved as reported, the teledermatology service has net costs that are on average £83.37 more than the conventional service. The top line shows the response to changes in the travel distance and costs saved, and this is less than the response to increased activity. In this example the teledermatology service would become cost-effective if activity were increased by 70%. However, this would depend on other specialities being able to access the equipment.

maintenance, training, duplication of files, office space and line rental. In rural areas the digital lines may be lacking and therefore the authors assumed that these would be introduced at a relatively high cost. With an assumed maximum of 260 consultations per year, the cost of a consultation was estimated to lie between US$257.50 and US$322.50. This cost would be very sensitive to the activity rate but the authors did not feel that there would be scope for other specialities to use the system and therefore bring the unit cost down. The conclusion was that telepsychiatry would not be economically viable. However, the authors did not attempt to link costs to patient outcomes (or staff ratings of satisfaction), nor did they take account of the value of staff time savings.

Chen et al[6] took issue with the above study on the grounds that it ignored time savings, focused only on costs and also did not recognize that costs will always be high in the short term. In addition they argued that a more holistic approach may be appropriate rather than a tele*speciality*, although this view is not shared by all proponents of telepsychiatry.[7] In another reaction to the article Smith[8] claimed that telepsychiatry has the benefit of improving continuity of care, with the effect of enabling patients to be discharged from hospital sooner and of remaining in the community longer.

Tang et al[9] described a telepsychiatry service for geriatric patients in residential homes in Hong Kong. This was a notable study because it was in an urban setting as opposed to most telepsychiatry services that are based in rural areas. (The distance between the home in the study and the clinic was only 3 km.) The usual mode of care involved psychiatry team members visiting residential homes each month with urgent care provided at the accident and emergency department or outpatient clinic. The video link was operational 5 days per week and was used by other teams. It replaced the monthly visits to the home but initial contacts were still made in person, as were urgent assessments (although these were arranged via the link). Over a 10-month period 1001 contacts via the link were made including 149 for psychiatry assessments. Patients and staff were generally satisfied with the service which enabled care to be delivered more promptly than under the existing system. The authors estimated the cost per contact via the link to be HK$92. Included in this cost were set-up and maintenance costs and the line charges. However, training costs, keeping two sets of records and office space for the system were not included. This compared with a saved travel cost of $HK106. The authors gave the high volume of contacts (including those by other specialities) as the reason for the low cost per consultation. This is interesting since it may be that telepsychiatry is cheaper in *urban* areas than in rural areas due to the higher prevalence of mental disorders, even though it makes sense to assume that telepsychiatry is of greater benefit in rural areas. The authors made the important point that cost-effectiveness results cannot easily be transferred from location to another.

A telepsychiatry service in rural Queensland, described by Kennedy and Yellowlees,[10] aimed to provide clinical consultations, aid with discharge planning, provide clinical advice to general practitioners and to deliver training in best practice. Data on 124 patients were collected but only 32 of these used the service. The mean cost of a teleconsultation was A$145 compared to A$162 for a visit from the psychiatrist and A$326 for a visit from the psychiatry team. There were no improvements in quality of life or well-being, but on the other hand telepsychiatry did not prove detrimental to the patients. However, there was a large time commitment on the part of health-practitioners who would otherwise have simply referred the case to a private psychiatrist. The authors felt that over time the use of videoconferencing would not necessarily increase – rather the local health-practitioners would gain confidence in treating patients because of the video link. Another service in Queensland was shown to produce costs savings to the local health authority of more than A$100 000 per year and also savings in terms of patients transfers via airplane.[11]

The routine use of a telepsychiatry service in Alberta, Canada – with a main centre providing consultations to patient in five remote areas – was shown to have comparable costs to the standard service of a psychiatrist visiting patients if the number of teleconsultations was 224 per year.[12] However, that was based on the assumption that a psychiatrist would only make one consultation per visit. The authors recognized that in reality the number may be greater, which would reduce the variable cost of a psychiatrist consultation and which would in turn make it harder for the telepsychiatry service to produce cost savings. The authors also assessed the views of patients regarding the service.[13] Overall satisfaction was good and patients were happy to use the equipment. The authors estimated the time cost to the patient of using the service as being C$30 per consultation. This compared with a cost of C$240 if travel time was included in the absence of telepsychiatry. This indicates that access can be greatly improved via telepsychiatry if travel time acts as a disincentive. In another study that examined the value of travel-time savings in Newfoundland and Labrador (where there is a shortage of child psychiatrists), Elford et al[14] asked parents of children who were receiving care from a child psychiatrist via a video link how they would otherwise have travelled to the clinic and where they would have stayed. The mean saving in travel and accommodation costs was C$428, which slightly exceeded the cost per patient of the telepsychiatry equipment (C$419). However, the data on saved travel and accommodation costs were very skewed and in fact there were savings for only nine out of the 30 patients in the study. The authors, as in other studies, stressed the fact that the cost of the services was particularly sensitive to the level of activity.

A further use of telepsychiatry is in the training of staff. One programme in Western Australia was used to deliver training in cognitive behavioural therapy over 16 sessions.[15] Although overall costs were 45% higher for the video-training compared with face-to-face training, there were savings in clinical time and therefore the knock-on effects for patients may be important.

Conclusions

Two of the key aims of telepsychiatry services are to improve access to psychiatry services for patients and to produce savings in time and costs. With these aims in mind the evaluation of telepsychiatry should necessarily consider the health economic implications. However, very few economic evaluations have been undertaken and those that have, have lacked methodological rigour. Studies have tended to have small sample sizes, which means that the power to generate definitive answers is lacking, have predominantly taken a cost-minimization perspective where costs are not linked to patient outcomes, have measured costs narrowly and have not explored the implications for the broader mental health care system. It is not therefore possible to determine whether telepsychiatry is an efficient alternative to existing methods of care provision based on the current literature.

What is clear from the small number of economic evaluations of telepsychiatry is that the level of activity is the main factor influencing its efficiency. One solution to potentially low rates of use is to open up the system to other specialities, such as those focusing on the physical and social condition of patients. This would seem to be a good use of the technology in that patients with mental illness frequently also have physical health problems as well as social difficulties.

Health care policy-makers and decision-makers at a local level need robust information regarding the 'cost-effectiveness' of a wide range of services and modes of service delivery. This level of information is unfortunately lacking in many areas including telepsychiatry. Proponents of telepsychiatry should also stress the need for comprehensive evaluations which assess the broad cost implications of telepsychiatry and which link cost data with patient outcome data in order to determine the worth of this form of care delivery.

References

1   Beecham J, Knapp M. Costing psychiatric interventions. In: Thornicroft G, ed. *Measuring Mental Health Needs*, 2nd edn. London: Gaskell, 2001:200–224.
2   McCrone P, Weich S. The costs of mental health care: paucity of measurement. In: Tansella M, Thornicroft G, eds. *Mental Health Outcome Measures*, 2nd edn. London: Gaskell, 2001:145–165.
3   Netten A, ed. *Unit Costs of Health and Social Care*. Canterbury, UK: Canterbury University, 2001.
4   Frueh BC, Deitsch SE, Santos AB, et al. Procedural and methodological issues in telepsychiatry research and program development. *Psychiatric Services* 2000;**51**:1522–1527.
5   Werner A, Anderson LE. Rural telepsychiatry is economically unsupportable: the Concorde crashes in a cornfield. *Psychiatric Services* 1998;**49**:1287–1290.
6   Chen DT, Blank MB, Worrall BB. Defending telepsychiatry. *Psychiatric Services* 1999;**50**:266.
7   Szeftel R. Defending telepsychiatry. *Psychiatric Services* 1999;**50**:267–268.
8   Smith HA. Defending telepsychiatry. *Psychiatric Services* 1999;**50**:266–267, discussion 267–268.
9   Tang WK, Chiu H, Woo J, Hjelm M, Hui E. Telepsychiatry in psychogeriatric service: a pilot study. *International Journal of Geriatric Psychiatry* 2001;**16**:88–93.
10 Kennedy C, Yellowlees P. A community-based approach to evaluation of health outcomes and costs for telepsychiatry in a rural population: preliminary results. *Journal of Telemedicine and Telecare* 2000;**6**(suppl 1):155–157.
11 Trott P, Blignault I. Cost evaluation of a telepsychiatry service in northern Queensland. *Journal of Telemedicine and Telecare* 1998;**4**(suppl 1):66–68.
12 Simpson J, Doze S, Urness D, Hailey D, Jacobs P. Evaluation of a routine telepsychiatry service. *Journal of Telemedicine and Telecare* 2001;**7**:90–98.
13 Simpson J, Doze S, Urness D, Hailey D, Jacobs P. Telepsychiatry as a routine service: the perspective of the patient. *Journal of Telemedicine and Telecare* 2001;**7**:155–160.
14 Elford DR, White H, St John K, Maddigan B, Ghandi M, Bowering R. A prospective satisfaction and cost analysis of a pilot child telepsychiatry service in Newfoundland. *Journal of Telemedicine and Telecare* 2001;**7**:73–81.
15 Rees CS, Gillam D. A comparison of the cost of cognitive-behavioural training for mental health professionals using videoconferencing or conventional, face-to-face teaching. *Journal of Telemedicine and Telecare* 2001;**7**:359–360.
16 Wootton R, Bloomer SE, Corbett R, et al. Multicentre randomized control trial comparing real time teledermatology with conventional outpatient dermatological care: societal cost-benefit analysis. *British Medical Journal* 2000;**320**:1252–1256.

4

Telepsychiatry and Doctor–Patient Communication – an analysis of the empirical literature

Edward Alan Miller

Introduction

Telepsychiatry involves the delivery of psychiatric and other mental health services when there is geographical separation between patients, mental health providers and other professionals. Although a number of different forms of communication (e.g. voice, sound, still picture, video and text transmission) and potential uses (e.g. continuing education, supervision, psychometric testing, psychotherapy, psychiatric assessment and consultation) are included in the telepsychiatric rubric, most of the enthusiasm for telepsychiatry is in the area of full motion, interactive video consultation between remote rural patients, tertiary care specialists (e.g. psychiatrists and psychologists) and/or other mental health personnel (e.g. psychiatric nurses, social workers, counsellors and community mental health workers). Because mental health personnel tend to be concentrated in populated regions, rural areas are typically underserved. Telepsychiatry may therefore be an efficient way to improve rural access to high-quality mental health care.

In contrast to user acceptance and satisfaction, few general conclusions have been reached with regard to telepsychiatry and doctor–patient communication.[1,2] Although some believe that telemedicine will alter doctor–patient relations,[3–6] there is, in fact, little agreement beyond the assertion that doctor–patient communication using telemedicine is indeed different. As Wootton and Darkin[7] observed, there is as of yet, no consensus as to whether telemedicine enhances or damages the therapeutic relationship or the traditional practice of medicine. This is a sentiment shared by Bashshur,[8] who pointed out that it has yet to be determined whether telemedicine facilitates or inhibits patient communication of their discomfort, symptoms and socio-emotional state, or, similarly, whether it encourages or inhibits doctors' communication of treatment instructions or expressions of empathy and caring. While some argue that over-the-screen therapy might one day be psychologically equivalent to face-to-face encounters,[9] others point out that telepsychiatry 'lacks the richness and intimacy of human contacts' and that 'those expecting a video conference to be a fully equivalent substitute for a face-to-face meeting are often disappointed'.[2] McLaren and Ball[10] suggested that telepsychiatry provides a particular challenge to telcommunication technology because 'complex emotional information needs to be transmitted and received but this is often complicated by the emotional state of the patient and the psychopathology'.

This lack of concurrence on the relational aspects of telemedicine is one reason why so many believe that changes in the nature and content of doctor–patient communication should represent an important component of any telemedicine evaluation.[8,11] The need for research is also clear if one acknowledges that although the adoption of advanced medical diagnosis and treatment technologies has become an inexorable feature of health care, interpersonal communication between doctors and patients 'provides the basis for establishing comfort and trust, for exchanging information that will be used to make health care decisions and for negotiating patient and physician decision making roles'.[12] This is especially true for mental health services where communication between mental health providers and patients is the primary means through which diagnoses are made and treatment plans effected.

In general, telemedicine may influence the extent of patient and physician participation during the medical encounter, either facilitating movement towards patient-centred and consumerist patterns identified by scholars such as Moskop[13] and Haug and Lavin,[14] or reinforcing traditional paternalistic patterns first described by Parsons[15] and Freidson[16] and later elaborated on by researchers such as Waitzkin.[17]

With paternalistic interactions, in particular, an asymmetrical relationship between doctor and patient allows physicians to dominate a medical encounter interaction, making decisions that either:

▶ reflect the patient's best interests (Parsons)

▶ protect their professional status and authority (Freidson)

▶ conform with society's expectations about appropriate behaviour (Waitzkin).

In this type of interaction, physicians mainly exhibit what has been referred to as 'doctor-centered' behaviours (e.g. giving directions, asking closed questions). Such behaviours are designed to gather sufficient information to make a diagnosis and consider treatment options in the least time possible.[18] For their part, patients are expected to agree with and follow whatever medical advice has been given.

Behavioural patterns are significantly different, however, when patients play a more active decision-making role. At the extreme are those patients who act purely as consumers, unilaterally making treatment decisions based on information provided by their providers. More common, however, are patients who act as neither passive bystanders nor sole decision-makers but instead as collaborators, bringing complementary strengths and resources to their interactions with physicians.[18] In doing so, patients place the biomedical focus of their doctors into context, bringing not only intimate knowledge of their physical state and well-being to the encounter but also knowledge of their psycho-social situations, including their personality, culture, living arrangements and relationships. Physician behaviour that encourages patient participation includes asking more open-ended questions, ensuring and confirming patient comprehension, requesting patient opinions and making statements of concern, agreement and approval.[18]

By influencing the way doctors and patients interact, telemedicine may also affect consultation outputs. These include:[19]

- process outcomes – during the medical encounter itself (e.g. patient assertiveness or provider empathy)

- short-term outcomes – immediately after medical encounter completion (e.g. satisfaction, tension release or knowledge acquisition)

- intermediate outcomes – within a few weeks or months after consultation (e.g. treatment compliance, psychological well-being, recall or understanding)

- long-term outcomes – recorded over longer periods of time (e.g. health status, symptom resolution, physiological status or survival).

A variety of behaviours have been correlated with outcomes such as these. Patients of physicians who engage in more information giving and positive talk, for example, report higher satisfaction and compliance, better recall and understanding and more favourable health status ratings and clinical outcomes.[20,21] Patients of physicians who encourage more active patient involvement also experience better results. In view of the association between certain communicative behaviours and medical encounter outcomes, it is important to understand whether telemedicine encourages such behaviours and, if not, how it may be configured to do so.

By altering consultation behaviour telemedicine may also affect trust, which can facilitate patient disclosure and cooperation, while reducing the likelihood of complaints, disputes and lawsuits.[22] As Mechanic[23] has observed, public distrust in medicine has increased over the last 20 years as a result of growing privatization and the proliferation of managed care. Although a variety of regulatory interventions have been pursued by professional and government organizations in order to enhance trust, patient-centred care models, which advise physicians to give patients time to tell their stories, listen intently without distractions, maintain eye contact and provide feedback, are particularly promising in this regard. As with medical encounter outcomes, however, it is unclear whether telemedicine facilitates or hinders behaviours such as these.

Doctor–patient interaction via telemedicine may also have important ethical and legal implications. Patients commonly have privacy and security concerns, which in today's health care environment primarily refer to third party access to electronic medical information.[24] However, privacy is a wide-ranging concept, which in addition to informational privacy (i.e. the releasing of personal files and data) also includes psychological privacy (i.e. the revealing of intimate attitudes, beliefs and feelings), social privacy (i.e. the ability to control social contacts) and physical privacy (i.e. the ability to control physical accessibility).[25] The nature of these may be different with two-way, interactive video, compared to conventional face-to-face encounters. Unlike in-person encounters, for example, video consultations often include multiple providers and technicians. As a consequence, patients may feel that that they are more susceptible to social and physical privacy violations with telemedicine. Unlike face-to-face medicine, moreover, video consultations can easily be recorded. While this may allow for a more complete medical record, it also increases the risks associated with third party access. In combination with virtually non-existent standards for ensuring privacy and confidentiality in the electronic transmission and storage of personal medical information,[26] patients may be more anxious about their privacy with telemedicine than with conventional in-person medicine. Because a number of USA states have higher confidentiality standards for psychiatric records, patient privacy and confidentiality is a particularly important issue for mental health care providers.[1]

From the physician's perspective malpractice liability is also an important legal issue, which generally occurs when a professional–patient relationship has been established and standards of care are violated. By changing the relationship between patients and providers, it is likely that telemedicine will challenge traditional malpractice principles.[5] The more fluid temporal boundaries of care and the simultaneous involvement of multiple providers and other personnel are particularly relevant. Because of jurisdictional and other issues, moreover, telemedicine may also alter traditional thinking about the standard of care. Exactly how it will do so is unclear since the only area in which specific telemedicine standards have been established in the USA is teleradiology, a non-interactive telemedicine application.[26] Given generally ambiguous care standards and unspecified changes in the doctor–patient relationship, it has yet to be determined whether current legal criteria apply to consultations taking place via two-way, interactive video. Regardless of any legal changes, however, telemedicine may still expose providers to more litigation because the impersonal nature of the service may compromise efforts to establish rapport with clients.[27] This is a non-trivial concern as malpractice experience has been associated with the communication behaviour of certain groups of providers.[28]

In summary, understanding how telepsychiatry affects doctor–patient communication is important for a number of reasons. Not only do communication behaviours reflect underlying decision-making roles but they may also affect consultation outcomes. Patient trust and privacy concerns are also intimately associated with doctor–patient interaction, not to mention practitioners' malpractice exposure. Given the likely significance of telepsychiatry for doctor–patient communication, further research in this area should certainly be a priority. To this end, a comprehensive survey has been performed of existing studies of doctor–patient communication via telemedicine.

Methods

Peer-reviewed articles assessing the nature and content of doctor–patient communication via telepsychiatry were identified from a search of the MEDLINE database. Combinations of the following key words were used: telemedicine, doctor–patient relations, communication, satisfaction, acceptance, surveys, qualitative methods, remote consultation, psychiatry, mental health, psychology and telepsychiatry. Approximately 150 articles were identified, collected and examined for other possible sources from their references. These other sources were also collected, resulting in a total of approximately 200 references.

Studies without any communication findings, along with essays, editorials and other non-peer-reviewed pieces were excluded from further analysis. Acceptable studies had to include some findings pertinent to the study of communication during two-way interactive video consultations, whether between provider and patient or between provider and provider. However, they did not have to focus exclusively on communication. In fact most focused more broadly on overall performance and satisfaction with the general attributes of telemedicine.

Sixty-one articles met the criteria for inclusion. Because multiple articles described the results of a single study, 57, not 61, were included in the review. The communication findings were then grouped into 23 categories. In addition to general communicative efficacy, specific categories included patients' and providers' expression, understanding and comfort, participant relations, embarrassment, anxiety and miscellaneous affect, audio and video quality, non-verbal behaviour, technology and other system attributes, multiple providers' and patients' involvement, privacy and encounter length, outcomes and care quality, satisfaction, video versus in-person consultation, and assessment and diagnosis. After coding each study's findings according to these categories, a positive or negative rating was assigned to each individual result based on a set of predetermined criteria, as follows:

1. For results reported using sample percentages, more than 50% had to rate a particular aspect favourably in order for a given finding to receive a positive rating.

2. For results reported using mean scores on survey or questionnaire items, the average study participant had to rate a given item higher than the mid-point on the particular scale used in order for a given finding to receive a positive rating (e.g. more than 5 on a 10-point scale).

3. For results reported using comparisons between telemedicine and other modes of health service delivery, the performance of telemedicine had to equal or exceed that which had been recorded for conventional in-person encounters in order for a given finding to receive a positive rating.

4. For results reported using qualitative research techniques (e.g. interviews, observation), investigators had to come to unambiguously favourable conclusions regarding the particular aspect of doctor–patient communication assessed in order for a given finding to receive a positive rating.

Using the mid-point as the cut-off for questionnaire results (i.e. >50% of sample respondents, average score >5 on a 10-point scale) is a common practice employed in literature reviews. Moreover, employing more stringent criteria (i.e. >75% of sample respondents, average score >7.5 on a 10-point scale) would not have altered my conclusions appreciably as comparatively few findings fell within the 50–75% or 5–7.5 range.

Using the above criteria, 550 individual findings were rated. Because a single study might include multiple measures of the same communication concept (e.g. patient comfort), each study could contribute multiple findings to a particular category (e.g. comfort with the video equipment used, comfort in relation to live consultations or overall comfort). Some findings could not be categorized as either positive or negative, usually because they were descriptive rather than evaluative in nature (e.g. such as those describing encounter structure and content).

Results

Two basic types of studies were identified, based on their general methodology. These were:

1. post-encounter surveys of telepsychiatry encounter participants (29 studies)

2. qualitative analyses of telepsychiatry encounters themselves, including participant and non-participant observation, in-depth interviews, case reports and content analysis (28 studies).

Eighteen of these studies[30-47] have been summarized previously.[29] The remaining studies are summarized in Tables 4.1 and 4.2 for post-encounter surveys and qualitative analyses, respectively.

Practically all research into the effects of telepsychiatry on doctor–patient communication is relatively recent and only 10 of the 61 articles surveyed were published before 1995. Most of these investigations originated in the US (23 studies) and the UK (16). Others originated in Australia (7), Canada (6), Finland (2) and France (2). Norway and South Korea also contributed one entry each. Studies took place in a number of locations. While specialists generally consulted from a variety of tertiary centres located in urban areas, patients and/or referring providers were located in a variety of remote sites, including rural and suburban hospitals and medical centres (20), clinics and physicians' offices (10), their own homes or schools (4), and in the case of two studies, prisons. Ten studies simulated the telepsychiatry experience by having mental health personnel and patients interact via a video link within the same facility. Most studies utilized PC- or video-based telemedicine systems (21 and 23, respectively) using ISDN lines (31) at 128 kbit/s (20) or greater (17).

Most studies examined encounters between off-site psychiatrists and on-site patients, although some also involved remote providers, including other psychiatrists (4 studies), nurses (13), general practitioners (11), on-site psychometric raters (2), social workers, case managers and counsellors (8). The persons most frequently consulted were general psychiatrists (36 studies) followed by child psychiatrists (8), psychologists (8) and psychiatric nurses (1). The purposes included psychiatric consultation and assessment (43), psychotherapy and counselling (11), family therapy (4), follow-up and care planning (2).

Twice as many studied telepsychiatry in an outpatient (34 studies) rather than an inpatient (17) setting. Although most recruited adults (35), others focused on teenagers and children (12), their parents (8), the elderly (3), prisoners (2) and medical residents (1). Most studies focused on patients with a variety of mental and psychiatric problems (31). Others, however, focused more narrowly on one or more of the following conditions: problematical and disruptive behaviour (10), schizophrenia (8), depression and bipolar disorder (8), schizoaffective disorder (4), anxiety and panic disorder (3), obsessive-compulsive disorder (1) and transsexualism (1).

Approximately half reported the length of their study periods. These ranged from one day in a small number of studies to 14 that extended over a year or more. Sample sizes displayed considerable variability as well, ranging from 7–230 and from 1–199 patients/clients in post-encounter surveys and qualitative investigations, respectively. Qualitative investigations, however, generally employed fewer participants. While close to two thirds of qualitative studies recruited less than 30 patients/clients, approximately two thirds of post-encounter studies recruited 30 or more. Most researchers, did not report their response or participation rates. Of the 11 studies that did, however, most tended to be reasonable (i.e. >50%). Of 31 studies reporting the number of participating providers, the majority (65%) employed only one or two. A small number, however, reported using 25 or more (6).

Fifteen post-encounter studies reported using a comparison group (i.e. 52%). Only three employed randomization. Two of these randomly allocated patients to a video and in-person control, while a third randomly assigned patients to one of three groups: observer in-person/rater over video, both in-person, and both over video. Although randomization was not indicated, five other studies also compared patients receiving video and in-person consultations, while an additional seven compared video and in-person assessment of the same patients.

Ten qualitative studies also reported using a comparison group. In only one instance, however, was randomization indicated, where clients were randomly assigned to one of three therapy groups: in-person, video and hands-free audio. The remaining studies used a variety of quasi-experimental alternatives. These included comparing the same subjects in a variety of consultation modes (4 studies), comparing video patients to in-person controls (3), comparing video patients to conventional cases reported elsewhere in the literature (1) and recording practitioners' insights from both their video and in-person experiences (1).

All post-encounter surveys relied on multi-item questionnaires. Most investigators, however, did not describe their questionnaires in detail. Of those who did, varying numbers of items were reported, ranging from 3 to 14. Qualitative investigations, however, employed a variety of research techniques, and often more than one in the same study. These included participant and non-participant observation (11 studies), in-depth interviews (6), case reports (11), questionnaires (8) and content analysis (6).

From the 57 studies reviewed, 550 findings were abstracted from post-encounter surveys of patients (239 findings), consultants (49) and local providers (46) and qualitative analyses of medical encounter behaviour (216). Overall, there were more than three times as many positive results as negative results (Table 4.3). For all but one of the 23 categories the number of findings rated positively exceeded the number of findings rated negatively. Particularly striking in this regard (i.e. categories with 15 or more positive than negative results) were patient expression, patient comfort, participant relations, outcome/care quality, satisfaction, assessment/diagnosis, and video versus in-person consultation. Non-verbal behaviour was the only area for which the number of positive findings (6) did not exceed the number of negative findings (22). Other areas with comparatively high levels of negative findings (>35%

Table 4.1. Telepsychiatry and the doctor–patient relationship: findings using psychiatric assessment, post-encounter surveys and self-report measures

Authors	Location	Consultation/equipment	Methods	Communication/other findings
Glueckauf et al (2002)[48]	Five Midwest states. 22 rural Midwestern homes (peripheral sites). Purdue University Indianapolis (central site)	Family intervention counselling with off-site psychologist. 5 sessions following initial in-person assessment. Various scales used: issue-specific measures, home and school functioning, therapeutic alliance and compliance. ISDN	Over 2 years. Surveys at pre-/post-test and 6-month follow-up. Compared home-based video and speaker-phone with in-person counselling. 22 teenagers with seizure disorders and psychosocial/education difficulties, and their parents. Two-step random assignment. Another 17 families dropped out	Teenagers and parents reported significant reductions in issue-specific severity and frequency across video, speakerphone and in-person modes. Parents reported increases in prosocial behaviours that were not maintained at the 6-month follow-up, while teachers reported no increase in prosocial behaviours. Neither parents nor teachers observed substantial change in teen problem behaviour. Both parents and teenagers reported high levels of therapeutic alliance across all three counselling conditions though teenagers reported lower levels than their parents. While teenagers also reported lower alliance levels in the video than speakerphone and office-based modes, parents reported the same levels across all three. Mode of service delivery did not influence treatment adherence (i.e. attendance, homework completion)
Bose et al (2001)[49]	London, UK. Grove Medical Centre (peripheral site). Ladywell Unit (central site)	Psychotherapy with off-site psychiatrist and on-site general practitioner. Video-system, ISDN, 128 kbit/s	Over 4 months. Six-item survey. At post-encounter. 13 non-psychotic patients previously seen in person. 29 video sessions	Most patients (>75%) indicated that they had achieved their aims, could see and hear all they needed to hear, would like to use video again, and that the closeness of the interaction was just right. Some had trouble seeing or felt that the interaction was too distant (25% each). None felt the interaction was too close
Elford et al (2001)[50]	Newfoundland, Canada. Western Memorial Regional Hospital, Corner Brook (peripheral site). Janeway Child Health Centre, St John's (central site)	Non-emergency psychiatric consultations with off-site child psychiatrist and on-site telepsychiatry nurse. PC-based, ISDN and digital lines, 336 kbit/s	Post-encounter survey. Child psychiatry. 30 patients (aged 5–16 years) accompanied by their parents. 94% patient participation rate. Five psychiatrists.	*Psychiatrist:* All 'satisfied' or 'very satisfied' with video. Most (84%) felt video was as good as face-to-face. None inconvenienced by system. Follow-up deemed acceptable for most cases (92%). *Parents/adolescents:* Most (>83%) liked or preferred using the system, would use it again and preferred it to travelling. On average, they rated overall satisfaction and comfort highly (>3, 5= highest). Comfort increased during the course of the interview. While parents rated the ease of giving information and seeing/ hearing highly, adolescents did so for ease in talking and understanding. Most (80%) thought video was just as good or better than in-person interview. *Children:* All liked video and most (56%) liked 'television doctor' better than 'real' doctor

Table 4.1. – *continued*

Authors	Location	Consultation/equipment	Methods	Communication/other findings
Kopel et al (2001)[51]	New South Wales, Australia. Rural areas (peripheral sites). Children's Hospital at Westmead (central site)	Consultations between off-site child psychiatrists and on-site rural clinicians. 384 kbit/s	Over 12 months. Four-item scale. At post-encounter. Child adolescent psychiatry. 84 new patients and parent/carers (60% response rate). 20 rural clinicians (74% response rate over 136 consultations). Eight child psychiatrists (100% response rate over 136 consultations)	Both patients and rural clinicians rated the following highly (>78% at top two scale points): service quality, received service wanted, service met needs, would recommend, amount of help, service helped with problem, would return, convenience, comfort, as good as in-person visit and overall satisfaction. Most (90%) patients and rural clinicians rated sound, visual and overall quality as good/excellent, while most consultants (>72%) rated them as fair/poor. Most participants (>85%) felt not at all/slightly anxious, self-conscious/embarrassed or interfered with by the equipment. Most patients and rural clinicians (91%) rated satisfaction almost or as good as in-person, while most consultants (80%) rated it as only adequate. While most rural clinicians (87%) rated ease of use as good/excellent, fewer consultants did (49%) with the remainder rating it fair/poor (52%)
Simpson et al (2001)[52,53]	Alberta, Canada. Five hospitals serving small towns (peripheral sites). Alberta Hospital Ponoka (central site)	546 routine telepsychiatry consultations. Video system, ISDN, 336–384 kbit/s	Over 2 years. Post-encounter surveys and phone interviews. 230 patients responded to the survey (61% response rate); 31 interviewed by telephone (14% response rate). 20 general practitioners surveyed (24% response rate). Interviews also with 3 of 11 psychiatrists using system and all 5 site coordinators	*Patient surveys:* Most (>95%) rated the equipment as good in relation to sound, picture, ease of use and room used. Most (>88%) indicated that they were able to present the same information as in person, felt comfortable with their ability to interact with doctor and satisfied with session. *Patient interviews:* Most (77%) identified consultants as the source of information received, including course of action or referral (39%) and emotional reassurance (32%). Most (90%) satisfied with service received. Most (>80%) agreed/strongly agreed that they would rather see a doctor over television than travel or wait, that they would use video again and that they would recommend it to a friend. Few would rather see a psychiatrist over video than in person. *Personnel:* All GPs were satisfied/very satisfied with referral/scheduling, consultation report and follow-up. All psychiatrists believed the system was acceptable and thought patients were comfortable. Some felt in-person contact provided for more non-verbal cues and sense of presence. Others felt communication adequate

Table 4.1. – *continued*

Authors	Location	Consultation/equipment	Methods	Communication/other findings
D'Souza (2000)[54]	South Australia. 15 rural hospitals (peripheral sites). Glenside Hospital, Adelaide (central site)	Psychiatric assessment and daily follow-up with off-site psychiatrist, on-site nurse and second rater. Brief Psychiatric Rating Scale (BPRS) given over video. A second behavioural scale was also completed but faxed	Post-encounter survey. 28 adult inpatients assessed initially and 4 weeks after discharge. Patients averaged 5.3 teleconsultations and 10 days hospitalization. One psychiatrist, one primary nurse and one trained rater	There was evidence for improved outcomes in the management of acute psychiatric inpatients. Average inpatient stay was much shorter than stays in Adelaide, which may be due to family and GP presence, and patient being cared for in familiar surroundings. Significant improvement in mean total BPRS and behavioural scores and good inter-rater reliability (0.95) for the latter. High patient ratings (>3.4, 5 = satisfied): got service wanted, met needs, helped problem, satisfied with help, overall satisfaction, consider using again and would recommend to friend. Although 67% were satisfied with confidentiality, 26% raised forms of dissatisfaction
Elford et al (2000)[55]	Newfoundland, Canada. Janeway Child Health Centre. Two rooms in same facility	Non-emergency psychiatric assessment with 'on/off-site' child psychiatrist. PC-based, ISDN and digital lines, 336–384 kbit/s	Over 3 months. Post-encounter survey. Child psychiatry. Compared video to in-person assessment for 23 patients (aged 4–16 years) and their parents. 68% patient participation rate. Five psychiatrists	*Psychiatrists*: Video was rated as an adequate alternative to in-person assessment and did not interfere with diagnosis. Comfort grew with use. All would use it again. Most (91%) said video went moderately/very well. Compared to in-person doctors felt that assessments did not go as well with video, nor did they feel they communicated as well or felt as understood. They also would liked to have changed or improved things more with video. No difference in non-technical difficulties or patient management. Initial sound quality rated negatively. Technical problems interfered with 10 video assessments. In most cases (96%) diagnosis and suggested treatment were the same for both video and face-to-face. *Children/parents*: Young children viewed video positively (would use again), while 29% preferred video and 29% face-to-face. Most (82%) adolescents and parents found it 'just as easy' to talk to the doctor using video, while 39% preferred video and 54% in person. Some parents found it easier to talk and hear in person; others noted lack of eye contact and poor sound quality with video. No difference in parents' rating of: their or their children's ability to talk/say all they wanted, comfort and doctors' understanding, and usefulness. Most parents would use it again (83%) and preferred it to travelling (91%)

Table 4.1. – *continued*

Authors	Location	Consultation/equipment	Methods	Communication/other findings
Kirkwood et al (2000)[56]	Scottish Highlands. Building 10 km from central site (peripheral site). Craig Dunain Hospital, Inverness (central site)	Consultations with on-/off-site clinical psychologist. Assessment tools covered intellectual functioning, verbal memory and attention/ concentration. PC-based, ISDN, 128 kbit/s	Four-item survey. At post-encounter. 26 patients with a history of alcohol abuse. Compared face-to-face and video assessments given on same day by same person	On average, patients rated sound and visual quality, and overall satisfaction with video highly (>7.5, 10 = high). Most (85%) said they would use video again. What they liked best included everything (5 patients), feeling relaxed and at ease (8), no effort to use equipment (5) and access to professional (3). Criticisms included difficulty in understanding words/general sound quality (6) and delays in communication (3). Video sessions were significantly longer than in-person sessions. Similar results generally achieved when assessments were performed in person or over video. Worse performance on some video assessments (Quick Test IQ, Story Recall) may have been due to poorer audio and visual clarity. Better performance on some video assessments (Motor Speed) may have been due to reduced performance anxiety when interviewer was not in the room. Lack of picture clarity made it difficult to view facial expressions
Mielonen et al (2000)[57]	Oulu, Finland. Two primary care centres (peripheral sites). Oulu University Hospital (central site)	Psychiatric inpatient care planning consultations between off-site psychiatrist/ psychiatric nurse and on-/off-site community psychiatric nurse/social worker/general practitioner. Video system, ISDN, 384 kbit/s	Over 11 months. Post-encounter survey. Compared 14 video to 20 in-person consultations. 124 participants: patients (14), health care staff (14) and nursing students (5) at hospital, and primary care workers (35), social workers (13) and relatives (13) at primary care centre. 90% response rate	Most health personnel that had used video felt it as good (47%) or almost as good (48%) as in-person meetings. Most health workers (86%), patients (84%) and relatives (92%) that had used video preferred to use it for their next meeting. Only 20% of relatives, ward staff and primary care staff that had conventional meetings were willing to use video again. Most often cited reason for preferring video was reduced travel time and ease and speed of consultations. The majority (>50%) rated content and interaction of videoconference as good/excellent for management and information concerning the purpose of the conference, ease of expressing opinions and participant collaboration. The majority rated usefulness and quality of results of video as good/excellent, and the audio, visual and overall technical quality as good/moderate. Working process for video and in-person meetings was different

Table 4.1. – *continued*

Authors	Location	Consultation/equipment	Methods	Communication/other findings
Ball et al (1999)[58]	UK and France. Community mental health team for the elderly	Researchers scored written material from the Mini-Mental Health Status Examination (MMHS). These included copying interlocking pentagrams and writing a sentence of their own choosing. PC-based, ISDN, 128 kbit/s	Compared MMHS exam scoring across three modes: face-to-face, fax and video. 99 written responses from the records of discharged elderly patients. Three raters scored 33 MMSEs in each mode. Two assessors in UK, one in France	Relative to in-person (0.71) but not over video (0.47). Results suggest that where the criteria for scoring are relatively loose and the assessor may use other clues from the task (i.e. as with sentences) both fax and video allow for reliable scoring. But when the rules are tighter and there is less room for the assessor to use other clues (i.e. as with pentagrams), fax provides adequate images but video may not. There may be dangers in uncritical acceptance of scoring done using video equipment
Chae et al (1999)[59]	South Korea. Patients' home or halfway house (peripheral sites). Koyang Community Mental Health Center (central site)	Psychiatric assessment with off-site psychiatrist and on-site nurse. Assessment tool used: Brief Psychiatric Rating Scale. Analogue videophone, ordinary telephone lines, 33 kbit/s	Over 3 months. Four-item survey. At post-encounter. Patients with schizophrenia randomly selected from those treated at mental health centre. Compared 15 low bandwidth video to 15 face-to-face assessments	No difference in total acceptance between video (14.1) and in person (13.7) assessment among patients. Although more felt comfortable in person (87%) than with video (73%), more felt at ease expressing themselves (73% vs. 60%) and rated their relationship with their doctors as good (87% vs. 47%) with video. Most found no difference in the interview's usefulness (73%). Controlling for other factors, results showed higher overall acceptance with interviews for less severely ill and patients assessed over video. Agreement for the total assessment score for the videophone (0.82) was significantly higher than for face-to-face interviews (0.67), possibly due to low correlation in one item (excitement, −0.06). Low correlation for anxiety item with video (0.22) was probably due to technology limitations. Concluded lower – as reliable as higher-bandwidth systems

Table 4.1. – continued

Authors	Location	Consultation/equipment	Methods	Communication/other findings
Doze et al (1999)[60,61]	Alberta, Canada. Five hospital-based mental health clinics (peripheral sites). Alberta Hospital Ponoka (central site)	Psychiatric consultations between off-site psychiatrist, on-site general practitioner, and/or mental health nurse or counsellor (available at three sites). Video system, ISDN, 336–384 kbit/s	Over 9 months. Post-encounter surveys and follow-up phone interviews. 90 patients, 31 general practitioners and 7 psychiatrists. 63% (57) of patients completed evaluation forms, 54% (46) agreed to telephone interview although 14 could not be reached	*Patient survey:* Benefits included less travel time, stress from travel, absence from work and delay accessing psychiatrist, more feelings of confidentiality/privacy, choice and control, improved quality and reduced hospitalization. Perceived disadvantages included impersonal interaction and less sensitivity in interviews. Most (>80%) felt that the quality of the equipment/room was good, that they were able to present the same information as in person, that they felt comfortable interacting with the psychiatrist, and that they were satisfied with the session. *Patient interview:* Most (>81%) strongly agreed/agreed that they would rather use video than travel or wait to see a psychiatrist, but were evenly divided on whether they preferred video or in-person consultations. Most would use video again (93%) or recommend it to a friend (97%). *Personnel:* 95% of GPs thought availability had improved. Some commented on the ability to support the patient and talk with the psychiatrist. For psychiatrists the benefits included seeing patients before conditions became severe, educating GPs and avoiding hospitalization. Most patients, GPs and psychiatrists were satisfied with video. Most rated picture and audio quality as good
Freir et al (1999)[62]	Scottish Highlands. Portree Hospital on the Isle of Skye (peripheral site). Craig Dunain Hospital, Inverness (central site)	Consultations with off-site psychologist. Treated using cognitive behavioural approaches. Video system, ISDN, 128 kbit/s	Post-encounter survey of 27 adults and 7 children (or their parents)	Most complained about poor picture and sound quality. They sometimes felt distracted by the quality of communication with the psychologist. Patients were still satisfied. 88% said that they would accept further treatment using video, but about 33% preferred face-to-face consultations

Table 4.1. – *continued*

Authors	Location	Consultation/equipment	Methods	Communication/other findings
Ball and Puffet (1998)[63]	London, UK. Inner city old-age psychiatric service	Psychiatric assessment by off-site assessor and on-site aid using the CAMCOG test. PC-based, ISDN, 128 kbit/s	Compared video and in-person assessment for 8 of 11 elderly subjects initially enrolled in the study. Two doctors	Despite a variety of technical problems, reasonable correlations between video and in-person assessments were recorded overall (0.72) and for most individual items in the scale (e.g. orientation, language, attention, praxis). Mean in-person (88.6) and video (88.3) scores were quite close. Unlike previous studies, an aide provided assistance at the remote site. Concluded that the CAMCOG test can be used reliably over a video system without major modification
Mielonen et al (1998)[64]	Oulu, Finland. Two regional health centres and two educational institutions (peripheral sites). Oulu University Hospital (central site)	Videoconferencing for family therapy, occupational counselling, patient consultation and teaching. Video system, ISDN, 128–384 kbit/s	Over 2 years. Three-item survey. At post-encounter. 37 mental health personnel. Some general observations also made	On average, mental health personnel rated audio quality (8.0), picture quality (7.5) and general quality of video interaction (7.5) highly (>midpoint, 10 = excellent). Personnel found adjustable camera, zooming and possibility of switching picture between pre-set camera positions important. Appreciated remote control and viewing 'outgoing screen'. Taking turns speaking when using video helped to structure the interaction. Patients and families were less negative about video than expected. Staff attitudes improved with increased participation and use
Bear et al (1997)[65]	Boston, Massachusetts. Medical Center of Central Massachusetts (peripheral site). Massachusetts Department of Mental Health (central site)	Emergency psychiatric assessment by on-/off-site assessors for purposes of involuntary commitment. Eight scales	Compared video to in-person assessment for 12 individuals. One on-site and one off-site psychiatrist	High inter-rater agreement (0.85) found in the mean ratings made by the on- and off-site assessors. In none of the evaluations did the on- or off-site psychiatrists feel that additional information had been observed directly but not over the video link

Table 4.1. – *continued*

Authors	Location	Consultation/equipment	Methods	Communication/other findings
McLaren et al (1996)[66]	London, UK. Community mental health centre (peripheral site). Teaching hospital (central site)	Psychiatric consultation with on-/off-site psychiatrist. PC-based, monochrome picture	Over 2 months. Post-encounter survey. Compared video and live consultations. Three questionnaires used. Although 15/26 outpatients agreed to participate only 7 had both video and live consultations	On average, patients rated video more positively than psychiatrists, both overall and across all categories, including being comfortable, being self-conscious, raising personal issues, seeing the other, hearing the other, other seemed too far, other seemed too close, and interview seemed impersonal. *Patients:* On average rated effect of video highly in all categories (>midpoint, 7 = very). Also rated efficacy of video higher than in-person interviews in terms of being informed, thinking doctor paid attention, feeling better and overall. Low patient participation probably due to videotaping. Patients were reluctant to use telephone when video equipment failed. *Psychiatrist:* Rated video's effect highly in all categories but raising personal issues, seeing/hearing the other and others seemed far away. Exhibited less confidence in judging key symptoms with video. Difficult to detect crying, see facial expressions, or hear changes in patient tone or volume
Salzman et al (1996)[67]	Massachusetts. Department of Mental Health facility (peripheral site). Massachusetts Mental Health Center (central site)	Psychiatric consultation with on- and off-site assessors. Patients rated on the Brief Psychiatric Rating Scale. PC-based	Compared video to in-person assessment. Seven severely ill hospitalized psychotic patients. One on- and one off-site psychiatrist	Found high inter-rater agreement (0.92) with video and in-person assessments of the same patients. Observed that the only frequent rating disagreement was on the self-neglect item. This was because some patients' self-neglect was not visible through the camera. Patients enjoyed using the video system
Ball et al (1993)[68]	London, UK. Guy's Hospital. Acute psychiatric unit. Two rooms in adjacent wards	Psychiatric assessments by off-site assessor. Tool used: Mini-Mental State Examination (MMSE). PC-based, monochrome camera, 2 Mbit/s	Compared face-to-face and video assessment of 11 adult inpatients with schizophrenia (6), depression (5) and movement disorder (1). One psychiatrist	High correlation observed in the test scores achieved in the video and face-to-face conditions (0.89). Re-scoring of illegible material raised the correlation (0.92). Concluded that standardized cognitive testing can be carried out using low-cost videoconferencing technology in adult populations with acute psychiatric illness. Higher scores by 6 patients with video may be due to added attention given to novel situation

Table 4.2. Telepsychiatry and the doctor–patient relationship: findings using qualitative methods (observation, interviews, case reports, and content analysis)

Authors	Location	Consultation/equipment	Methods	Communication/other findings
Hill et al (2001)[69]	Honolulu, Hawaii. Mainland videoconferencing site (peripheral site). Tripler Army Medical Center, Hawaii (central site)	Family therapy sessions with on-site psychiatrist and off-site family members. Video system	Two case reports. Patients with bipolar disorder and schizoaffective disorder hospitalized in inpatient psychiatric unit	Purpose of each session was to facilitate social support and mend family disconnections. Believed that high clarity images (e.g. tears, emotional displays, body language, facial expressions) provided by video system were critical in developing a virtual interactive social presence among participants. Asserted that participants can communicate in ways similar to in-person. Concluded that skilled clinicians can create an atmosphere of trust and comfort and encourage exploration of important issues
Simpson (2001)[70]	Scotland. Lerwick Health Centre, Shetland (peripheral site). Royal Cornhill Hospital, Aberdeen (central site)	Videoconferencing therapy sessions with off-site psychologist. PC-based, ISDN 128 kbit/s	Over 12 months. Post-encounter survey including self-completed qualitative scale. Post-therapy interview and improvement rating. Therapeutic alliance scale. 10 clients with previous face-to-face contact, 12 sessions	The psychologist and all but one client were highly satisfied. Clients were able to develop a positive therapeutic relationship with therapist and all reported improvement from therapy. Clients obtained some new understanding and felt therapist understood them and that they worked together. Some clients felt it enhanced the therapeutic relationship (less confrontational, self-conscious), although a few felt it impersonal and isolating. Most clients rated image and audio quality adequate. They did not feel distracted by technology, and found video easy to communicate with and useful. Client satisfaction increased with use and was higher for those with simpler problems. Many felt it gave them space and confidentiality (e.g. therapist did not live in local community). After initial technical problems, the therapist found clients engaged and were able to express their feelings and difficulties openly. Lack of picture clarity sometimes made it difficult to identify facial expressions, particularly when clients were tearful

Table 4.2. – *continued*

Authors	Location	Consultation/equipment	Methods	Communication/other findings
Turner (2001)[71]	State prison hospital (peripheral site). Large academic medical centre (central site)	Consultation with off-site psychiatrist. Video system, 768 kbit/s	Over 18 months. Multiple methods, including surveys, observation and analysis of treatment recommendations. 43 consultations involving 14 patients in prison hospital, all taking psychotropic medication. One psychiatrist	On average, psychiatrist ranked appropriateness of system highly (8.8, 1–10 scale), while patients ranked information exchange (30) and comfort (24) highly (>midpoint, 7–35 scale). Not all of the psychiatrist's recommendations were followed by prison staff. This might be due to lack of credibility and relationships between the psychiatrist and hospital staff. Compared to in-person sessions a number of information sources were removed, including contact with other health personnel, patient's family and broader surroundings (e.g. living conditions). Only context available with telemedicine was provided by the interview itself and what little could be seen and heard in the background. This can affect therapeutic efficacy and credibility with ancillary personnel
Day and Schneider (2000)[72]	Illinois. Psychological Services Center at the University of Illinois at Urbana-Champaign. Two rooms in the same facility	Cognitive behavioural therapy with 'off-site' psychotherapist over five sessions. Video system, direct line	Over 2 years. Transcript analysis, ratings of working alliance, therapist interviews and surveys. Clients randomly allocated to in-person, video and hands-free audio. 26/27 clients per group. All 10 therapists were doctoral students. Each saw from 3 to 30 clients, some in each mode	Results indicate that video/audio modes may substitute and in some cases improve upon in-person therapy. No difference in working alliance found (therapist exploration, client hostility and participation) across the three modes although some therapists felt disconnected with video/audio. Although some therapists were frustrated with the audio mode, others indicated that it kept them from appearance-based judgements, forced them to refine their listening skills, and sometimes made their clients and/or themselves more relaxed, open and comfortable. Therapists felt that some approaches, types of problems and clients were better suited to distance modes than others. Seven therapists liked in-person therapy best, two preferred audio and one all modes equally. High client and therapist satisfaction was reported with no difference across modes. Both clients and therapists seemed able to adjust to whatever situation they encountered. Concluded that in some cases distancing effect of audio/video may promote honesty, feelings of safety, which may serve some groups well (e.g. schizophrenics, agoraphobics)

Table 4.2. – *continued*

Authors	Location	Consultation/equipment	Methods	Communication/other findings
Deitsch et al (2000)[73]	South Carolina. Ralph H. Johnson Veterans Administration Medial Center (peripheral site). Dorn Veterans Administration Medical Center (central site)	Group therapy session between one off-site leader and two on-site leaders. PC-based, ISDN, 384 kbit/s	Case report from one session. Four Vietnam veterans with post-traumatic stress disorder and co-morbid major depression	All patients were able to use the video equipment, believed the session was as helpful as a usual session, felt comfortable communicating with the remote therapist, would use it again to save travel time and rated the quality as good/very good. The group familiarized themselves with camera controls, gaining a sense of control. Camera views were adjusted appropriately according to the dynamics of the discussion. All were willing to discuss personal, sensitive and painful issues after initial experimentation and assurances of privacy. They seemed to forget about technology during session
May et al (2000)[74]	Northwest England. Two general practices in Carnforth (peripheral sites). Community mental health centre in Morecambe (central site)	Consultations with off-site psychiatrist and on-site general practitioner. PC-based, ISDN, 128 kbit/s	Over 12 months. Semi-structured informal interviews analysed using discourse analysis. 22 patients with anxiety and depression. 13 general practitioners and psychiatrists. Low-cost videophone	Some users were positive, others ambivalent. Patients viewed it as a means of obtaining additional 'expert advice'. GPs saw it as potential barrier to good doctor–patient relationship in psychiatry. Both patients and GPs noticed that video modified normal interaction (missed body language and facial expressions). Need to adjust to technology where image and audio quality is variable. May be difficult to uncover underlying psychology when mediated by videophone. Psychiatrist found it difficult to help people relax over video. Some felt that it increased convenience and had potential to reduce the stigma of mental health encounters

Table 4.2. – continued

Authors	Location	Consultation/equipment	Methods	Communication/other findings
Schopp et al (2000)[75]	Missouri. Rural hospitals/clinics (peripheral site). University of Missouri-Columbia (central site)	Neuropsychological assessment with off-site psychologist and on-site psychometrist. Used two tests: Brief Symptom Inventory and Full-Scale IQ. T1 links, 768 kbit/s	Post-encounter surveys. Open-ended interviews with providers and referral sources. Compared 49 neuropsychology outpatients with 49 matched in-person controls. Seven neuro-psychologists, two interns, one psychometrist	High mean patient ratings (>5.2, 7 = very much) indicated for: global satisfaction, how relaxed or tense they felt, ease of communication, perceived psychologist caring and whether they would want to meet again under the same condition (in person, over video). No difference across modes in any rating but desire to repeat their experience, which was higher for video. Providers gave significantly higher satisfaction ratings for in-person than video contacts. Several clients noted that it was interesting to take part in a novel high-tech. clinic and that it made it easier to access high-quality care close to home. Some clients had concern for confidentiality during their interviews although psychologists expressed more frustration with even modest connection, indistinct audio, and audio/visual desynchronization problems than their brain-injured clients. Telehealth sessions were less expensive than alternative scenarios in which the psychologist or client travelled from their respective sites to the other. Referral sources indicated that there were no perceptible difference in psychologists' reports or recommendations for in-person or telehealth groups

Table 4.2. – continued

Authors	Location	Consultation/equipment	Methods	Communication/other findings
Hufford et al (1999)[76]	Indianapolis, Indiana. Three family homes (peripheral sites). Family Assessment and Intervention Laboratory, Indiana University (central site)	Family intervention counselling with off-site psychologist. Various scales used: issue severity, frequency, and change, intervention priority, audio-visual, and working alliance. Video system, ISDN	Mixed methods. Post-encounter surveys and content analysis. Three adolescents (aged 11–19 years) with epilepsy and at-risk/problematical behaviour and their mothers. Six sessions. Compared in person (1st and 6th session), speakerphone (2nd and 4th), and video (3rd and 5th) counselling. Two clinical psychology doctoral students served as co-therapists	Ratings indicated that family comfort with all three modes was moderately high, while their perceived level of distraction was low. Mothers, however, reported being less comfortable and more distracted than their children. Content analysis indicated that both mothers and children experienced higher comfort in the video and office than audio-only modes. Positive responses focused on the convenience and more relaxed feeling of being at home generally, and picture quality and comfort felt from seeing therapists over video specifically. Negative responses focused on the audio quality (hearing specific words) of the speakerphone and video modes. Content analysis also indicated fewer distractions during office than home-based counselling sessions (i.e. from relatives, fatigue, anxiety, friends). Family members reported similarly high levels of alliance with their counsellors in all three modes, along with substantial and equivalent reductions in problem severity and frequency and substantial problem improvement over time
Manchanda and McLaren (1998)[77]	London, UK. General practice (peripheral site). Guy's Hospital (central site)	Cognitive behavioural therapy sessions with off-site therapist. PC-based, ISDN, 128 kbit/s	Case report of a course of therapy for one patient with mixed anxiety and depressive disorder. 12 sessions	Client experienced positive clinical and social outcomes. System was acceptable to both client and therapist. The 'impersonal nature' of video may have facilitated discussion by making client less self-conscious and inhibited. A collaborative therapeutic relationship was established although certain non-verbal behaviours were missing/difficult to see (eye contact, touching and body language – nodding, leaning, positioning). Certain postures became exaggerated to compensate. Handshake may be a display of dominance by therapist and its absence may not be so bad. Client did not complete all assessments; video may thus affect compliance

Table 4.2. – continued

Authors	Location	Consultation/equipment	Methods	Communication/other findings
Mannion et al (1998)[78]	Galway, Ireland. Island of Inishmore (peripheral site). University College Hospital (central site)	Psychiatric consultations with off-site psychiatrist and on-site nurse if patient desires. PC-based, ISDN, 384 kbit/s	Over 8 months. Based on experience with nine patients with depression, panic disorder, bipolar affective disorder and schizophrenia	Video acceptable/satisfactory to both patients and staff. Most patients were comfortable with video and it did not prove to be a barrier to establishing rapport. All health professionals who used the system found it satisfactory. One woman expressed reservations about discussing personal issues over the system
Rendon (1998)[79]	New York City. Local school (peripheral site). Child Psychiatric Clinic, Lincoln Hospital (central site)	16-session cognitive behaviour protocol with off-site psychiatrist. PC-based, ISDN, 128 kbit/s	Case report. Child psychiatry. Cognitive behaviour therapy. Single child, 10 years old, identified by school as particularly disruptive	Although video and audio quality was not perfect, the system was sufficient for psychotherapy. Psychiatrist taught child how to use the computer. Sessions conducted weekly with a regimented sequence thereafter. By the end the child was no longer disruptive and had become attached to therapy. Video may help reduce resistance, non-compliance and drop-out among certain children
Montani et al (1997)[80,81]	Meylan, France. Centre Hospitalier Universitaire. Two rooms in same facility	Consultation and assessment with 'off-site' psychologist and 'on-site' observer. Assessments included: Mini-Mental State Examination (MMSE) and Clock Face Test (CFT). Closed circuit television, coaxial cable	Over 4 months. Mixed methods, including two psychometric tests, observation and content analysis. Compared video and in-person consultation for 15 elderly patients without a psychiatric history (100% participation rate). Sessions occurred 8 days apart	Both clients and therapists preferred in-person sessions although video was judged acceptable. Video sessions were significantly shorter, possibly due to the inhibiting effects of the medium. Patients' scores were lower with video. But there was high correlation with the MMSE (0.95) although not with the CFT (0.55). Patients had particular problems registering and/or recalling three words from the MMS, and arranging digits around the clock face. This may be due to a decline in concentration due to more distant interviewer presence or 'unsynchronized' eye contact. The content of the spontaneous phrase was less positive emotionally and more descriptive with video. Felt greater patient participation and presence in person. Physical distance of video appeared to bring psychological distance, which, for some patients, hindered communication. Some felt ill at ease or intimidated by equipment, and manoeuvring the equipment distracting. Eye contact was distorted and silence not tolerated well. Video altered some conventional rituals; the atmosphere was different in the two rooms

Table 4.2. – continued

Authors	Location	Consultation/equipment	Methods	Communication/other findings
Yellowlees (1997)[82]	South Australia. Adult Education College. New South Wales (peripheral site). Glenside Hospital Adelaide (central site)	Psychiatric assessment with off-site psychiatrist and on-site case manager and relatives under the provisions of a Mental Health Act. Video system ISDN, 128 kbit/s	Case reports. Participant observation. Case 1: long-standing schizo-affective psychosis; Case 2: paranoid schizophrenia. One psychiatrist	Assessments in both cases were accepted as valid by a magistrate. Medication was prescribed in both cases and a medical report supporting an invalidity pension was also provided after the telemedicine assessment in the second. Although the first patient had delusional symptoms with ideas of reference from television, she readily accepted the author talking to her from the television as real. Audio/visual quality were adequate to make the assessments
Myhill (1996)[83]	South Australia. Regional hospital (peripheral site). Glenside Hospital (central site)	Psychiatric consultation with off-site psychiatrist and on-site mental health nurse and drug/alcohol counsellor. Video system, 128 kbit/s	Single case report. Post-encounter impressions by consulting psychiatrist. 36-year old patient with suicidal/homicidal thoughts. Recently admitted to hospital. Two sessions, with/without patient	Video did not interfere with depth of rapport or communication of emotion during session. Degree to which patient felt uncomfortable or withheld expressions of emotion seemed no different than in person. Depth of emotion expressed by patient was profound. Distress was obvious and presence of other physically present therapists important for consoling patient. Problems arose when the interview was interrupted by subsequent users. Authors discuss the need for teleconferencing 'etiquette' to account for delays and other technical difficulties
McLaren et al (1993)[84]	London, UK. Acute psychiatric unit. Two rooms in adjacent wards	Consultation and assessment with off-site psychiatrist. PC-based, monochrome camera, 2 Mbit/s link	Case reports. Two psychiatric inpatients selected because they were not straightforward candidates for psychotherapy. Patient A had overdosed/self-destructive behaviour; Patient B had paranoid illness/delusions. Two psychiatrists	*Patient A*: Doctor reacted negatively to patient and felt frustrated because of difficulty hearing him due to technical problems and patient mumbling. Felt distanced from patient and had urge to climb into the system to get closer. *Patient B*: Doctor talked with patient but system did not enable him to 'get under the surface of the problem.' Indicated that it was difficult to appreciate non-verbal cues, including eye narrowing, pupil dilation and body movements. Authors were not sure whether difficulties experienced were due to subject or technological characteristics

Table 4.2. – *continued*

Authors	Location	Consultation/equipment	Methods	Communication/other findings
Jerome (1986)[85,86]	London, Ontario. Woodstock General General Hospital (peripheral site). University of Western Ontario (central site)	Consultation between off-site therapist and on-site child psychiatric team, including assessment and crisis interviews. Interactive television	Over 10 months. Participant observation. Compared video to live interviews. Range of child psychiatric and family difficulties. (100% participation rate)	Consensus among personnel and patients that live interviews were superior. Valuable diagnostic information unavailable due to technical difficulties. Could not focus on individual when general view was on the entire family. Fewer hypotheses were generated. The system was considered a 'second-best' option to in-person contact. On-site visits important for establishing rapport and team cohesion, but contributed to negative attitude toward television link. Patients enjoyed the novelty of the situation, but experienced emotional distance from themselves and their examiners. Nonetheless, link was useful for consultation, treatment and assessment. Had 50% reduction in clinic time compared to in-person visits
Straker et al (1976)[87]	New York City. Wagner Child Health Station, East Harlem (peripheral site). Mount Sinai School of Medicine (central site)	Consultation between off-site child psychiatrist and on-site nurse and community health worker. Also used for psychiatric conferences and training. Dedicated coaxial cable television connection	Over 2 years. Participant and other observation. Child psychiatry. 58 conferences that discussed 138 problems cases. 34 consultations with 30 inner city children and their mothers. 69% of appointments were kept	Very intense relationship developed between psychiatrist and nurse associates. Most families (87%) accepted psychiatrist's recommendations where most referrals by clinic nurse prior to the system had been refused. One possible reason is that their first exposure to the psychiatrist took place in a less threatening and intimidating environment (i.e. their own clinic, neighbourhood and caregivers) than in-person contact at an unfamiliar medical centre. Kept 'psychiatrist and his imagined dangerous powers at a safe distance'. Not sure if anything was lost – could observe mother–child interaction and contact had been intimate and effective. All mothers responded positively to 'being on television'. Observed heightened self-esteem among mothers, which had not been noticeable during in-person contacts

Table 4.2. – *continued*

Authors	Location	Consultation/equipment	Methods	Communication/other findings
Dwyer (1973)[88]	Boston, Massachusetts. Medical station, Logan Airport (peripheral site). Massachusetts General Hospital (central site)	Consultation with off-site psychiatrist, psychiatric resident or medical student. Some group therapy. Closed circuit television, microwave transmission	Over 2.5 years. Participant and other observation. About 150 patients seen 2–20 times. Clients included airport staff and their families, junior high staff/ students, prisoners, juveniles. Some psychiatric disorders but most situational crises. About 30 psychiatrists and 30 residents/medical students	Most medical staff at first sceptical but became positive about its feasibility and acceptability with use. Initial anxiety led some to complain loudly about visual and audio quality, while neglecting simple controls to remedy these problems. Concluded that a high degree of personal contact is possible with interactive television although more research needs to examine what may be missing and how it can be replaced (e.g. handshake). Some patients found it easier to communicate than if doctor was in same room with them (i.e. schizophrenics, adolescents, young children). The rare patient with initial anxiety proceeded normally with interview
Solow et al (1971)[89]	New Hampshire. Claremont General Hospital (peripheral site). Dartmouth Medical School, Hanover (central site)	Consultation between off-site psychiatrist and on-site family physician. Closed-circuit television, two microwave relay stations	Over 12 months. Participant and other observation. 142 new patients and 57 follow-up consultations. 60% had no prior psychiatric contact. 40% with psychotic illness; rest with emotional disorders	Television presented no difficulties for psychiatric consultation. Diagnostic and therapeutic effectiveness approximated face-to-face interviewing. Not a significant barrier to establishing rapport or perceiving emotional nuances. Patient acceptance was high. Did not produce additional anxiety in paranoid patients. Both patients and psychiatrist quickly lost awareness of system. Some mild distraction from quality of audio and visual signals. Also served an educational function for on-site physicians
Wittson. et al (1961)[90,91]	Omaha, Nebraska. Nebraska Psychiatric Institute. Two rooms within the same facility	Group therapy sessions with 'off-site' therapist. Closed-circuit television	Observation. Psychiatric inpatients. Two therapists led four groups each, two televised and two non-televised. The groups, which had 5 or 6 patients each, met 6 times	Found that choice of therapist and selection of group members had greater effect than use of television, which they concluded was 'neither a problem nor an asset'. Few patients had privacy concerns or referred to the system after the first session. System did not affect establishment of rapport or attitude of most participants toward therapy. But no relationship of trust in therapist or willingness to discuss problems emerged in an atypical group with 'anti-social' predilections. Instead, they used the system to increase their resistance by excluding the therapist from some of the discussion by whispering with one another. Reported that procedures were modified several times to make important cues (facial expressions, gestures) clearer to them

Table 4.3. Frequency of positive and negative communication findings

Category (no. of studies)	Positive findings (no.)	Negative findings (no.)
Communicative efficacy (19)	20	6
Patient understanding (5)	4	1
Provider understanding (5)	7	2
Patient expression (15)	19	2
Provider expression (6)	6	1
Patient comfort (20)	24	2
Provider comfort (7)	7	0
Participant relations (25)	31	6
Embarrassment (9)	10	3
Anxiety/nervousness (9)	13	3
Miscellaneous affect (7)	12	4
Audio quality (14)	16	13
Video quality (23)	21	9
Non-verbal behaviour (23)	6	22
Technology/system attributes (25)	33	19
Multiple providers (12)	12	2
Patient involvement (6)	6	0
Privacy (8)	5	3
Shorter encounter length (4)	3	1
Outcomes/care quality (24)	51	9
Satisfaction (23)	53	3
Favoured video consultation (18)	27	12
Assessment/diagnosis (24)	29	12
Total	415	135

of total findings) included audio quality, technology/system attributes (i.e. the equipment, room and machine–human interface) and privacy. While the majority of findings abstracted from post-encounter surveys of patients (85%), local providers (74%) and consultants (61%) were rated positively, comparatively fewer qualitative (67%) study findings were rated favourably using the criteria described above. Post-encounter results also indicated that patients tended to view telepsychiatry more favourably than providers.

Discussion

Studies of doctor–patient communication in telepsychiatry are evenly divided between post-encounter surveys of consultation participants and qualitative investigations using observation, interviews, case reports, questionnaires and content analysis. Virtually all were published after 1994. More than half were either US or UK based. Most studies focused on consultation and assessment by psychiatric consultants serving adult psychiatric outpatients with a variety of conditions, including schizophrenia, depression, bipolar and schizoaffective disorder. Approximately three quarters of abstracted findings favoured telepsychiatry, with all but one of the 23 categories analysed, non-verbal behaviour, reporting more positive than negative results.

The evidence of the present study overwhelmingly favours communication by telepsychiatry, especially when assessed through post-encounter surveys of consultation participants. However, it should be noted that patients routinely report high levels of satisfaction with the care that they receive.[92] Participant ratings may therefore be skewed in favour of telemedicine. This is suggested by the present findings, which show that the proportion of positive results abstracted from post-encounter surveys of telepsychiatry participants (81%) exceeds the proportion of positive findings abstracted from qualitative investigations (67%). It appears that conclusions about the relationship between telepsychiatry and doctor–patient communication might differ depending on whether they were based on participant ratings or researcher judgements using qualitative data. Post-encounter assessments of encounter participants, therefore, need to be supplemented with qualitative investigations of actual encounter behaviour in order to obtain a better understanding of the effects of telepsychiatry on the doctor–patient relationship.

While the results of further qualitative investigations may or may not reinforce the conclusions drawn from post-encounter surveys, they will almost certainly provide information unavailable to researchers relying solely on retrospective participant assessments. It was primarily the qualitative studies identified for this review, for example, which revealed the problematical nature of non-verbal communication via telepsychiatry. In particular, these studies indicate that separation between consultation participants sometimes compromises the richness and complexity of visual and auditory information as reflected in non-verbal behaviours such as voice quality and tone, eye contact, gaze, posture, laughter, facial expressions, body positioning, proximity, touch, activity (e.g. chart reviewing, computer usage) and other cues that modify the meaning of verbal utterances (e.g. hesitations). In fact, it has been in the area of telepsychiatry, where studies highlight the importance of non-verbal cues for expressing emotion and affect, that the effect of telemedicine on non-verbal communication has primarily been explored. But as McLaren and Ball[10] observed, 'the tasks which would be expected to be most sensitive to the medium of communication (i.e. non-verbal communication) are tasks in which the expression and perception of emotion are important'. Cukor et al,[41] for example, concluded that although most clinical information was carried on the audio channel, important non-verbal cues – nods, blinks, facial expressions and body language – were missing, possibly making video a potentially ineffective tool for interpersonal communications. Gosh, McLaren and Watson[43] came to a similar conclusion, noting that while neither participant seemed inhibited or uncomfortable in exploring issues, useful body language and appearance information was largely absent, while the therapist was unable to perform certain supportive gestures such as supplying their patients with tissues. They went on to suggest that videoconferencing 'has a voyeuristic sense of promoting detachment or dissociation from the other participant, thereby impairing an essential clinical tool – empathy'.[43] In some instances, visual information was lost when doctors checked their notes or leaned forward to convey intimacy or empathy with their patients.[45,47] In others, missing information made it difficult for patients to show side effects or symptoms.[45] In certain cases, however, missing information actually facilitated interaction by removing potentially distractive behaviours from view.[47] In one study, consultants actually found it easier to detect certain clinical signs (i.e. tongue tremors) using video.[44]

In addition to highlighting the effect of telemedicine on non-verbal behaviour, qualitative analyses also generate other important insights unavailable to those relying exclusively on post-encounter surveys. Day and Schneider,[72] for example, concluded that the distancing effect of teletherapy may promote honesty and feelings of safety, which may serve certain populations, such as schizophrenics and agoraphobics, well. Kavanagh and Yellowlees[46] came to a similar conclusion in arguing that the ability of patients to walk out of the room or out of the sight of the camera may create a less threatening environment, allowing interviews to continue where they may have otherwise ended prematurely. While Gosh et al[43] found that transmission delays led study participants to use shorter sentences and to wait before replying, McLaren et al[47] found psychiatric patients to be less inhibited in discussing their problems over video than during conventional in-person encounters. Although video may be more impersonal than face-to-face consultations, it is more personal than consultations that take place entirely over the telephone. As Cukor et al[41] observed with respect to psychiatric consultations, the added value of the video channel is the creation of a 'social presence' that allows consultation participants to share a virtual space and to feel comfortable discussing complex issues. This is a finding that has been replicated by others, including Ball et al,[45] who found that patients appeared more anxious in non-visual modes than when visual cues were present. Compared to in-person consultations, however, important sources of information may still be unavailable, including contact with other health personnel, the patient's family and broader surroundings (e.g. living conditions). Turner,[71] for example, argued that the only context available with telepsychiatry is provided by the interview itself and what little can be seen and heard in the background. Not only might this compromise therapeutic efficacy but it may also lessen consultant credibility with ancillary and other personnel at the remote site. This result parallels findings from the broader communication literature, which indicate that the impressions people form of remote others are different from and less positive than the impressions they form of face-to-face others.[93]

Taking heed of lessons such as these, Cukor and Baer[2] drew on human factors insights to propose a 'how-to-guide' for conducting telepsychiatry consultations, including suggestions related to knowing when to start talking, maintaining eye contact and avoiding rapid movements. They also proposed encouraging prior participant contact where possible, teaching participants how to operate the equipment, not wearing anything unusual or flashy, eliminating distracting objects, lighting and unnecessary institutional differences, along with a variety of other norms of appropriate behaviour, such as avoiding lengthy pauses, acting naturally, and being well prepared and organized. They also emphasized the importance of audio quality, which is a continual source of irritation and distraction when functioning poorly. That audio quality and participant familiarity and comfort with the technology should not be taken for granted is reinforced by the present study, which found comparatively high numbers of negative findings (i.e. >35% of total findings) for these two aspects of the telemedicine experience.

Not only might telepsychiatry guidelines be produced using insights drawn from other literatures, but they may also be generated by applying qualitative research techniques to particular settings. The use of focus groups to help develop guidelines for the use of telepsychiatry technology in Queensland, Australia is a recent example.[94] Another possibility is to use qualitative-methods to acquire in-depth knowledge regarding the nature and content of participant behaviour during actual encounters between mental health providers and patients. A particularly well-suited technique for this purpose is verbal content analysis, which identifies and quantifies communication events and is commonly used by researchers studying doctor–patient communication during conventional face-to-face consultations. Only three examples, however, could be identified in the telemedicine literature. These include studies examining consultation behaviour in three rural clinics in West Texas,[95] in a nursing home in northern Sweden,[96] and in an acute psychiatric unit in London.[45] This last telepsychiatry example, in particular, found no verbal content differences between four consultation modes (i.e. face-to-face, video, telephone and hands-free-telephone).

Given the relative newness of the field and the fact that most studies have focused more broadly on telemedicine system attributes, it is understandable that only three studies have used such a comparatively resource-intensive research strategy. The dearth of such studies, however, contrasts markedly with the long tradition of using interaction analysis techniques to study the way doctors and patients communicate during conventional medical encounters. Not only have face-to-face researchers used the findings of verbal content studies to develop theoretical models of the doctor–patient relationship but they have also developed multiple instruments for quantifying communication events, the results of which have been correlated with patient, provider and system attributes and health outcomes (see Miller[97] for an overview).

In general, interaction analysis systems describe and categorize communication behaviours. Most employ an exhaustive taxonomy for classifying verbal events or utterances. A verbal utterance is 'the smallest meaningful and distinguishable speech segment, conveying only one thought or relating to one item of interest'.[98] The Roter Interaction Analysis System, for example, uses 34 categories to describe physician behaviour and 28 categories to describe patient behaviour. These can be grouped into broader categories for analysis, including instrumental behaviours (e.g. information-giving or question-asking), affective behaviours (e.g. positive talk or negative talk) and social conversation.[18] Systems may also keep track of non-verbal behaviours such as eye contact, facial expressions, voice tone, physical proximity, hand gesturing, body positioning and touch. In addition to the behaviours measured (instrumental/affective, verbal/non-verbal), particular instruments may also be distinguished by their relevance to various patient types and medical settings. They also differ in their observation strategies. Coding, for example, may be accomplished using videotape, audiotape, direct observation or literal transcripts. Although most of the 44 verbal content analysis instruments included in a recent review had not been adequately tested for their validity, the majority had been shown to be reliable.[99]

Future telepsychiatry research should employ instruments similar to the interaction analysis systems used to study conventional doctor–patient communication. It would be inappropriate, however, to adopt such systems wholesale without first developing instruments specific to the telemedicine experience. The importance of developing context-appropriate instruments has been demonstrated by researchers such as Ong et al[100] who applied the Roter Interaction Analysis System to an oncological setting, rather than the primary care setting for which it had originally been developed. Not only did it fail to provide an option for classifying the communication behaviours of third party participants, a common occurrence during oncological, not to mention telemedicine consultations, but it also tracked certain behaviours which were rarely used.

To ensure the appropriate use of interaction analysis to study doctor–patient communication via telemedicine a research strategy grounded in three types of analyses should be used, a strategy which Inui and Carter[101] refer to as developmental/descriptive, subexperimental/aetiological and interventional studies. The purpose of developmental/descriptive studies is to expand on the repertoire of theories, measures and experience available to serve as the basis for empirical research. Because they primarily rely on observation, interviews, archival analysis and 'thick' (i.e. in-depth) description, developmental studies provide empirical data unconstrained by existing categories. As such, they can be used to substantiate or adapt existing medical communication categories to the telemedicine context and to develop new ones when appropriate, a task critical to the design of telemedicine appropriate interaction analysis instruments. Such instruments may, in turn, be used to undertake subexperimental/aetiological investigations, which are primarily cross-sectional in nature and rely on frequency distributions, correlations and regression for analysis. By characterizing the communication process and assessing cause and affect theories linking telemedicine system attributes, communication behaviours and health outcomes, subexperimental/aetiological investigations should play an extremely important role in the development of effective interventions aimed at improving doctor–patient communication under telemedicine. The efficacy of such promising suggestions, including educational strategies (e.g. teaching, instructions or information), behavioural strategies (e.g. skill-building or reminders) and affect-oriented strategies (e.g. relationship-building),[102] should be assessed by randomized clinical trials.

Conclusion

With more than 75% of the abstracted findings being rated positively and with all but one of the 23 communication categories reporting more positive than negative results, the present review strongly favours doctor–patient communication via telepsychiatry. However, further research is necessary if the nature and content of the communication process is to be fully understood. This will help us to understand the interpersonal dynamics associated with telepsychiatry and its effects on patients' outcomes, and will also allow us to develop and implement technological improvements and adjustments to facilitate communication between providers and patients. In addition, it will represent another step toward formulating and promulgating behavioural norms that aid telepsychiatry transactions, while furthering the development of educational and other strategies to reduce any trepidation associated with this comparatively new medium. Understanding the relationship between telepsychiatry and doctor–patient communication will also shed light on the distribution of decision-making power between consultation participants as well as any effect telepsychiatry may have on patient trust and privacy, and the malpractice exposure of psychiatrists and other mental health personnel. Together, these insights should provide payers and policy-makers with further evidence regarding telepsychiatry's ability to promote high-quality care that maximizes value for money.

References

1 American Psychiatric Association. *APA resource document on telepsychiatry via videoconferencing (Approved by APA board of trustees 7/98)*. Available at http://www.psych.org/pract_of_psych?tp_paper.cfm [last checked 20 August 2002].

2 Cukor P, Baer L. Human factors issues in telemedicine: a practical guide with particular attention to psychiatry. *Telemedicine Today* 1994;**2**(2):9,16–18.

3 Field MJ, ed. *Telemedicine: a guide to assessing telecommunications in health care*. Washington, DC: National Academy Press, 1996.

4 Ostbye T, Hurlen P. The electronic house call. Consequences of telemedicine consultations for physicians, patients, and society. *Archives of Family Medicine* 1997;**6**:266–271.

5 Kuszler PC. Telemedicine and integrated health care delivery: compounding malpractice liability. *American Journal of Law and Medicine* 1999;**25**:297–326.

6 Collins B, Sypher H. Developing better relationships in telemedicine practice. Organizational and interpersonal factors. *Telemedicine Today* 1996;**4**(2):27–42.

7 Wootton R, Darkins A. Telemedicine and the doctor–patient relationship. *Journal of the Royal College of Physicians of London* 1997;**31**:598–599.

8 Bashshur RL. On the definition and evaluation of telemedicine. *Telemedicine Journal* 1995;**1**:19–30.

9 Seeman MV, Seeman B. E-psychiatry: the patient–psychiatrist relationship in the electronic age. *Canadian Medical Association Journal* 1999;**161**:1147–1149.

10 McLaren P, Ball CJ. Interpersonal communications and telemedicine: hypotheses and methods. *Journal of Telemedicine and Telecare* 1997;**3**(suppl 1):5–7.

11 Anonymous. Telecommunications infrastructure: the human dimension. *Telemedicine Journal* 1995;**1**:351–356.

12 Barnsley J, Williams AP, Cockerill R, Tanner J. Physician characteristics and the physician–patient relationship. Impact of sex, year of graduation, and specialty. *Canadian Family Physician* 1999;**45**:935–942.

13 Moskop JC. The nature and limits of the physician's authority. In: Staum MS, Larsen DE, eds. *Doctors, Patients, and Society: power and authority in medical care*. Waterloo, Ontario: Wilfrid Laurier University Press, 1981:29–44.

14 Haug M, Lavin B, eds. *Consumerism in Medicine: challenging physician authority*. Beverly Hills, CA: Sage Publications, 1983.

15 Parsons T. Illness and the role of the physician: a sociological perspective. *American Journal of Orthopsychiatry* 1951;**21**:452–460.

16 Freidson E, ed. *Profession of Medicine: a study of the sociology of applied knowledge*. New York: Dodd, Mead and Co, 1970.

17 Waitzkin H, ed. *The Politics of Medical Encounters: how patients and doctors deal with social problems*. New Haven: Yale University Press, 1991.

18 Roter DL, Hall JA, eds. *Doctors Talking with Patients/Patients Talking with Doctors: improving communication in medical visits*. Wesport, CT: Auburn House, 1992.

19 Beckman H. Kaplan SH, Frankel R. Outcome based research on doctor–patient communication: a review. In: Stewart M, Roter D, eds. *Communicating with Medical Patients*. Newbury Park: Sage Publications, 1989:223–227.

20 Hall JA, Roter DL, Katz NR. Meta-analysis of correlates of provider behavior in medical encounters. *Medical Care* 1988;**26**:657–675.

21 Kaplan SH, Greenfield S, Ware JE Jr. Assessing the effects of physician–patient interactions on the outcomes of chronic disease. *Medical Care* 1989;**27**(suppl 3):110–127.

22 Mechanic D. Public trust and initiatives for new health care partnerships. *Milbank Quarterly* 1998;**76**:281–302.

23 Mechanic D. The functions and limitations of trust in the provision of medical care. *Journal of Health Politics, Policy and Law* 1998;**23**:661–686.

24 Starr P. Health and the right to privacy. *American Journal of Law and Medicine* 1999;**25**:193–201.

25 Parrot R, Burgoon JK, Burgoon M, LePoire BA. Privacy between physicians and patients: more than a matter of confidentiality. *Social Science and Medicine* 1989;**29**:1381–1385.

26 Joint Working Group on Telemedicine, Department of Commerce. *Telemedicine Report to Congress*. Available at http://www.ntia.doc/gov/reports/telemed/index.htm [last checked 17 October 2002].

27 Sanders JH, Bashshur RL. Challenges to the implementation of telemedicine. *Telemedicine Journal* 1995;**1**:115–123.

28 Levinson W, Roter DL, Mullooly JP, Dull VT, Frankel RM. Physician–patient communication. The relationship with malpractice claims among primary care physicians and surgeons. *Journal of the American Medical Association* 1997;**277**:553–559.

29 Miller EA. Telemedicine and doctor–patient communication: an analytical survey of the literature. *Journal of Telemedicine and Telecare* 2001;**7**:1–17.

30 Gustke SS, Balch DC, West VL, Rogers LO. Patient satisfaction with telemedicine. *Telemedicine Journal* 2000;**6**:5–13.

31 Mekhjian H, Turner JW, Gailiun M, McCain TA. Patient satisfaction with telemedicine in a prison environment. *Journal of Telemedicine and Telecare* 1999;**5**:55–61.

32 Callahan EJ, Hilty DM, Nesbitt TS. Patient satisfaction with telemedicine consultation in primary care: comparison of ratings of medical and mental health applications. *Telemedicine Journal* 1998;**4**:363–369.

33 Baigent MF, Lloyd CJ, Kavanagh SJ, et al. Telepsychiatry: 'tele' yes, but what about the 'psychiatry'? *Journal of Telemedicine and Telecare* 1997;**3**(suppl. 1):3–5.

34 Blackmon LA, Kaak HO, Ranseen J. Consumer satisfaction with telemedicine child psychiatry consultation in rural Kentucky. *Psychiatric Services* 1997;**48**:1464–1466.

35 Clarke PH. A referrer and patient evaluation of a telepsychiatry consultation-liason service in South Australia. *Journal of Telemedicine and Telecare* 1997;**3**(suppl. 1):12–14.

36 Huston JL, Burton DC. Patient satisfaction with multispecialty interactive teleconsultations. *Journal of Telemedicine and Telecare* 1997;**3**:205–208.

37 Zarate CA, Weinstock L, Cukor P, et al. Applicability of telemedicine for assessing patients with schizophrenia: acceptance and reliability. *Journal of Clinical Psychiatry* 1997;**58**:22–25.

38 Baer L, Cukor P, Jenike MA, Leahy L, O'Laughlen J, Coyle JT. Pilot studies of telemedicine for patients with obsessive-compulsive disorder. *American Journal of Psychiatry* 1995;**152**:1383–1385.

39 Dongier M, Tempier R, Lalinec-Michaud M, Meunier D. Telepsychiatry: psychiatric consultation through two-way television: a controlled study. *Canadian Journal of Psychiatry* 1986;**31**:32–34.

40 Zaylor C. Clinical outcomes in telepsychiatry. *Journal of Telemedicine and Telecare* 1999;**5**(suppl 1):59–60.

41 Cukor P, Baer L, Willis BS, et al. Use of videophones and low-cost standard telephone lines to provide a social presence in telepsychiatry. *Telemedicine Journal* 1998;**4**:313–321.

42 Gammon D, Sorlie T, Bergvik S, Hoifodt TS. Psychotherapy supervision conducted by videoconferencing: a qualitative study of users' experiences. *Journal of Telemedicine and Telecare* 1998;**4**(suppl 1):33–35.

43 Ghosh GJ, McLaren PM, Watson JP. Evaluating the alliance in videolink teletherapy. *Journal of Telemedicine and Telecare* 1997;**3**(suppl 1):33–35.

44 McLaren PM, Blunden J, Lipsedge ML, Summerfield AB. Telepsychiatry in an inner-city community psychiatric service. *Journal of Telemedicine and Telecare* 1996;**2**:57–59.

45 Ball CJ, McLaren PM, Summerfield AB, Lipsedge MS, Watson JP. A comparison of communication modes in adult psychiatry. *Journal of Telemedicine and Telecare* 1995;**1**:22–26.

46 Kavanagh SJ, Yellowlees PM. Telemedicine. Clinical applications in mental health. *Australian Family Physician* 1995;**24**:1242–1247.

47 McLaren P, Ball CJ, Summerfield AB, Watson JP, Lipsedge M. An evaluation of the use of interactive television in an acute psychiatric service. *Journal of Telemedicine and Telecare* 1995;**1**:79–85.

48 Glueckauf RL, Fritz SP, Ecklund-Johnson EP, Liss HJ, Dages P, Carney P. Videoconferencing-based family counseling for rural teenagers with epilepsy: phase 1 findings. *Rehabilitation Psychology*. 2002;**47**:49–72.

49 Bose U, McLaren P, Riley A, Mohammedali A. The use of telepsychiatry in the brief counseling of non-psychotic patients from an inner-London general practice. *Journal of Telemedicine and Telecare* 2001;**7**(suppl 1):8–10.

50 Elford DR, White H, St John K, Maddigan B, Ghandi M, Bowering R. A prospective satisfaction study and cost analysis of a pilot child telepsychiatry service in Newfoundland. *Journal of Telemedicine and Telecare* 2001;**7**:73–81.

51 Kopel H, Nunn K, Dossetor D. Evaluating satisfaction with a child and adolescent psychological telemedicine outreach service. *Journal of Telemedicine and Telecare* 2001;**7**(suppl 2):35–40.

52 Simpson J, Doze S, Urness D, Hailey D, Jacobs P. Telepsychiatry as a routine service: the perspective of the patient. *Journal of Telemedicine and Telecare* 2001;**7**:155–160.

53 Simpson J, Doze S, Urness D, Hailey D, Jacobs P. Evaluation of a routine telepsychiatry service. *Journal of Telemedicine and Telecare* 2001;**7**:90–98.

54 D'Souza R. Telemedicine for intensive support of psychiatric inpatients admitted to local hospitals. *Journal of Telemedicine and Telecare* 2000;**6**(suppl 1):26–28.

55 Elford R, White H, Bowering R, et al. A randomized, controlled trial of child psychiatric assessments conducted using videoconferencing. *Journal of Telemedicine and Telecare* 2000;**6**:73–82.

56 Kirkwood KT, Peck DF, Bennie L. The consistency of neuropsychological assessments performed via telecommunication and face to face. *Journal of Telemedicine and Telecare* 2000;**6**:147–151.

57 Mielonen ML, Ohinmaa A, Moring J, Isohanni M. Psychiatric inpatient care planning via telemedicine. *Journal of Telemedicine and Telecare* 2000;**6**:152–157.

58 Ball C, Tyrrell J, Long C. Scoring written material from the Mini-Mental State Examination: a comparison of face-to-face, fax and video-linked scoring. *Journal of Telemedicine and Telecare* 1999;**5**:253–256.

59 Chae YM, Park HJ, Cho JG, Hong GD, Cheon KA. The reliability and acceptability of telemedicine for patients with schizophrenia in Korea. *Journal of Telemedicine and Telecare* 2000;**6**:83–90.

60 Doze S, Simpson J, Hailey D, Jacobs P. Evaluation of a telepsychiatry pilot project. *Journal of Telemedicine and Telecare* 1999;**5**:38–46.

61 Doze S, Simpson J, eds. *Evaluation of a Telepsychiatry Pilot Project.* Edmonton: Provincial Mental Health Advisory Board and Alberta Heritage Foundation for Medical Research, 1997.

62 Freir V, Kirkwood K, Peck D, Robertson S, Scott-Lodge L, Zeffert S. Telemedicine for clinical psychology in the Highlands of Scotland. *Journal of Telemedicine and Telecare* 1999;**5**:157–161.

63 Ball C, Puffett A. The assessment of cognitive function in the elderly using videoconferencing. *Journal of Telemedicine and Telecare* 1998;**4**(suppl 1):36–38.

64 Mielonen ML, Ohinmaa A, Moring J, Isohanni M. The use of videoconferencing for telepsychiatry in Finland. *Journal of Telemedicine and Telecare* 1998;**4**:125–131.

65 Bear D, Jacobson G, Aaronson S, Hanson A. Telemedicine in psychiatry: making the dream reality. *American Journal of Psychiatry* 1997;**154**:884–885.

66 McLaren PM, Laws VJ, Ferreira AC, O'Flynn D, Lipsedge M, Watson JP. Telepsychiatry: outpatient psychiatry by videolink. *Journal of Telemedicine and Telecare* 1996;**2**(suppl 1):59–62.

67 Salzman C, Orvin D, Hanson A, Kalinowski A. Patient evaluation through live video transmission. *American Journal of Psychiatry* 1996;**153**:968.

68 Ball CJ, Scott N, McLaren PM, Watson JP. Preliminary evaluation of a Low-Cost VideoConferencing (LCVC) system for remote cognitive testing of adult psychiatric patients. *British Journal of Clinical Psychology* 1993;**32**:303–307.

69 Hill JV, Allman LR, Ditzler TF. Utility of real-time video teleconferencing in conducting family mental health sessions: two case reports. *Telemedicine Journal* 2001;**7**:55–59.

70 Simpson S. The provision of a telepsychology service to Shetland: client and therapist satisfaction and the ability to develop a therapeutic alliance. *Journal of Telemedicine and Telecare* 2001;**7**(suppl 1):34–36.

71 Turner JW. Telepsychiatry as a case study of presence: do you know what you are missing? *Journal of Computer-Mediated Communication* 2001;**6**(4). M. Available at http://www.ascusc.org/jcmc/vol6/issue4/turner.html [last checked 20 August 2002].

72 Day SX, Schneider P. The subjective experience of therapists in face-to-face, video, and audio sessions. In: Bloom JW, Waltz GR, eds. *Cybercounseling and Cyberlearning: strategies and resources for the Millennium.* Alexandria, Virginia: American Counseling Association. ERIC/Counseling and Student Services Clearinghouse at the University of North Carolina, 2000:203–218.

73 Deitsch SE, Frueh BC, Santos AB. Telepsychiatry for post-traumatic stress disorder. *Journal of Telemedicine and Telecare* 2000;**6**:184–186.

74 May C, Gask L, Ellis N, et al. Telepsychiatry evaluation in the north-west of England: preliminary results of a qualitative study. *Journal of Telemedicine and Telecare* 2000;**6**(suppl 1):20–22.

75 Schopp L, Johnstone B, Merell D. Telehealth and neuropsychological assessment: new opportunities for psychologists. *Professional Psychology: Research and Practice* 2000;**31**:179–183.

76 Hufford BJ, Glueckauf RL, Webb PM. Home-based, interactive videoconferencing for adolescents with epilepsy and their families. *Rehabilitation Psychology* 1999;**44**:176–193.

77 Manchanda M, McLaren P. Cognitive behaviour therapy via interactive video. *Journal of Telemedicine and Telecare* 1998;**4**(suppl 1):53–55.

78 Mannion L, Fahy TJ, Duffy C, Broderick M, Gethins E. Telepsychiatry: an island pilot project. *Journal of Telemedicine and Telecare* 1997;**4**(suppl 1): 62–63.

79 Rendon M. Telepsychiatric treatment of a schoolchild. *Journal of Telemedicine and Telecare* 1998;**4**:179–182.

80 Montani C, Billaud N, Tyrrell J, et al. Psychological impact of a remote psychometric consultation with hospitalized elderly people. *Journal of Telemedicine and Telecare* 1997;**3**:140–145.

81 Montani C, Billaud N, Couturier P, et al. 'Telepsychometry': a remote psychometry consultation in clinical gerontology: preliminary study. *Telemedicine Journal* 1996;**2**:145–150.

82 Yellowlees P. The use of telemedicine to perform psychiatric assessments under the Mental Health Act. *Journal of Telemedicine and Telecare* 1997;**3**:224–226.

83 Myhill K. Telepsychiatry in rural South Australia. *Journal of Telemedicine and Telecare* 1996;**2**:224–225.

84 McLaren PM, Ball CJ, Watson JP. Assessment for psychotherapy by interactive television suitable for transmission through telephone links. *Psychiatric Bulletin* 1993;**44**:104–105.

85 Jerome L. Telepsychiatry. *Canadian Journal of Psychiatry* 1986;**31**:489.

86 Jerome L. Assessment by telemedicine. *Hospital and Community Psychiatry* 1993;**44**:81.

87 Straker N, Mostyn P, Marshall C. The use of two-way TV in brining mental health services to the inner city. *American Journal of Psychiatry* 1976;**133**:1202–1205.

88 Dwyer TF. Telepsychiatry: psychiatric consultation by interactive television. *American Journal of Psychiatry* 1973;**130**:865–869.

89 Solow C, Weiss RJ, Bergen BJ, Sanborn CJ. 24-hour psychiatric consultation via TV. *American Journal of Psychiatry* 1971;**12**:1684–1687.

90 Wittson CL, Affleck DC, Johnson V. Two-way television in group therapy. *Mental Hospitals.* 1961;**12**:22–23.

91 Wittson C, Benschoter R. Two way television: helping the Medical Center reach out. *American Journal of Psychiatry* 1972;**129**:624–627.

92 Hall JA, Dornan MC. Meta-analysis of satisfaction with medical care: description of research domain and analysis of overall satisfaction levels. *Social Science and Medicine* 1988;**27**:637–644.

93 Storck J, Sproull. Through a glass darkly: what do people learn in videoconferences? *Human Communication Research* 1995;**22**:197–219.

94 Kennedy C, Yellowlees P. Guidelines for using videoconferencing in mental health services. *Journal of Telemedicine and Telecare* 2000;**6**:352–353.

95 Street RL, Wheeler EJ, McCaughan WT. Specialist-primary care provider–patient communication in telemedical consultations. *Telemedicine Journal* 2000;**6**:45–54.

96 Savenstedt S, Bucht G, Norberg L, Sandman PO. Nurse–doctor interaction in teleconsultations between a hospital and a geriatric nursing home. *Journal of Telemedicine and Telecare* 2002;**8**:11–18.

97 Miller EA. Telemedicine and doctor–patient communication: a theoretical framework for evaluation. *Journal of Telemedicine and Telecare* 2002;**8**:311–318.

98 Ong LM, De Haes JC, Hoos AM, Lammes FB. Doctor–patient communication: a review of the literature. *Social Science and Medicine* 1995;**40**:903–918.

99 Boon H, Stewart M. Patient–physician communication assessment instruments: 1986 to 1996 in review. *Patient Education and Counseling* 1998;**35**:161–176.

100 Ong LML, Visser MRM, Kruyver IPM, et al. The Roter Interaction Analysis System (RIAS) in oncological consultations: psychometric properties. *Psycho-oncology* 1998;**7**:387–401.

101 Inui TS, Carter WB. Design issues in research on doctor–patient communication. In: Stewart M, Roter D, eds. *Communicating with Medical Patients.* Newbury Park: Sage Publications, 1989:197–210.

102 Roter DL, Hall JA, Merisca R, Nordstrom B, Cretin D, Svarstad B. Effectiveness of interventions to improve patient compliance: a meta-analysis. *Medical Care* 1998;**36**:1138–1161.

5

E-therapy: Opportunities, Dangers and Ethics to Guide Practice

Robert C. Hsiung

Introduction – opportunities and dangers

Mental health professionals have discovered the new world of the Internet. Exploring it presents not only opportunities, but also dangers. Although hypothetical and improbable as a whole, each step of the scenario shown in Box 5.1 is plausible. The Internet is a double-edged sword. For example:

▶ The patient may feel safer and less inhibited and therefore be more revealing online than in person. However, visual, auditory and olfactory channels of information are limited, so the therapist has less data with which to work. In some cases, the net effect will be positive, but in others it will be negative.

▶ Using text-based modalities such as email makes it easier to record communications. Having a transcript to refer to can help the patient – and provide additional incentive for the therapist to provide good care[1] – but it also makes it easier for the patient to violate the privacy of the therapist by releasing that text to others.

▶ The Internet gives each therapist access to more patients and each patient access to more therapists. Efficiency should result from this freer 'market'. However, regulatory bodies still need to be able to regulate. The market should not be so free that quacks can make fraudulent claims and harm patients with impunity.

The clinical and legal principles that will guide the practice of e-therapy will emerge as experience is gained, research is conducted and legislation is passed. Ethical principles are also needed in this uncharted territory. A 'map' of the ethical hazards will not only help guide the pioneers (giving therapists a better idea of how to treat patients and patients a better idea of how to expect to be treated), but also reassure the public (both lay and professional) that a safe route can be found.

The basic values of professional ethics are beneficence, non-maleficence and, at least in much of the western world, autonomy. Therapists should help and not hurt. Patients should be able to decide what treatments to undertake. The more closely e-therapy develops in accordance with these basic ethical values, the more widely it will be accepted.

Box 5.1.   One scenario

Therapist A receives his Illinois licence, rents an office, and opens for business. His practice, however, is slow to grow. He decides to diversify into e-therapy. He creates a Web page as a virtual shingle: 'Online Therapy Services, Inc. Get help by secure real-time chat. Email now for more information'. Patient A, at work in California and taking advantage of the fast Internet connection in his office, sees the page and sends an email: 'I'm having an affair with my boss's wife. It's starting to get complicated! Can you help me?'

Therapist A replies and says he charges $100 an hour. Patient A accepts, but reluctantly, since he considers that steep. They start having chat meetings, and Patient A tells Therapist A about his passionate feelings for his boss's wife. They focus on his dissatisfaction in his marriage. To fill Therapist A in on the history of the affair, Patient A emails him the last 3 years of entries from his (electronic) diary. Therapist A spends 2 hours reviewing and commenting on them and enters that time into his automatic billing software.

Therapist A is then unexpectedly called away because of an illness in his family. That same day, the boss's wife calls Patient A at home and gives him an ultimatum: if he doesn't leave his wife, she'll end their affair.

Patient A immediately sends Therapist A an email asking him what he should do. Therapist A uses a regional Internet service provider, however, and doesn't have access where he is. Not getting a response, Patient A calls the California licencing board and asks for the phone number for Online Therapy Services, Inc. They have no such entity in their database. Increasingly desperate, he takes, in an attempt to calm himself, a handful of lithium tablets he was prescribed in the past. Meanwhile, the boss, a possessive type, has the company email server searched, as he does each week, for his wife's name, 'wife', 'love', 'sex' and 'affair'. It being the end of the month, Therapist A's billing software automatically sends Patient A an email bill for the month's chat sessions – plus $200 for dealing with the diary entries.

Patient A's wife sits down at their home computer to check her email and finds her husband's message to Therapist A about the boss's wife. The California licencing board initiates an investigation, determines that Therapist A has violated the California Business and Professions Code, and notifies the Illinois licencing board. Having taken too much lithium at once, Patient A gets dizzy, falls down some stairs, and breaks his leg. The boss is informed of Patient A's initial email to Therapist A about the boss's wife and fires him. And even though Therapist A is not online, his automatic billing service sends an email bill to Patient A – for $200 more than Patient A expects.

Ethical guidelines have long existed for the provision of mental health services in person. Traditionally, they have been specific to particular disciplines in particular countries. For example, the American Psychiatric Association[2] has annotated the seven principles of the American Medical Association, and the American Psychological Association Ethics Committee has issued its own detailed principles.[3]

Ethical guidelines have been developed for the provision of health information online[4-9] and the development of electronic health records.[10] The provision of *treatment* online has, however, its own issues.

Ethical guidelines

In 1996, Shapiro and Schulman proposed an ethics standard that stated that 'email facilitated therapeutic communication' should be discouraged except for general questions, should not take place repeatedly between the same therapist and patient, and therefore would not create a therapist–patient relationship.[11]

The potential drawbacks of e-therapy have long been recognized.[12,13] Methods of communicating emotions over the Internet are very basic. The therapist may be unaware of conditions or cultural issues that affect the patient. There is no consensus on how to train an e-therapist. Appreciating, let alone checking, the qualifications of the therapist may be difficult. A person who is unlicenced may promote themselves as competent. It may be important for the therapist to determine whether the patient is a minor. Screening of patients for suitability for e-therapy may be inadequate. The therapist has no way of knowing who is in the room with the patient. While communicating with the therapist, the patient may be interrupted – or, if in a public area, observed – by others. Messages may be intercepted. The patient may be in a state of emotional distress and unable to understand security issues. The patient may accidentally send a message meant for the therapist to someone else (or vice versa). The patient may use their office computer for e-therapy, unaware that their employer has a right to all employee email. Following a duty-to-warn mandate may be difficult if the patient has given no identifying information. Technical failures may make reliability difficult to achieve. It may not be possible to assist the patient in locating local support. It may be easier for abusive therapists to hide their intentions – and even their identity. It may be more difficult for the patient to access formal complaint procedures and for the exploitative therapist to be traced by authorities. A path through these many ethical shoals is only now beginning to emerge.

King and Moreggi[14] had concerns about the lack of guidelines and a governing body, the possible inappropriateness of e-therapy for certain problems, and the potential for misdiagnosis. They observed that 'the Internet provides an arena where an individual can create a personality character, not unlike a writer imagining the main character in his new novel'. To some extent, however, we all create our characters, and 'as if' pseudoaffectivity was described long before the Internet.[15]

Holmes[16] felt that therapists were obliged to 'do what they can' to keep patients safe if, for example, they were suicidal. He acknowledged, however, that that would be possible only to the extent that identifying information had been supplied.

In 1997, the American Psychological Association Ethics Committee stated that therapists should follow the same guidelines when delivering services online as in person.[17] The National Board for Certified Counselors[18,19] and the American Counseling Association[20] developed standards specifically for online counselling, and the Australian Psychological Society[21] considered both educational and clinical online services. Kane and Sands reported guidelines for the clinical use of email with patients in general.[22]

The American Counseling Association Ethical Standards for Internet Online Counseling[20] included identifying the patient, contacting the patient in an emergency, informing the patient of how long records are kept, and seeking appropriate legal and technical assistance in developing e-therapy services.

Rosik and Brown[23] proposed a number of specific measures to promote ethical practice. Encryption should be used whenever communicating with or about a patient by email unless the patient has explicitly waived that option. The patient should be informed that confidential or sensitive information should not be sent via office email, even with encryption. All patient-related email should contain a notice that the message is confidential. When treatment teams are involved, each staff member should have their own email address. Consent should be in written form and obtained prior to using email. Technology-specific disclosures should include: the lack of confidentiality guarantees; the inclusion of electronically transmitted information in the record; how electronic records will be stored and who will have access to them; the differences between e- and traditional therapy; the advantages, disadvantages and experimental nature of e-therapy; normal response times; ways to confirm the therapist's identity and qualifications; security measures in place; and the probable right of a parent to the records of a child who is a minor. Responses should be written by the therapist. Arrangements during the therapist's absences should be made. The patient should be notified of any prohibited topics. The therapist should consider obtaining training and education in e-therapy. The therapist should have a plan for handling emergencies and technical failures. If the therapist advertises e-therapy services, they should be fully described.

Suggested principles of professional ethics

In 2000, the International Society for Mental Health Online (ISMHO) and the Psychiatric Society for Informatics (PSI, now the American Association for Technology in Psychiatry) endorsed a set of Suggested Principles of Professional Ethics for the Online Provision of Mental Health Services.[24-26] The goal of these principles was to guide both the therapists who provide and the patients who receive such services. The principles were to be broad enough to apply to the entire continuum of clinical mental health services that might be provided online, from email exchanged between office sessions to real-time videoconferencing between therapists and patients who never met in person. The principles were also to be general enough to have international application. Since their endorsement, a small number of additional changes have been made. 'Regulatory' issues were considered to be subsumed under 'legal' ones, the possibility that patients might feel safer online was added, 'competence' was broadened to include not just the types of problems addressed but also the use of the Internet to address them, 'requirements to practice' were specified as 'legal,' third-party coverage was mentioned and minor changes in wording were made. Box 5.2 shows the most recent version.

Limitations

The ISMHO/PSI principles were developed by a small, self-selected group comprising mainly psychiatrists and clinical psychologists in the USA. This might have limited its perspective. In addition, the very fact of undertaking the development of these principles could imply an underlying bias in favour of e-therapy.

Other limitations stem from the scope of these principles. They are ethical, as

---

Box 5.2. Suggested principles of professional ethics for the online provision of mental health services

---

A. *Informed consent*
    Informed consent is one of the foundations of ethical health care today. Before the patient consents to receive online mental health services, he or she should be informed about the process, the therapist, the potential risks and benefits, safeguards and alternatives.

1. Process
a. Possible misunderstandings
    The patient should be informed that when interacting online with the therapist, less information about each may be available to the other, so misunderstandings may be more likely. With text-based modalities such as email, non-verbal cues are relatively lacking, and even with videoconferencing, bandwidth is limited.
b. Turnaround time
    One issue specific to the provision of mental health services using asynchronous (not in 'real time') communication is that of turnaround time. The patient should be informed of how soon after sending an email, for example, he or she may expect a response.
c. Privacy of the therapist
    Privacy is more of an issue online than in person. The therapist has a right to his or her privacy and may wish to restrict the use of any copies or recordings the patient makes of their communications. See also B6 below on the confidentiality of the patient.
2. Therapist
    When the patient and the therapist do not meet in person, the patient may be less able to assess the therapist and to decide whether or not to enter into a treatment relationship with him or her.
a. Name
    The patient should be informed of the name of the therapist. The use of pseudonyms is common online, but is insufficient in a clinical context.
b. Qualifications and how to confirm them
    The patient should be informed of the qualifications (e.g. having a degree or being licenced, certified or registered) of the therapist. The therapist may also wish to provide supplemental information such as areas of special training or experience. So that the patient can confirm the qualifications, the therapist should provide the telephone numbers or web page URLs of the relevant organizations.
3. Potential benefits
    The patient should be informed of the potential benefits of receiving mental health services online. This includes both the circumstances in which the therapist considers online mental health services appropriate and the possible advantages of providing those services online. An example of the latter is that the patient might feel safer and therefore less inhibited.
4. Potential risks
    The patient should be informed of the potential risks of receiving mental health services online, for example, that misunderstandings might interfere with evaluation or treatment or that confidentiality might be breached.
5. Safeguards
    The patient should be informed of safeguards (such as the use of encryption) that are taken by the therapist and could be taken by himself or herself against the potential risks. Extra safeguards should be considered when family members, students, library patrons, etc., share a computer.
6. Alternatives
    The patient should be informed of alternatives to receiving mental health services online.
7. Proxies
    Some patients are not in a position to consent themselves to receive mental health

services. In those cases, consent should be obtained from a parent, legal guardian or other authorized party – and the identity of that party should be verified.

B. *Standard operating procedure*
    The mental health professions have evolved a standard service delivery framework. When treatment is provided online, that framework need not – indeed, should not – be discarded.

1. Competence
    The therapist should remain within the boundaries of competence determined by his or her education and training, both in regard to the types of problems addressed and the online provision of services.

2. Legal requirements to practice
    The therapist should meet any legal requirements (e.g. have a degree or be licenced, certified or registered) to provide mental health services where he or she is located. In fact, the legal requirements where the patient is located may also need to be met for it to be legal to provide services to that patient. See also A2b above on qualifications.

3. Structure of the online services
    The therapist and the patient should agree on the frequency and mode of communication, the method for determining the fee, the estimated total cost to the patient (third-party coverage may or may not apply), the payment procedure, etc.

4. Evaluation
    The therapist should adequately evaluate the patient when providing any mental health services online. The patient should understand that evaluation could potentially be helped or hindered by communicating online.

5. Multiple treatment providers
    When the patient receives mental health services from others at the same time, either online or in person, the therapist should carefully consider the potential effects of his or her interventions in the overall treatment context.

6. Confidentiality of the patient
    The confidentiality of the patient should be protected. Information about the patient should be released only with his or her permission. The patient should be informed of any exceptions to this general rule.

7. Records
    The therapist should maintain records of the services provided. If those records include copies or recordings of communications with the patient, the patient should be informed.

8. Existing guidelines
    The therapist should of course follow the laws and other existing guidelines (such as those of professional organizations) that apply to him or her.

C. *Emergencies*
    When mental health services are provided online, the therapist can be a great distance from the patient. This may limit the ability to respond to an emergency.

1. Procedures
    The procedures to follow in an emergency should be discussed. These procedures should address the possibility that the therapist might not immediately receive an online communication (perhaps because of technical problems) and might include trying to call the therapist, an answering service or a local backup.

2. Local backup
    When the therapist and the patient are in fact geographically separated, the therapist should identify and obtain the telephone number of a qualified local health care provider. A local backup who already knows the patient, such as his or her primary care physician, may be preferable.

opposed to clinical or legal, in nature. Adequately evaluating the patient is an ethical issue, but how to evaluate a particular patient online – and whether doing so is even possible – is a clinical question. Meeting requirements to practise is an ethical issue, but what specific requirements need to be met given a particular therapist and a particular patient is a legal question (and varies depending on the discipline and jurisdiction and may change over time). Whether a given service is a clinical one, i.e. constitutes e-therapy, is another legal question. There is currently no consensus regarding the meaning of terms like 'consultation' – in some cases it might be a clinical service, in other cases not. Maintaining records of services provided is an ethical issue, but the form in which they should be maintained (e.g. in electronic form or on paper, as transcripts or as summaries) is an administrative question.

These are principles, not a blueprint. It remains to be determined how to put them into practice given particular therapists, patients and practice settings. Research will need to be conducted, experience will need to be gained and clinical judgement will need to be applied. Some issues remain unresolved. First, verifying the identity of a proxy is not a simple matter; the signature of a parent or guardian could be requested, but could easily be forged. Second, a person who is unlicenced could promote themselves as competent not by claiming false credentials for themselves, but by claiming the actual credentials ('stealing' the identity) of a qualified therapist. Third, there is the question of how or even whether to work with a patient who insists on anonymity.

What about enforcement? These principles were designed to guide and to influence through education. The more clear therapists are about what to provide and patients are about what to expect, the higher the standard of care will be. These principles could, however, be enforced. Professional organizations could endorse some or all of these principles and require compliance as a condition of membership (i.e. discipline members who violate them). Similarly, government agencies could require compliance as a condition of licensure, certification or registration. Finally, courts could look to these principles for guidance in legal proceedings. Boulding has discussed the complementary nature of self-regulation and legal enforcement.[27]

Further development

These principles are a work in progress – as e-therapy itself is still evolving. Additional input has been and continues to be sought from other interested parties (including readers of this chapter). The author has created a message board for discussion of 'distance' mental health services, including these principles.[28] There has been technical discussion, for example, about how to allow users to confirm a credential by simply clicking a button and about different methods of encryption. There has also been discussion about more general issues, such as the reluctance of 'mainstream' physicians to use the Internet to communicate with patients. It has not, however, developed into an active forum for ongoing discussion by current or prospective e-therapists or e-patients. No further revisions of the principles have yet been proposed or made.

Conclusions

Traditional principles of professional ethics can be extended to e-therapy. The wheel does not need to be reinvented, though it does need to be modified for this new terrain.

Comprehensive principles of professional ethics can be developed by groups that cross disciplinary and national boundaries. Although there are of course differences between the traditions and current practices of different professionals in different countries, ethical principles are derived from cultural values, and principles derived from values common to a number of cultures should be applicable in those cultures.

These principles should help guide both the therapists who provide and the patients who receive e-therapy (Box 5.3). These individuals will then be able to benefit from

---

Box 5.3. Another scenario

Therapist B, in California, decides to diversify into e-therapy. He is aware of the ISMHO/PSI guidelines and creates a virtual shingle: 'Therapy Services Online, Inc. Get help by secure real-time chat. Therapist B, PhD Licenced in California. Email now for more information, but keep in mind that email may be intercepted by hackers, read by employers, or misunderstood by the recipient. Please therefore think twice about what you say, how you say it, and where you say it from.' Patient B sees Therapist A's Web page, but doesn't see Therapist A's name or qualifications and moves on. Next, he sees Therapist B's Web page. Heeding its advice, he sends an email: 'There's something I'm concerned about, and I wonder if you can help me with it. Can we chat to discuss this further?' He starts corresponding with other e-therapists, too.

Therapist B and Patient B have a chat meeting, and Therapist B says he charges $100/hour spent chatting or responding to email. Patient B accepts, but makes a mental note not to email Therapist B unnecessarily. Therapist B says Patient B can expect email to be responded to within 12 hours. Therapist B asks if Patient B has a primary care physician. Patient B does, Doctor B, and gives Therapist B his name and telephone number. Therapist B instructs Patient B to call Doctor B if he can't contact Therapist B in an emergency.

They start having chat meetings. Patient B tells Therapist B about his passionate feelings for his boss's wife. Therapist B asks about other concurrent therapy relationships, and Patient B tells him about the other e-therapists. Therapist B explains how too many cooks can spoil the broth, and Patient B accepts that and terminates with the others. Therapist B asks what Patient B had been discussing with them, and Patient B says one issue was his feelings of commitment to his wife. They discuss both his satisfactions and dissatisfactions in his marriage.

To fill Therapist B in on the history of his affair, Patient B emails him entries from his diary. Not wanting to pay Therapist B to go through irrelevant material, Patient B is selective about what he sends. Therapist B spends 30 minutes reviewing and commenting on the diary entries and enters that time into his automatic billing software.

Therapist B is then unexpectedly called away. The boss's wife calls Patient B at home and gives him an ultimatum.

Patient B immediately sends Therapist B an email, but, aware of the risks of using his home computer, first unchecks the default 'save a copy' feature. Not getting a response within 12 hours, he decides Therapist B must be having technical problems and calls Doctor B, as previously discussed. Doctor B advises him not to take any lithium and prescribes a benzodiazepine instead. Feeling more relaxed, Patient B reflects on his situation and considers his options. Therapist B's automatic billing service sends an email bill to him for the month's chat sessions plus $50 for dealing with the diary entries. Patient B grumbles to himself about the extra charge, but feels confident that he will find his way and looks forward to continuing to work with Therapist B when they are able to connect again.

---

the opportunities of this new treatment modality, and others will then be reassured that e-therapy can be conducted ethically. To paraphrase King and Moreggi,[14] e-therapy may be controversial today but commonplace tomorrow.

Acknowledgements

This chapter is based, with permission, on Hsiung RC. Suggested principles of professional ethics for e-therapy. In: Hsiung RC, ed. *E-therapy: case studies, guiding principles, and the clinical potential of the Internet.* New York: WW Norton, 2002:150–165. The members of the joint International Society for Mental Health Online/Psychiatric Society for Informatics committee that developed the Suggested Principles were Martha Ainsworth (co-chair), Michael Fenichel, Denis Franklin, John Greist, John Grohol, Leonard Holmes, Robert C. Hsiung (co-chair), Martin Kesselman, Peggy Kirk, Judy Kraybill, Russell Lim, Roger Park-Cunningham, Richard N. Rosenthal, Jeanne N. Rust, Gary Stofle, Nancy Tice, Giovanni Torello, Mark Vardell and Willadene Walker-Schmucker.

References

1   Murphy LJ, Mitchell DL. When writing helps to heal: E-mail as therapy. *British Journal of Guidance and Counselling* 1998;**26**:21–32.
2   American Psychiatric Association. The principles of medical ethics with annotations especially applicable to psychiatry. Available at http://www.psych.org/apa_members/medicalethics2001_42001.cfm [last checked 11 September 2002].
3   American Psychological Association Ethics Committee. Ethical principles of psychologists and code of conduct. *American Psychologist* 1992;**47**:1597–1611.
4   Health on the Net Foundation. 1997. Health on the Net code of conduct (HONcode) for medical and health Web sites. Available at http://www.hon.ch/HONcode/Conduct.html [last checked 9 September 2002].
5   Boyer C, Selby M, Scherrer JR, Appel RD. The Health on the Net Code of Conduct for medical and health Websites. *Computers in Biology and Medicine* 1998;**28**:603–610.
6   Rodriguez JC. Legal, ethical, and professional issues to consider when communicating via the Internet: a suggested response model and policy. *Journal of the American Dietetic Association* 1999;**99**:1428–1432.
7   Asmonga DD. IHC eyes E-health Code of Ethics. *Journal of the American Health Information Management Association* 2000;**71**:14–16.
8   Hi-Ethics. Ethical principles for offering Internet health services to consumers. Available at http://www.hiethics.com/Principles/index.asp [last checked 9 September 2002].
9   Internet Healthcare Coalition. eHealth Code of Ethics. Available at http://www.ihealthcoalition.org/ethics/ehealthcode0524.html [last checked 11 September 2002].
10 International Medical Informatics Association. A code of ethics for health informatics professionals. Available at http://www.imia.org [last checked 11 September 2002].
11 Shapiro DE, Schulman CE. Ethical and legal issues in e-mail therapy. *Ethics and Behavior* 1996;**6**:107–124.
12 Hughes RS. Cybercounseling and regulations: quagmire or quest? In: Bloom JW, Walz GR, eds. *Cybercounseling and Cyberlearning: strategies and resources for the Millennium.* Alexandria, VA: American Counseling Association, 2000:321–338.
13 Robson D, Robson M. Ethical issues in Internet counselling. *Counselling Psychology Quarterly* 2000;**13**:249–257.
14 King SA, Moreggi D. Internet therapy and self-help groups – the pros and cons. In: Gackenbach J, ed. *Psychology and the Internet: intrapersonal, interpersonal, and transpersonal implications.* San Diego, CA: Academic Press, 1998:77–109.

15   Deutsch H. Some forms of emotional disturbance and their relationship to schizophrenia. *Psychoanalytic Quarterly* 1942;**11**:301–321.

16   Holmes LG. Delivering mental health services on-line: current issues. *Cyberpsychology and Behavior* 1998;**1**:19–24.

17   American Psychological Association Ethics Committee. 1997. APA statement on services by telephone, teleconferencing, and Internet. Available at http://www.apa.org/ethics/stmnt01.html [last checked 9 September 2002].

18   Bloom JW. The ethical practice of webcounseling. *British Journal of Guidance and Counselling* 1998;**26**:53–59.

19   National Board for Certified Counselors. The practice of Internet counseling. Available at http://www.nbcc.org/ethics/webethics.htm [last checked 11 September 2002].

20   American Counseling Association. Ethical standards for Internet on-line counseling. Available at http://www.counseling.org/resources/internet.htm [last checked 11 September 2002].

21   Australian Psychological Society. 1999. Considerations for psychologists providing services on the Internet. Available at http://www.aps.psychsociety.com.au/ [last checked 11 September 2002].

22   Kane B, Sands DZ. Guidelines for the clinical use of electronic mail with patients. *Journal of the American Medical Informatics Association* 1998;**5**:104–111.

23   Rosik CH, Brown RK. Professional use of the Internet: legal and ethical issues in a member care environment. *Journal of Psychology and Theology* 2001;**29**:106–120.

24   International Society for Mental Health Online and Psychiatric Society for Informatics. ISMHO/PSI suggested principles of professional ethics for the online provision of mental health services. http://www.ismho.org/suggestions.html [last checked 9 September 2002].

25   International Society for Mental Health Online and Psychiatric Society for Informatics. 2000. Available at ISMHO/PSI suggested principles of professional ethics for the online provision of mental health services. Available at http://www.dr-bob.org/psi/suggestions.3.13.html [last checked 11 September 2002].

26   Hsiung RC. Suggested principles of professional ethics for the online provision of mental health services. *Telemedicine Journal and E-health* 2001;**7**:39–45.

27   Boulding ME. Self-regulation: who needs it? *Health Affairs* 2000;**19**:132–139.

28   Tele-Psycho-Babble. Available at http://www.dr-bob.org/babble/tele [last checked 9 September 2002].

6

Cybermedicine in Psychiatry and Psychology – a personal recollection*†

Warner V. Slack

Introduction

During the 1960s, when I was at the University of Wisconsin in Madison, two lines of reasoning evolved in my mind. The first led to the philosophy that, in the vernacular of the times, was called 'patient power,' arguing that patients who want to should be encouraged to make their own clinical decisions and helped to do so.[1-3] For centuries, the medical profession had perpetrated paternalism as an essential component of medical care, thereby depriving patients of the self-esteem that comes from mutual respect. The assumption was that the doctor knew best. Patient power questioned this. As George Bernard Shaw once wrote, 'Do not do unto others as you would that they should do unto you. Their tastes may be different.'[4]

My second line of reasoning led to the conclusion that the computer could be used wisely and well in the practice of medicine. This was also controversial for its time, and those of us who were entering this new field were confronted by concerns about the computer in medicine under any circumstances – concern about the potential encroachment of this new technology on the practice of medicine and the traditional rapport between doctor and patient. Would these machines result in the de-humanizing processes that had been associated with the Industrial Revolution? Would modern times destroy the art of medicine? The debate was frequently lively, and a commonly asked question was 'Will your computer replace the doctor?' A rejoinder that I found useful, and one which is still apt today, was that any doctor who could be replaced by a computer deserved to be.

---

*Portions of this chapter were adapted from Slack WV. *Cybermedicine: how computing empowers doctors and patients for better health care*, revised and updated edition. San Francisco: Jossey-Bass, 2001, with the permission of the publisher.

†Author's note: Shortly after the Second World War, the eminent mathematician Norbert Wiener, then at the Massachusetts Institute of Technology in Cambridge Massachusetts, drew upon the Greek word kybernetes, meaning 'pilot' or 'Governor', to coin the English word 'cybernetics', which he defined as the science of communication between people and machines. More recently, the word cyberspace has come to mean the worldwide computer-based network that has already so greatly enhanced communication. As a derivative of cybernetics, 'cybermedicine' is my word for the use of computing to enhance communication in the field of medicine, computing that improves the quality of medical care while reducing the financial costs and improving the relationship between doctor and patient.[1]

Patient–computer dialogue

It was there in Madison in 1965 that my colleagues and I had the idea that we could program a computer to interact directly with a patient, to engage in meaningful dialogue, to explore medical problems in detail, and to do so in a personalized, dignified and considerate manner – an idea that had not been tried before.[5] There were theoretical reasons for pursuing this idea – could the computer model the clinician as an interviewer? – but there were practical reasons as well. The traditional time-consuming method of taking and recording detailed medical histories involves serious problems for the busy clinician, particularly in regions that are short on doctors.

I hoped that the computer-based interview would be helpful to the doctor in the care of the patient, that using the computer would be of interest to the patient (perhaps even enjoyable), and that pooled responses from many interviews would help us to learn more about the importance of the questions in the interview and to study the process of clinical interviewing. In the back of my mind was the idea that perhaps the computer could actually help patients to help themselves.

We used a Laboratory Instrument Computer (LINC) for our study.[6] This small, general-purpose digital computer was developed at the Massachusetts Institute of Technology in 1962; it was a pioneering machine, and in many respects was the forerunner of today's personal computers. It found widespread use in neurophysiology laboratories, where it could be programmed to study the nervous system of experimental animals. The LINC had a small memory and was very slow by today's standards, and there was a flicker on the screen that became increasingly noticeable as more characters were displayed. There was reason, therefore, to keep the questions short, but this electronically imposed succinctness had a beneficial effect on my writing.

The LINC was in great demand, and as a neurology resident with little authority, I was given late night and early morning hours to program. Still, within a few months we had an allergy interview written and working well. But I found myself continuing to make revisions, and eventually I had to admit that I was procrastinating. It had been fun to talk about the computer and to argue with the sceptics, but to try it with a real patient – *for the first time* – that was another matter.

The time came, however, when it was now or never. I approached a patient, an older man who was recovering from a heart attack and about to go home, and asked if he would give us a hand. He agreed. Fortunately, there was a free hour at lunchtime for us to try our first interview. He sat down in front of the machine; I turned it on, turned down the lights in the room (the dim characters on the screen were easier to read in the dark), pressed the start button, and stepped back to observe.

The question 'HAVE YOU EVER HAD HIVES?' appeared on the screen. The characters flickered, the lights on the console flashed on and off, and the LINC's speaker emitted an eerie, high-pitched sound. Although we had the computer, its owners were still doing a cat brain experiment next door, and on the other side of the partition, people were walking in and out, and a cat was meowing. It was a scene reminiscent of Kafka's *Castle* or Koestler's *Darkness at Noon*. Clearly, these were not the best circumstances for *any* medical interview, let alone one conducted by a computer.

However, my patient seemed oblivious to his surroundings. He responded appropriately to the questions and soon it was clear that he was having fun and there was rapport between man and machine. He laughed out loud at some of the comments from the computer. Some I had intended to be funny; some I had not. And he talked out loud to the machine, sometimes in praise and sometimes in criticism. Of course, he never would have said this to me face-to-face, a doctor with a white coat and an engraved nametag. It occurred to me that perhaps for the first time in his experience as a patient, he was in control of the interview. Here was patient power at work.

In a formal study with the program, we found that patients communicated more relevant medical information to the computer than they had to their doctors (Fig. 6.1). At the end of the interview, the computer asked each patient what he or she had thought of the experience. As we had hoped, almost all the patients found their interaction with the computer both interesting and enjoyable.[1,5]

Encouraged by our early results, we carried out further studies of computer-based medical interviews in our laboratories at the University of Wisconsin and, more recently, at Beth Israel Deaconess Medical Center in Boston. Our programs have addressed a wide variety of medical problems and have been well received by patients

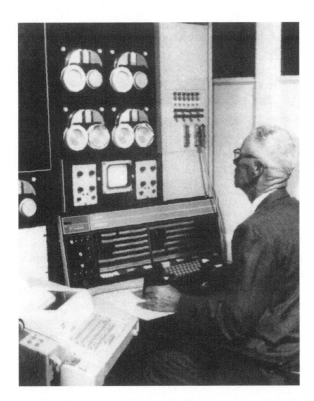

Fig. 6.1. The LINC (Laboratory Instrument Computer) in use in a medical interview in 1968. (Reproduced from Slack WV, Van Cura LJ. Patient reaction to computer-based medical interviewing. *Computers in Biomedical Research* 1968;**1**:527–531 with permission.)

and physicians alike.[7-16] In our experience, and the experience of others,[17-19] concern about the computer as a depersonalizing influence has been unfounded. Most patients who have had the opportunity to engage in dialogue with the computer have found it to be enjoyable, interesting and informative.

Over the years, we have incorporated into our programs a number of provisions designed to enhance rapport and to yield control to the patient. The debate about patient power in the traditional setting would continue into the twenty first century, but all would agree during the decades of debate that when it came to dialogue with the computer, the patient should be in charge.

A psychiatric interview

In 1968, Maxie Maultsby and I ventured into a field that was more controversial than our other computer interviews at the time. We developed a computer-based psychiatric interview, designed as a general review of behavioural problems, and introduced it to 69 volunteers who had been scheduled for psychiatric evaluation.[20] As with other computer histories, the patients reacted favourably. They indicated a slight preference for the computer as an interviewer in comparison with doctors in their experience. Some patients responded yes to preferring the doctor *and* yes to preferring the computer, apparently not wanting to hurt the feelings of either and nicely demonstrating that human beings are not always Aristotelian in their logic. They also found the computer to be more thorough.

The consensus among the nine participating psychotherapists was that routine computerized psychiatric histories, if available, would add a valuable dimension to their diagnostic evaluations.

Research with the computer as a psychiatric interviewer continued at the University of Wisconsin under the direction of John Greist,[21] and the field became increasingly active with studies of the computer in psychiatry and psychology in institutions throughout the world, as well as in our Center for Clinical Computing in Boston.[22-25]

Emotionally laden topics and the computer interview

In traditional psychotherapy, topics of major psychological importance are thought to be the most unpleasant and hence the most difficult to discuss. For psychotherapy to be effective, the reluctance to unearth or discuss such difficult topics should be removed. This tenet is held whether the reluctance is interpreted as resistance to abreaction – bringing emotionally laden topics from the unconscious to open discussion (in accordance with the psychoanalytic concepts of Freud) – or the weakening of a conditioned response in the absence of reinforcing stimuli (in accordance with the behaviourist concepts of John Watson and B.F. Skinner). Furthermore, it is generally assumed that this resistance must be removed by means of the relationship established between patient and therapist.

Under some circumstances, however, disinhibition with such communication can occur in the absence of the human clinician, including the psychotherapist. This has been our experience with patient–computer dialogue, with both our psychiatric and medical interviews.[7,8,16,20] Even when patients are eager for their doctor to be informed, direct communication about emotionally charged issues is sometimes difficult, and indirect communication by means of the computer can be easier.

Our original observation about disinhibition (and perhaps abreaction) with the computer has been corroborated by others: in one study, patients undergoing treatment for alcoholism found it easier to report high levels of alcohol consumption to the computer than to a psychiatrist;[26] and in other studies, patients were more likely to communicate with the computer about problems such as impotence, attempted suicide and being fired from a job.[27,28] In addition, Steven Locke, our coworkers and I have demonstrated that a computer-based screening interview could elicit more HIV-related factors in the health histories of potential blood donors than the standard questionnaire and interviewing methods currently in use at the Red Cross.[29]

Psychotherapy

The most common use of the computer in the psychotherapeutic setting has been to collect information directly from the patient to help the psychologist and psychiatrist with both diagnosis and treatment. But the computer has also been used for psychotherapy, more commonly as an adjunct to the human therapist, but sometimes as a therapist on its own. Computer-based psychotherapy is still in its infancy – most of the work has been research projects in academic medical centres, rather than in clinical practice – but the future is bright.

In one of the earliest ventures, in the mid 1960s, Joseph Weizenbaum,[30] Kenneth Colby[31] and their colleagues wrote computer programs (Weizenbaum's was called ELIZA after Shaw's heroine in *Pygmalion*) that took messages typed by the user, rephrased them with words of similar meaning, and responded in a manner suggestive of the non-directive psychotherapy first proposed by Carl Rogers.[32]

Since then, a number of good programs have been developed and studied, and a wide variety of theoretical approaches have been employed. John Greist and his colleagues at the University of Wisconsin employed cognitive behavioural therapy in their program,[33] based on principles first elucidated by Aaron Beck and his coworkers.[34] In a comparative study, the computer performed impressively – as well as the human therapist in reducing scores on tests of depression. Computer-based cognitive behavioural therapy has also been used with some reported success for patients with early Alzheimer's disease and stuttering problems.[35,36]

Interactive voice response systems, with the telephone as the medium of therapeutic interaction between patient and computer, show great promise as a means of reaching a large number of people; they can be accessed from the patient's home or mobile phone at any time of day or night. In a large, randomized controlled trial, Lee Baer, John Greist, Isaac Marks, and their colleagues have studied this approach using principles of behaviour therapy for patients with obsessive-compulsive disorders, and the results have been encouraging.[37] They have also studied a similar program using cognitive behavioural therapy for depression with promising preliminary results.[38]

In addition, there is growing use of the Internet for 'on-line therapy', whereby patients and psychotherapists communicate with each other by means of chat groups, newsgroups and email.

Talking therapy

In 1971, I teamed up with my brother, Charles, who is a psychologist. We wanted people to be able to talk during a computer interview. We had the idea that the computer could facilitate talking therapy and that it could encourage people to talk out loud about matters of importance to them. Although there are important theoretical and practical differences between the various schools of talking therapy, all are based on the premise that the presence of the therapist and the relationship that results are essential to the therapeutic process. Charles and I questioned this.

In the late 1950s, in the Psychology Department at Harvard University during that wild psychedelic era of Timothy Leary and friends, Charles had experimented with soliloquy.[39] He had equipped a tape recorder with a device that emitted repetitive clicks in response to sustained sound. It also tallied the number of clicks. Charles then employed teenagers from Cambridge Massachusetts to help him with his study. As long as subjects in the experiment talked into the microphone, they could hear and see the counter adding up points at a steady rate, but whenever they stopped talking for more than a normal pause, the counter ceased to give points. At the end of each experimental session of talk, each subject was paid according to the number of points accumulated during the session. The system worked well in initiating and maintaining talk without a human listener in the room. Portions of the resulting tape recordings were indistinguishable from those of interpersonal interviews, and some of the participants said they felt better for having talked this way.

In the meantime, James Webb at Ohio University showed that people would talk alone when encouraged to do so by a standardized series of prerecorded (auditory) non-directive statements presented in a fixed sequence whenever there was a pause in the subject's speech.[40] Expanding on this technique, Michael Dinoff and his colleagues at the University of Alabama promoted talk on the part of experimental subjects (including hospitalized patients) in response to 15 requests from a prerecorded, videotaped interviewer who appeared on a screen whenever the person paused for 2 seconds.[41] With this 'talking alone' research, however, the stimuli promoting talk were presented in a predetermined sequence without branching; no use was made during the interviews of information provided by the person. In most clinical situations, by contrast, information obtained from the patient is used in subsequent conversation.

Computer-based speech-understanding systems would of course be useful in studies of talking therapy. Such systems, however, are currently limited in capabilities, and not yet readily available except in rudimentary form. Some systems can 'comprehend' single words and short phrases, but sustained, protracted speech remains a difficult problem.[42,43] Furthermore, Charles and I had the idea that the computer did not *have* to understand what was being said to help people help themselves. In other words, the computer could facilitate beneficial soliloquy.

Computer-assisted soliloquy

There are problems with talking therapy as traditionally practised in the USA. Typically, many sessions are required for treatment; few patients can afford the cost, and third-party payers – particularly those in the business of managed care – are reluctant to finance long-term therapy. Furthermore, hard-to-control variables, so important to the art of human discourse, lend uncertainty to scientific study and to our knowledge of how or whether desired goals are achieved through clinical conversation. Standards of comparison for controlled studies are difficult to establish. Therapists, even within the same school of thought, differ from each other and are themselves inconsistent. Furthermore, the interested therapist may bias the session, unwittingly communicating by verbal and non-verbal cues, and thus evoke responses that conform to expectations.

As an alternative to interpersonal dialogue, we have studied computer-assisted soliloquy – an approach to talking therapy that is more easily subjected to the rigours of scientific investigation than the traditional dialogue between therapist and patient.

Charles and I have three hypotheses. First, that the presence of a therapist is not essential in talking therapy, because patients will talk aloud alone about matters of psychological importance; second, that speaking out, as opposed to thinking quietly, is important to the effectiveness of psychotherapy; and third, that the doctor–patient relationship, although for the most part beneficial, can sometimes inhibit frank disclosure. In the latter case, soliloquy can be more effective in the process of disinhibition than dialogue with a therapist. In a preliminary study,[44-46] performed to test these hypotheses, we used an interactive computer to facilitate soliloquy and found that volunteers talked to the computer with ease and personal revelation, as judged by the Gendlin scale.[47]

Computer-assisted soliloquy in a study of anxiety

In a more recent experiment, designed to study the effectiveness of soliloquy with a specific emotional problem, Douglas Porter, Peter Balkin, Hollis Kowaloff, Charles, and I programmed a computer to conduct an automated interview that would address the symptoms of anxiety.[48] In doing so, we did our best to improve the interviewing process on the basis of our experience with earlier programs.

As with our earlier study, the computer communicated with text on the screen (explanations, questions, requests, comments and advice), and the user responded at the keyboard and via a microphone beneath the screen. The computer was oblivious to the meaning of spoken words and the user was so informed. However, the machine could respond to the occurrence of speech at the microphone, to the durations of speech and silence, to the time elapsed between various points of reference in the interview, and to the time the user took to respond, as well as to entries on the keyboard, and it could use this information to direct the course of the interview. In addition, wires connected the user to a monitor, which transmitted the heart rate to the computer.[49]

The interview began with words of welcome followed by instructions about use of the keyboard, instructions on the use of the microphone, a request for the person's first name and for permission to use this during the interview. As a measure of anxiety at the beginning of the interview, the introductory section concluded with the Spielberger State anxiety measure, which consists of 20 questions designed to assess a person's level of anxiety at the moment.[50]

The computer then proceeded to the section on anxiety. Introductory comments ('Most people are nervous, tense or anxious, at least sometimes') were followed by questions about the occurrence of anxiety when alone, with friends, with strangers, in a crowd, at a party, at school (if the user was a student), at work and at home. Along the way, the computer encouraged the user to talk aloud about feelings ('Now tell yourself how you feel when you are anxious. Speak out loud, into the phone') and about each of the situations in which they had occurred. Next, the computer encouraged the user to try to become anxious ('Make a mental list of the circumstances most likely to make you anxious … now list them to yourself out loud'). The section concluded with a repeat presentation of the State anxiety measure.

The computer then turned to the subject of relaxation ('You have talked about being anxious … now the idea is to dwell on a more comfortable state … relaxation'). The computer asked about the user's ability to relax under the circumstances that had been discussed in the section on anxiety, and then encouraged talking aloud about relaxation. ('Talk a bit about being at ease with strangers … say a little more if you can.') Then it encouraged the user to talk aloud about circumstances most conducive to relaxation and experiences with relaxation (as opposed to anxiety), and to develop and discuss strategies for relaxation in the future. The interview ended with a repeat of the State anxiety measure, a request for suggestions about the program and thanks.

As a control, we developed a 'thinking interview' that encouraged the user to think quietly, as indicated by pressing a button instead of talking aloud. Otherwise, the wording and manner of presentation were identical in the two interviews. A control interview of this quality – identical in all respects except for the variable being studied – is rare in studies of interviewing.

Forty-two men between the ages of 20 and 30 years (none of whom were currently receiving psychotherapy) were recruited through colleges and graduate schools in the Boston area and paid to participate in the study. During preliminary sessions, the volunteers were divided into two matched groups – the talking group and the thinking group – on the basis of comparable scores on the computer-administered State anxiety and Taylor Manifest Anxiety[51] measures and on the basis of comparable past experience with computers. At the end of the session, each volunteer was asked, by written questionnaire, about his reaction to the interviews.

Results of the soliloquy study[48]

The two measures of anxiety improved in the experimental group but not in the control group. Both the mean heart rate and the State anxiety scores of the 21 volunteers in the talking group went down significantly between the beginning and the end of the interview. In the thinking group, by contrast, the drop in scores and heart rate was not significant. Furthermore, the talking group spent more time talking aloud than the thinking group spent thinking quietly. During the relaxation section of the talking interview, the time devoted to talking was found to correlate significantly with both the drop in anxiety scores and the drop in heart rate – the more time spent talking, the greater the change. During the relaxation section of the thinking interview, by contrast, there was no significant correlation between the time devoted to thinking and changes in anxiety scores and heart rate. As judged by responses on the written questionnaire, the participants reacted favourably to the experiment in general, being equally well disposed to both the talking and the thinking interviews.

The participants in this study were not patients; they were paid volunteers whose mean State anxiety scores at the start of the study were substantially lower than they would have been among men with the clinical diagnosis of anxiety. It is possible that computer-assisted soliloquy would have produced more striking results among patients with the symptoms of anxiety.

Reflections on computer-assisted soliloquy

The primary approach with the soliloquy interview – to encourage each subject to speak first about anxiety, then about relaxation, and finally about personally developed strategies for replacing anxiety with relaxation – appears to have been effective under the experimental conditions of the study. Encouragement to talk about relaxation was more effective than encouragement to think about it, as judged by the time devoted to each and the reductions in heart rate and State anxiety scores in the talking group. The correlations between these reductions and the time devoted to talking aloud indicate that computer-assisted soliloquy was more beneficial than thinking quietly in promoting relaxation. It would seem that talking aloud helps to keep us on track – on mental course, so to speak – when we are developing strategies that could promote our mental health.

With the computer in this research, the variability and bias of the human interviewer are eliminated as independent variables, and standards for comparison, such as the thinking interview for comparison with the soliloquy interview, can be more readily established. In future, we plan to use the computer to study soliloquy further, both as an independent approach to therapy and as an adjunct to more traditional methods.

The future of cybermedicine in psychotherapy

It is important for computer programs designed for use by patients in psychiatry and psychology to be carefully evaluated. In developing our interactive programs for patients, I have tried to keep the following guidelines in mind: the programs should be easy to use; they should be truly interactive; they should be of immediate and if possible long-range benefit to the patient; they should have the patient in charge; they should protect confidentiality; they should be readily available to people of all socioeconomic backgrounds; they should be fast and reliable; and they should be studied for effectiveness and safety. To my knowledge, no program yet exists that achieves this ideal. Certainly none of ours do. On the other hand, a number of people in the field are making progress and I am optimistic.

References

1   Slack WV, ed. *Cybermedicine: how computing empowers doctors and patients for better health care*. San Francisco: Jossey-Bass, 1997.
2   Slack WV. Patient power: a patient-oriented value system. In: Jacques JA, ed. *Computer Diagnosis and Diagnostic Methods*: Proceedings of the Second Conference on Diagnostic Process held at the University of Michigan. Springfield, IL: Charles C Thomas, 1972:3–7.
3   Slack WV. The patient's right to decide. *Lancet* 1977;**2**:240.
4   Shaw GB. *Man and Superman: a comedy and philosophy*. Baltimore: Penguin, 1952 (originally published 1903).
5   Slack WV, Hicks GP, Reed CE, Van Cura LJ. A computer-based medical history system. *New England Journal of Medicine* 1966;**274**:194–198.
6   Clark WA, Molnar CE. The LINC: a description of the laboratory instrument computer. *Annals of the New York Academy of Science* 1964;**115**:653–668.
7   Slack WV, Van Cura LJ. Patient reaction to computer-based medical interviewing. *Computers and Biomedical Research* 1968;**1**:527–531.
8   Peckham BM, Slack WV, Carr WF, Van Cura LJ, Schultz AE. Computerized data collection in the management of uterine cancer. *Clinical Obstetrics and Gynecology* 1967;**10**:1003–1015.
9   Slack WV, Van Cura LJ. Computer-based patient interviewing. 1. *Postgraduate Medicine* 1968;**43**:68–74.
10 Slack WV, Van Cura LJ, Greist JH. Computers and doctors: use and consequences. *Computers and Biomedical Research* 1970;**3**:521–527.
11 Chun RWM, Van Cura LJ, Spencer M, Slack WV. Computer interviewing of patients with epilepsy. *Epilepsia* 1976;**17**:371–375.
12 Bana DS, Leviton A, Swidler C, Slack W, Graham JR. A computer-based headache interview: acceptance by patients and physicians. *Headache* 1980;**20**:85–89.
13 Bennett SE, Lawrence RS, Fleischmann KH, Gifford CS, Slack WV. Profile of women practicing breast self-examination. *Journal of the American Medical Association* 1983;**249**:488–491.
14 Leviton A, Slack WV, Bana D, Graham JR. Age-related headache characteristics. *Archives of Neurology* 1984;**41**:762–764.
15 Slack WV. A history of computerized medical interviews. *M.D. Computing: Computers in Medical Practice* 1984;**1**:52–59.
16 Slack WV. Patient–computer dialogue: a review. In: van Bemmel JH, McCray AT, eds. *Yearbook of Medical Informatics 2000: patient-centered systems*. Stuttgart, Germany: Schattauer, 2000:71–78.
17 Mayne JG, Weksel W, Sholtz PN. Toward automating the medical history. *Mayo Clinic Proceedings* 1968;**43**:1–25.
18 Lucas RW. A study of patients' attitudes to computer interrogation. *International Journal of Man-Machine Studies* 1977;**9**:69–86.
19 Dugaw JE Jr, Civello K, Chuinard C, Jones GN. Will patients use a computer to give a medical history? *Journal of Family Practice* 2000;**49**:921–923.
20 Maultsby MC Jr, Slack WV. A computer-based psychiatry history system. *Archives of General Psychiatry* 1971;**25**:570–572.
21 Greist JH, Gustafson DH, Stauss FF, Rowse GL, Laughren TP, Chiles JA. A computer interview for suicide-risk prediction. *American Journal of Psychiatry* 1973;**130**:1327–1332.
22 Coddington RD, King TL. Automated history taking in child psychiatry. *American Journal of Psychiatry* 1972;**129**:276–282.
23 Carr AC, Ghosh A, Ancill RJ. Can a computer take a psychiatric history? *Psychological Medicine* 1983;**13**:151–158.
24 Carr AC, Ghosh A. Response of phobic patients to direct computer assessment. *British Journal of Psychiatry* 1983;**142**:60–65.
25 Skinner HA, Allen BA. Does the computer make a difference? Computerized versus face-to-face versus self-report assessment of alcohol, drug, and tobacco use. *Journal of Consulting and Clinical Psychology* 1983;**51**:267–275.

26 Lucas RW, Mullin PJ, Luna CB, McInroy DC. Psychiatrists and a computer as interrogators of patients with alcohol-related illnesses: a comparison. *British Journal of Psychiatry* 1977;**131**:160–167.

27 Greist JH, Klein MH. Computer programs for patients, clinicians, and researchers in psychiatry. In: Sidowski JB, ed. *Technology in Mental Health Care Delivery Systems*. Norwood, CN: Ablex, 1980:161–182.

28 Kobak KA, Greist JH, Jefferson JW, Katzelnick DJ. Computer-administered clinical rating scales. *Psychopharmacology* 1996;**127**:291–301.

29 Locke SE, Kowaloff HB, Hoff RG, et al. Computer-based interview for screening blood donors for risk of HIV transmission. *Journal of the American Medical Association* 1992;**268**:1301–1305.

30 Weizenbaum JE. ELIZA: a computer program for the study of natural language communication between man and machine. *Communications of the Association of Computing Machinery* 1966;**9**:36–45.

31 Colby KM, Watt JB, Gilbert JP. A computer method of psychotherapy: preliminary communication. *Journal of Nervous and Mental Disease* 1966;**142**:148–152.

32 Rogers CR, ed. *Client-centered Therapy. Its current practice, implications and theory*. Boston: Houghton Mifflin, 1965.

33 Selmi PM, Klein MH, Greist JH, Sorrell SP, Erdman HP. Computer-administered cognitive-behavioral therapy for depression. *American Journal of Psychiatry* 1990;**147**:51–56.

34 Beck AT, ed. *Cognitive Therapy of Depression*. New York: Guilford Press, 1979.

35 Hoffmann M, Hock C, Muller-Spahn F. Computer-based cognitive training in Alzheimer's disease patients. *Annals of the New York Academy of Science* 1996;**777**:249–254.

36 Blood GW. A behavioral-cognitive therapy program for adults who stutter: computers and counseling. *Journal of Communication Disorders* 1995;**28**:165–180.

37 Baer L, Brown-Beasley MW, Sorce J, Henriques AI. Computer-assisted telephone administration of a structured interview for obsessive-compulsive disorder. *American Journal of Psychiatry* 1993;**150**:1737–1738.

38 Baer L, Greist JH. An interactive computer-administered self-assessment and self-help program for behavior therapy. *Journal of Clinical Psychiatry* 1997;**58**(suppl 12):23–28.

39 Slack CW, ed. *Timothy Leary, the Madness of the Sixties and Me*. New York: PH Wyden, 1974.

40 Webb JT. Interview synchrony: an investigation of two speech measures in an automated standardized interview. In: Siegman AW, Pope B, eds. *Studies in Dyadic Communication*. New York: Pergamon Press, 1972:115–133.

41 Dinoff M, Clark CG, Reitman LM, Smith RE. The feasibility of video-tape interviewing. *Psychological Reports* 1969;**25**:239–242.

42 Bergeron B, Locke S. Speech recognition as a user interface. *M.D. Computing* 1990;**7**:329–334.

43 Devine EG, Gaehde SA, Curtis AC. Comparative evaluation of three continuous speech recognition software packages in the generation of medical reports. *Journal of the American Medical Informatics Association* 2000;**7**:462–468.

44 Slack WV, Slack CW. Patient-computer dialogue. *New England Journal of Medicine* 1972;**286**:1304–1309.

45 Slack CW, Slack WV. The computer that listens to your troubles. *Psychology Today* 1975;**7**:62–65.

46 Slack WV, Slack CW. Talking to a computer about emotional problems: a comparative study. *Psychotherapy: Theory Research and Practice* 1977;**14**:156–164.

47 Gendlin ET. *Experiencing and the Creation of Meaning. A philosophical and psychological approach to the subjective*. New York: Free Press of Glencoe, 1962.

48 Slack WV, Porter D, Balkin P, Kowaloff HB, Slack CW. Computer-assisted soliloquy as an approach to psychotherapy. *M.D. Computing* 1990;**7**:37–42,58.

49 Slack WV. Computer-based interviewing system dealing with nonverbal behavior as well as keyboard responses. *Science* 1971;**171**:84–87.

50 Spielberger CD. The measurement of state and trait anxiety: conceptual and methodological issues. In: Levi L, ed. *Emotions: their parameters and measurement*. New York: Raven Press, 1975:713–725.

51 Taylor JA. A personality scale of manifest anxiety. *Journal of Abnormal Social Psychology* 1953;**48**:285–290.

Section 2: Real-time Telepsychiatry – diagnosis and patient management

7

Telepsychiatry in Canada and the United States

Doug Urness, Lydia Weisser, Robbie Campbell and Donald Hilty

Introduction

The development of telepsychiatry in Canada and the USA has been driven by the desire to improve access to psychiatric services. In both countries, approximately 25% of the population lives in rural areas. Travel for traditional face-to-face consultations can be arduous, not only because of distance, but also because of climate, terrain and traffic conditions.

Socially the health care systems of the two countries are quite different but there are similarities that work to promote the development of telepsychiatry. These include pressures to improve the quality of medical care, to improve access to medical care and to contain the costs of medical care. Telepsychiatry can help by improving the distribution of clinical expertise, reducing the need to travel and the travel costs for both patients and consultants, reducing the 'intensity of care' which tends to be higher in specialized urban health care environments, and by providing earlier interventions.[1] The telepsychiatry infrastructure also facilitates better access to educational programmes in rural areas. In addition, telepsychiatry fits the shift in treatment philosophy to a more patient-focused, less institutionally oriented system of care.

At the time of writing there were approximately 39 telepsychiatry programmes in the USA and approximately nine in Canada. A comprehensive survey of telepsychiatry programmes in the USA has been published elsewhere.[2] In this chapter we describe four established telepsychiatry programmes, two from each country.

Medical College of Georgia Telepsychiatry Programme

The Georgia State-wide Telemedicine Programme (GSTP) began in 1989 as a proposed solution to the maldistribution of health care resources within the state. The project was funded by the BellSouth Foundation and the Medical College of Georgia (MCG). A videoconferencing link was formed between the MCG (the hub site) and Dodge County Hospital (the remote site). The connection was via a T1 line (1.54 Mbit/s) and allowed videoconferencing as well as remote-controlled biomedical telemetry. The cost of the equipment was US$330 000. During the first year, 180 clinical consultations were conducted and high levels of satisfaction were expressed by both patients and clinicians.

During this time, the state government's Public Service Commission was attempting to find uses for a US$73 million surplus resulting from an overcharge by the BellSouth company to its customers that year. A state-wide distance learning and telemedicine network was proposed. This subsequently resulted in the passage of Senate Bill 144, the Georgia Distance Learning and Telemedicine Act of 1992 which led to the Georgia Statewide Academic and Medical System, the largest distance learning and health care network in the world at that time. Of the $50 million awarded initially, $8 million was allocated for telemedicine.

By December 1993, the original project had grown to seven sites including two county hospitals, a public health clinic, a rural primary care clinic serving three counties and two correctional facilities. Plans for expansion encompassed a total of nine secondary hub sites strategically placed throughout the state, as well as the inclusion of a second tertiary-care facility located at Emory University in Atlanta, Georgia. The network was designed to connect all 62 telemedicine and 375 distance learning sites. A T1 network was used for telemedicine and a ½ T1 (768 kbit/s) network for the distance learning sites. A flat fee of $1500 per month for 74 hours of utilization was negotiated with BellSouth for the telemedicine sites.

Telepsychiatry

In 1994, the MCG began to develop a comprehensive telepsychiatry programme which was funded by a $1.5 million grant. Since nearly two thirds of Georgia's 159 counties had (and still have) no psychiatrist, patients with mental health problems have traditionally been required to drive long distances or receive no care at all. The goals of the programme were: (i) to create a comprehensive mental health telemedicine system for underserved patients; and (ii) to foster an interdisciplinary collaboration between the GSTP, the MCG, and the Georgia Division of Mental Health, Mental Retardation and Substance Abuse (DMHMRSA).

A needs assessment questionnaire was sent to all clinical directors of state psychiatric hospitals, the executive directors of the 13 state mental health regions, the medical director of the DMHMRSA, and clinicians attending a mental health services medical management conference. The results revealed a strong interest in diagnostic consultations, child psychiatry services, pharmacology consultations and continuing medical education.

The implementation of service delivery was initially difficult because some clinicians were sceptical about embracing an 'unproven' technology. During the first two years, a total of 80 consultations were carried. From July 1997 to March 1999, nearly 800 telepsychiatry consultations took place. Common diagnoses included depression, anxiety, bipolar disorder, psychosis, dementia, post-traumatic stress disorder, substance abuse and borderline personality disorder.

During that period, the demand for child and adolescent psychiatry services grew. In addition to diagnostic assessment, pharmacological management and psychotherapy, a paediatric neuropsychiatry clinic began. The multidisciplinary team was composed of a child psychiatrist, paediatric neurologist, clinical social worker, psychiatric clinical nurse specialist and ancillary personnel such as a paediatric geneticist, speech pathologist, occupational therapist and physical therapist, as needed. Paediatric consultations increased from eight in 1997 to 102 in 1999.

Unfortunately, the key positions of lead telepsychiatrist and psychiatric clinical nurse specialist became vacant in 1999. Although there was coverage by part-time staff, there was a subsequent decrease in the overall number of consultations. Since its inception in 1991, however, nearly 2000 psychiatric consultations have been conducted (Fig. 7.1).

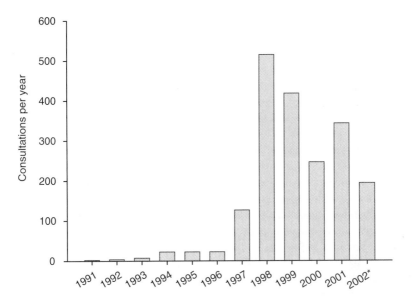

Fig. 7.1. Consultations in the Georgia Telepsychiatry Programme. There were 1923 telepsychiatry consultations between 1991 and 2002. The decrease in the number of consultations after 1999 was partly due to the departure of two key clinicians. *2002 data incomplete; first 9 months only.

Current status

In April 2001, budget cuts affecting the GSTP resulted in the transfer of management responsibilities from the MCG Telemedicine Center to the newly created Georgia Technology Authority (GTA). Several sites were closed because of under-utilization and prohibitive line and maintenance costs. At present, the MCG Telemedicine Center is exploring the use of lower bandwidth communications. One such project involves the installation of both ISDN and PSTN (conventional telephone system) based equipment in a remote primary care centre and a patient's house in a rural area. These will be used to deliver various clinical services including psychiatry.

Alberta Mental Health Board Telemental Health Service

The Alberta Mental Health Board Telemental Health Service was developed to improve access to psychiatric services in rural areas. A pilot telepsychiatry project involving six sites began in 1996. Most start-up funding came from internal sources. A partnership with the regional health authorities was necessary for site selection, cost sharing and evaluation. Receiving sites were rural towns with populations of approximately 5000. Videoconferencing equipment was located in renovated conference rooms located in local general hospitals, which generally had 20–30 acute care beds. Psychiatric inpatient units and specialty consultation were 1–3 hours travel time away. Travelling consultants made regular visits to four of the five receiving sites approximately every 2 weeks.

Telepsychiatry was a method of augmenting those visits and provided general practitioners with direct access to psychiatrists as opposed to clinic referrals which would be screened by therapists before psychiatric consultation occurred. Telecommunications were initially made using six switched-56 lines at 336 kbit/s. Subsequently a variety of connections have been used, including satellite links and ISDN at 384 kbit/s. Videoconferencing equipment consisted of room-based systems with dual 80-cm monitors.

The pilot project evaluation included an analysis of 109 consultations. Most of these were general psychiatry consultations, but there were psychogeriatrics and substance abuse consultations as well. Depression was the most common diagnosis (40%) and 32% of referral forms indicated suicidal ideation at the time of referral. There was a history of previous hospitalization in 41% of patients seen. Overall satisfaction with the telepsychiatry consultation was 84% for consumers, 90% for consultants and 96% for referring general practitioners. Telephone interviews with consumers indicated the urgency of the need for consultation and the value they placed on the service. The evaluation of the 6-month pilot project was important in justifying the transition to an operational service.[3]

Expansion

The pilot project received generally positive feedback. The numbers of referrals increased and there was strong organizational support for expansion, both internally and externally.[4] This led to an additional five sites being added to the service in 1998/1999. Subsequent growth in the number of sites has been through the Wellnet Provincial Telehealth Initiative, a partnership between the provincial government and private companies to facilitate the application of communication technology to health care. The telehealth component of the Wellnet initiative was stimulated by a C$14 million donation from a private anonymous donor with specific conditions that telehealth was to be implemented throughout the province, without disproportionate funding to urban areas. All sites were compatible whether Wellnet or the Alberta Mental Health Board funded them. Currently there are approximately 140 active telehealth sites in Alberta, of which 25 routinely receive telepsychiatry clinical services.

Telepsychiatry delivery model

The model of clinical care for the service is a type of shared care. This maintains continuity of care within a patient's home community by requiring a general practitioner's referral and involvement, encourages the involvement of local mental health clinic therapists and provides comprehensive initial assessments. Ongoing care, provided by the local health care professionals, is encouraged. Time allotments for consultations are generous, with initial assessments booked for 1.5 hours and follow-up visits for 45 minutes. Report preparation may require additional time. Approximately 75% of all consultations are initial assessments. Information from the provincial health care insurance plan indicates that in routine outpatient psychiatric practice only about 5–10% of visits are initial assessments.

The number of completed clinical telepsychiatry consultations has grown each year (Fig. 7.2). This growth in the service reflects the expanding network of telehealth sites and the increased number of psychiatrists providing clinical consultations.

Quality of care

The quality of care provided by the telemental health service was assessed using satisfaction questionnaires, telephone interviews, consultant logbooks and, to a limited extent, quality of life measures. In a study comparing preconsultation SF12 and Euroquol-5D scores between patients seen by telepsychiatry and those seen at two community mental health clinics, the telepsychiatry group had significantly lower SF12 mental composite subscale scores, and higher but less significant physical

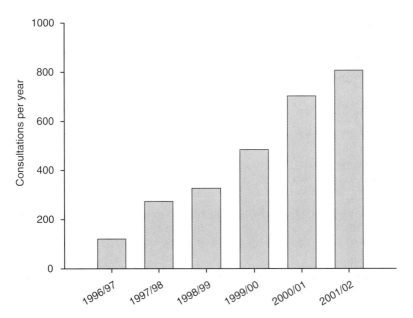

Fig. 7.2. Consultations in the Alberta Telemental Health Service. There were 2715 telepsychiatry consultations between 1996 and 2002.

composite scores (D. Urness et al, unpublished work). In a comparison of patient satisfaction in the two groups, all of whom saw the same psychiatrist, there was very good satisfaction in both groups with the community clinic group showing a trend to higher satisfaction. The two groups were drawn from the routine clinical population and had different demographics, which were not controlled for. In a separate telephone follow-up study involving a different group of 30 patients pre- and post-consultation (average 60 days), SF12 scores were compared and showed a significant improvement (D. Urness, unpublished work).

Cost

A detailed analysis of the costs of telepsychiatry has not yet been carried out. In the pilot study a cost comparison for providing the identical service in a face-to-face manner was conducted. This involved estimating the actual cost of running the telepsychiatry system, which is volume sensitive, and comparing this to the calculated cost of sending a psychiatrist to each of the sites where the consultation occurred. While this is not a situation that occurs in practice it is nonetheless a useful comparator. It was calculated that the break-even point (the workload at which both methods cost the same) was 140 consultations per year. Since that time equipment costs and telephone line charges have decreased. Other estimates of costs and effects on resource utilization are somewhat anecdotal. One rural hospital reported an 80% reduction in bed utilization for mental health reasons after the telepsychiatry programme began. Even though this may simply represent a correction to an average level of utilization, it demonstrates that telepsychiatry does not involve an element of increased case finding with subsequent increased pressure on hospital beds. Less than 5% of consultations result in direct hospitalization to the Alberta Hospital Ponoka, even though many referrals are for acutely decompensated individuals who were inpatients at their local hospital.

Factors in success

There has been a steady growth in the number of consultations. In the financial year 2001/02 there were 807 consultations. Educational and administrative applications have grown more rapidly, and in the same period comprised 8% and 26% of all system activities, with clinical activity at 63%.

Several factors have contributed to the success of the programme. The involvement of interested, capable and well-motivated people with good relationships with all stakeholders has been critical. Those sites with high referral rates tend to have site coordinators with clinical backgrounds in mental health and close linkages with community physicians. Support from senior management, particularly in ensuring stable funding, is critical. Encouragement from external organizations including regional health authorities, universities and government is also important. Future growth will depend on the support of these organizations particularly to support the recruitment of consultants and to plan for expanded volumes of referrals, which will affect traditional referral patterns.

Factors that inhibit programme growth include the difficulty in recruiting consultants, especially in the area of child and adolescent psychiatry. Currently there is no financial advantage in providing telepsychiatry services compared to traditional services. Funding for physician services is available through the routine provincial fee-for-service billing system, but a sessional billing system is generally preferable given the lower volume of services per hour and allowances for technical delays. Physicians who do provide services seem to enjoy the style of practice and are likely to represent innovative individuals. All current consultants participate on a part-time basis with one psychiatrist providing approximately 50% of all services.

Different models of clinical administration will require exploration as growth continues. Until now the programme has been a relatively independent service. The recent addition of forensic psychiatric services has involved a different model. Instead of day-to-day management by the telemental health service the forensic outpatient service will manage their referrals directly and supply their own manpower. The telemental health service has taken a supportive role in programme design, development of standards and protocols, and promotion of the programme. Funding will still come through the telemental health service and will be linked to evaluation activity.

Province of Ontario Telepsychiatry Delivery System

In the four years starting in 1997, the province of Ontario developed telepsychiatry services in small regions that were for the most part not connected to each other. These services were implemented as small pilot projects without a Province-wide telehealth policy. Such a policy has subsequently been passed by the government and the future may bring funding sources from a government implementation budget.

Despite the services developing in relative isolation, a number of lessons have been learned. They include:

- Telepsychiatry can be as effective as face-to-face services.

- Early intervention practices lead to improved compliance and outcomes with the effect of a decrease in waiting lists and preventing hospitalization.

- Site development takes approximately 1 year before a 3–6 h/week service can be delivered.

- Medical management of a clinic at a remote or distant site is easiest with a multidisciplinary team, as well as an affiliation with the local pharmacy and family practitioner.

- Medical record-keeping has involved keeping records at both sites. An electronic psychiatric record would be a major asset.

It also became clear that the farther away the remote community was, the greater the increase in access to psychiatric services. We found that for sites less than 160 km away, telepsychiatry cost about two thirds less than the conventional alternative; for sites more than 160 km away which required fly-in psychiatrists, telepsychiatry cost only one third as much as face-to-face visits.

First nation participation

Because the preliminary experience was very positive, a state-wide telepsychiatry service was planned. This was planned to include First Nation healers (i.e. traditional aboriginal healers) and their communities. It was recognized that it would be difficult to obtain the necessary bandwidth for telepsychiatry in remote areas. However the Ontario government agreed to connect First Nation and remote communities through the Smart Systems for Health (SSH) programme. It was also recommended that the First Nation sites with smaller communities should be able to include education and other teleservices in addition to health and that appropriate security, confidentiality and privacy issues relating to this kind of 'shared' 1–2 Mbit/s bandwidth would be addressed.

The Canada Health CHIPP Initiative

In Ontario four service delivery projects received funding under the Canadian Health Infostructure Partnership Programme (CHIPP). Three of the projects were to deliver telemedicine generally and our project, Project Outreach, represented a collaboration between the Universities of Toronto, Western Ontario, Ottawa and McMaster. The purpose of the project was to bring telepsychiatry services to the larger telemedicine networks and allow delivery of psychiatric services to remote and underserviced areas.

The project received C\$2.5M from Health Canada to match our \$2.5M in contributions in kind funding from our partners. This budget was to set up and run 20 remote and underserviced municipal sites and 20 remote and underserviced First Nation sites in the Ontario region. These sites are managed by the four departments of psychiatry where there is a concentration of psychiatrists. It should be noted that there is a shortage of psychiatrists in Ontario. This shortage is coupled with an Ontario-wide mandate that has transferred the management of long-term care facilities (psychiatric hospitals) to the Schedule 1 hospitals, thus providing an incentive for telepsychiatry.

The Ontario Psychiatric Outreach Programme is funded by the Ontario government which pays for drive-in and fly-in services, and more recently a telepsychiatry component to complement these services. Northern and remote communities have always been concerned that a provincial style management would interfere with traditional referral patterns and the introduction to telepsychiatry would inhibit psychiatrists from flying in rather than complement the service they have (see 'Next steps' below).

Telepsychiatry delivery model

A provincial wide CAT Model was used. The CAT Model refers to the Clinical, Administrative and Technical components of Project Outreach. The introduction of new technologies brings with it the addition of a technical team to an already highly functioning clinical team. This relationship needs cultivating to ensure that these new applications are understood and used to enhance the delivery of psychiatric services without compromising the quality of care.

Telepsychiatry utilization

The CHIPP grant enabled us to set up 20 municipal sites and 20 First Nation sites. In the first 9 months we established 20 municipal sites and saw a total of 511 patients in 622 teleconsultations, i.e. some patients were seen more than once for follow-up. The total connection time was 647 hours (Fig. 7.3). Each site averaged 3 hours of psychiatric service per week. For the most part this was a general psychiatry service. We are now moving towards specialty programmes that bring added usage, added access to specialties within psychiatry, and added benefits and outcomes for the communities.

From Figure 7.3 it can be seen that the 3 hours per week per site were reached within the first 6 months of operation. A maximum of 9 hours a week for a peripheral site, depending upon the population and specific needs, would be the maximum required for psychiatric services and 3 hours per week would be required to intervene with both educational and service components of the delivery system. We expect that we will use over 1000 hours of connection time in the first year of operation for the 20 municipal sites.

Connection costs

Prior to the introduction of SSH, our connection costs were approximately $1000 per site per month. The usage time was 3–6 hours per site per week on average and the cost was felt to be prohibitive. Connection costs fell dramatically when we changed from ISDN lines to IP network transmission. There are however various gateway and membership fees for individual hospitals or community clinics because the SSH only

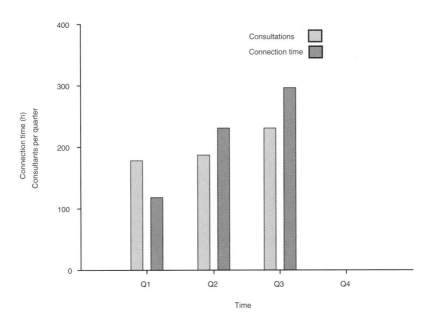

Fig. 7.3. Consultations in the first 9 months of the Ontario telepsychiatry project.

provides its bandwidth to a single point in the hospital. Routing systems and security measures beyond that point are the responsibility of each individual hospital.

Next steps

The use of telepsychiatry is expanding rapidly in Ontario. We are using telepsychiatry to train clerks and residents in the field. Telepsychiatry will be a major factor in staff retention and recruitment in remote communities. The electronic psychiatric record is being researched with regard to the special needs of psychiatry. With quick access to records, treatments can be more easily managed resulting in improved outcomes. Telepsychiatry is time- and cost-efficient and is welcomed by patients and their families as an acceptable medical intervention.

The University of California Davis Telepsychiatry Consultation-Liaison Service

The telepsychiatry consultation-liaison service (TCLS) at the University of California Davis provides increased access to specialist consultation for patients at approximately 60 sites in California. The TCLS has provided over 500 consultations since 1997. The TCLS developed as a result of several factors. First, the university telemedicine programme had successfully piloted services with rural hospitals (e.g. fetal monitoring through its obstetrics and gynaecology department). Second, as the programme developed, the rural sites began asking about psychiatric services. Third, leadership changed in the department of psychiatry, which enhanced collaboration with primary care and specialists through recruitment of faculty staff specializing in consulting services. The TCLS began with ad hoc consultations with one faculty, who subsequently invited others to help on specialized cases (e.g. child psychiatry). Others who were already consulting to sites 50–75 km away were invited to try teleconsultation for half of their trips, which was well received. Eventually, residents were given opportunities to learn and help these rural patients who would otherwise not receive consultation services.

Telepsychiatry delivery model

A consultation care model is used, whereby the psychiatrist evaluates the patient and offers suggestions to the primary care physician regarding the delivery of mental health services. Faculty staff, fellows and residents deal with adult, child and geriatric patients in rural and suburban/urban settings. The clinical care is a well-liked educational experience for trainees.

Clinical care

The TCLS is part of the University of California Davis Health System Telemedicine Programme.[5] The programme is based in Sacramento, at the only tertiary care facility in between the centre of California and the Oregon state border. The programme provides consultations to suburban/urban clinics (30–120 km away) and rural clinics (160–560 km away).

The TCLS was established in 1996. The service provides consultations for approximately 15 hours/week for adult patients by faculty, residents and medical students. In addition, child (4 hours/week) and geriatric patients (2 hours/week) are seen by faculty and fellows (child only).

The service's consultation model helps the primary care physician provide mental health services with initial and follow-up support on evaluation and treatment, and in doing so, helps the primary care physician develop skills and learn while doing the job.[6-8] Primary care providers are encouraged to join the consultation session for at least 5–10 minutes, particularly at the end of the evaluation when options for future treatment are discussed. If this is not possible, a brief report is faxed to the provider on the day of the consultation, or a telephone call is made if there is an urgent issue. Brief follow-up telephone consultations are also available for primary care providers.

Procedures, satisfaction and outcomes have been reviewed elsewhere (D.M. Hilty et al, unpublished work). All telemedicine clinics are equipped for videoconferencing using ISDN lines at 384 kbit/s. The cost of these videoconferencing units was US$8–12 000 and the hourly line charges for the rural sites were $30–60, depending on the distance.

Triaging generally involves emergency (1–3 day), urgent (4–7 day) or routine (8–30 day) delays. Patient consultations are scheduled hourly for adults and every 1.5 hours for children; follow-up appointments are scheduled for 30 minutes and 45 minutes, respectively. Telepsychiatric consultations occur for a variety of disorders often presenting in primary care practice, mainly depressive, anxiety and adjustment disorders.

Education

TCLS faculty staff have developed curricula, hands-on training for consultations, selective rotations, advanced required rotations and elective research rotations for residents in the department of psychiatry and the Combined Family Medicine and Psychiatry Programme. The regular curriculum (for the second-year psychiatry residents) and advanced curriculum (for fourth-year psychiatry residents) helps them acquire knowledge to prepare them for their telepsychiatry clinical experience. Foci include: (i) learning about rural health, telemedicine, and telepsychiatry; (ii) adapting consultation-liaison principles to outpatient and rural settings by telemedicine; and (iii) learning how to apply new technologies to clinical practice in general. Advanced senior resident clinical and research electives are available. Telepsychiatry education initiatives are part of a larger primary care education theme in the department of psychiatry, as curricula are in place for family medicine residents, internal medicine residents and primary care faculty. Didactics include lectures, difficult case discussions, CD-ROM case-based discussions on medical decision-making and continuing medical education courses.

Research

Evaluation shows that:

▶ Primary care physicians were satisfied with telepsychiatry, open trial with rural physicians more satisfied than urban physicians.

▶ Overall, approximately 70% of patients are adult (18–65 years) and 55% are female.

▶ More Medi-Cal (Medicaid) patients are seen by rural telemedicine (55%) and rural telepsychiatry (36%) than suburban/urban telepsychiatry and telemedicine (4–6%).

▶ The primary reason for telepsychiatry referrals was for diagnosis (34%), a new treatment plan (22%) or modification of a current treatment plan (20%).

▶ Alternative options for the rural telepsychiatry consultation are to provide care by mental health locally with delay (56%), to provide care locally by primary care physician in medical clinic without delay (26%) or to refer the patient out of the community for mental health outpatient services (9%).

▶ Satisfaction is high at 4.3–5.0 on a 5-point Likert scale for all variables for patients, primary care providers and psychiatrists; primary care provider satisfaction increases over time (D. Hilty et al, unpublished work).

Conclusion

The four telepsychiatry programmes described above demonstrate both similarities and differences, which reflect the contexts in which each programme evolved. Most of them developed in response to social pressures for improved access to specialty care, the availability of extraordinary or surplus funding, organizational motivation for innovation, and encouragement from larger organizations such as governments or other funding agencies. There was no strong assumption of or expectation for improvement in the quality of care other than the effects of earlier and more convenient consultation. Early evaluations of quality usually involved satisfaction questionnaires that have uniformly indicated high levels of satisfaction from patients, consultants and referral sources. Current research is addressing the issue of clinical outcomes, especially where the programmes involve strong academic links and research protocols involving controlled trials are facilitated.

Table 7.1 provides a summary of the features of each programme. The service models are similar in providing relatively standard forms of psychiatric care and subspecialty services which are available in traditional face-to-face settings. Some programmes focus more on a consultation-liaison model whereas others offer more ongoing care. All programmes offer some flexibility in providing both assessments and follow-up services. Some programmes also dedicate considerable time to research activities. Collaborative working relationships with health care providers in the patient's community are essential to all programmes.

Table 7.1. Features of four telepsychiatry programmes

	Medical College of Georgia Telepsychiatry Programme	Alberta Mental Health Board Telemental Health Service	Project Outreach (data based on 9-month period)	University of California, Davis Telepsychiatry Programme
Number of psychiatry consultations/year				
Adolescent/child	91	133	0	100
Adult/general	237	593	497	300
Forensic	0	0	1	0
Geriatric	12	60	0	75
Subspecialty services				
Brain injury	0	5	897 indirect consultations, e.g. case conferencing not involving direct patient contact	0
Substance abuse	0	12		Just starting
Psychological testing	0	4		0
Other	0	0		HIV: 60 consults
Civil commitment orders	No	Yes – rare		No
Health professional required at patient site during interview	No	No – encouraged	No – strongly encouraged	No – encouraged
Service activities				
Consultation liaison/shared care	Yes	Yes	Yes	Yes
Ongoing care	Yes	Yes	Yes	Yes
Case management	No	No	Yes	Yes
Other	No	No	No	No
Annual statistics				
Proportion of clinical consultations				
(%) initial assessments	19	70	20	50
(%) follow-up visits	81	30	80	50
No. of service delivery sites	1	AMHB = 11	20	60
No. of sites receiving clinical services	5	Regional health authority = ~ 28	20	45
Total no. of sites available to the programme	8	>100	20	Up to 100 if needed

Table 7.1. – *continued*

	Medical College of Georgia Telepsychiatry Programme	Alberta Mental Health Board Telemental Health Service	Project Outreach (data based on 9-month period)	University of California, Davis Telepsychiatry Programme
Consulting staff/% consultations provided				
Psychiatrists	2 + 2 residents/100%	6–10/96%	30/36%	5/60%
Other physicians	0	0	0/0%	3/30%
Psychologists	0	2–3/–4%	4/0%	2/5%
Registered nurse/allied professionals	0	0	50/64%	1/5%
Education sessions				
No. of sessions/year	0	78 (4122 participants)	18	1–2
Average no. of participating sites/session	0	12	2	40
Average no. of participants/room/session	0	4	10	5–15
No. of administrative meetings/year	4	300	99	10
Type of technology				
Network/bandwidth	T-1: 1.54 Mbit/s	PSTN: <128 kbit/s SW56: 336 kbit/s ISDN: 384 kbit/s IP: 384 kbit/s	IP SW56 ISDN Satellite (Bandwidth depends on each hub and remote site)	ISDN: 128 / 384 kbit/s IP: 384 kbit/s
Other technology used				
Videophone	No	Yes	No	No
Public Internet, email assessment or treatment	No	No	No	No
Telephone clinical contacts	No	Yes	No	Yes
Type of equipment				
Dual or single monitor	Dual	Dual	Single	Single
Monitor type/size	TV: <69 cm	TV: 69–81 cm	TV: <69 cm, 69–81 cm, >81 cm	PC: 43 cm TV: 69–81 cm
Far-end camera control	Yes	Yes	Yes	Yes

None of the programmes routinely requires a health care professional to be with the patient during adult psychiatry consultations, but this practice is generally encouraged and may be necessary for child or geriatric consultations.

Issuing civil commitment papers under state or provincial legislation is done in at least one of the programmes, although this is not a common practice. This may represent a function of selection factors in that patients requiring acute involuntary hospitalization typically present in obvious need of care and referring physicians simply do not require a psychiatric consultation to take action. In addition such patients may not consent to a telepsychiatry assessment if they know it may lead to involuntary hospitalization.

The costs of telepsychiatry programmes have been mentioned only briefly. The complexities of a thorough analysis are considerable and involve direct and indirect costs that need to be considered from the perspectives of patients, providers, health care organizations, payors and society. A comparison with routine care involves a detailed analysis of the costs of services offered through private offices, community clinics, outpatient departments and other settings. In addition rapidly changing equipment costs and the volume-sensitive nature of the costs make cost studies difficult to do.

The four telepsychiatry programmes described have all shown a pattern of expansion and clinical success which indicates that under the right circumstances such activities can thrive. Relative to the rural population, however, the proportion of psychiatric services delivered through telepsychiatry is small. Further demonstrations of clinical and programme successes will be necessary to narrow this gap and further reduce geographical barriers to receiving psychiatric services.

References

1   Bashshur RL, Mandil SH, Shannon GW. Telemedicine/telehealth: an international perspective. Executive summary. *Telemedicine Journal and e-Health* 2002;**8**:95–107.
2   Dahlin MP, Watcher G, Engle WM, Henderson J. *2001 Report on U.S. Telemedicine Activity.* Portland, OR: ATSP, 2001.
3   Hailey D, Jacobs P, Simpson J, Doze S. An assessment framework for telemedicine applications. *Journal of Telemedicine and Telecare* 1999;**5**:162–170.
4   Doze S, Simpson J, Hailey D, Jacobs P. Evaluation of a telepsychiatry pilot project. *Journal of Telemedicine and Telecare* 1999;**5**:38–46.
5   Nesbitt TS, Hilty DM, Kuenneth T, Siefkin A. Development of a telemedicine program: a review of 1000 videoconferencing consultations. *Western Journal of Medicine* 2000;**173**:169–174.
6   Pincus HA. Patient-oriented models for linking primary care and mental health care. *General Hospital Psychiatry* 1987;**9**:95–101.
7   Strathdee G. Primary care-psychiatry interaction: a British perspective. *General Hospital Psychiatry* 1987;**9**:102–110.
8   Katon W, Von Korff M, Lin E, et al. Collaborative management to achieve depression treatment guidelines. *Journal of Clinical Psychiatry* 1997;**58**(suppl 1):20–23.

8

Telepsychiatry in Australia

Anne Buist

Introduction

Delivery of psychiatric services in Australia has undergone significant change in the past two decades, as it has elsewhere in the western world. There has been a radical shift in the last 20 years, from the institution-based approach of the first half of the twentieth century to a community-based treatment regime. In Victoria (Fig. 8.1.) there has been an 11% decrease in acute adult mental health beds and a 72% decrease in extended care beds in hospital facilities, with an 82% increase in community residential beds since 1994.[1] These changes have occurred, however, at a time when health economics are coming under increased scrutiny. The risk that mental health service delivery, always a poor cousin of other areas of medicine, would be neglected remains a concern.

Increased awareness of human rights has enabled public acceptance of these changes, and is reflected in government regulations establishing strict criteria for

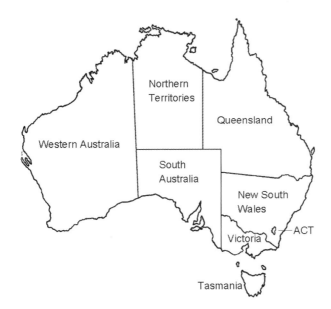

Fig. 8.1. Australian States and Territories.

people with mental illness to be held or treated against their will. These legal criteria have varied between the six Australian states and two territories. While there is some central, Federal/Commonwealth governance, each state or territory is essentially governed by separate health and legal systems (Fig. 8.1, Table 8.1).

One of the most crucial of the regulations relevant to service delivery in remote areas is the requirement for a qualified *psychiatrist* to see any person who is being detained.

Psychiatry has had difficulties in recruiting medical graduates, and those that do choose to train in psychiatry frequently move to the private system. Psychiatrists have gravitated to the main city centres, which within the structure of the Australian health system is relatively well funded and lucrative. Attracting psychiatric nurses also remains a challenge. Public psychiatry – where the majority of the seriously mentally ill are managed – has had to resort to recruiting overseas-trained doctors and nurses. This has been particularly important in maintaining the quality of care in rural areas. Many remote areas have no or few psychiatrists. Psychiatrists who come to work in rural areas from overseas require education and support as they work in an unfamiliar system and frequently work towards accreditation as an Australian psychiatrist. Rural areas thus offer a particular challenge for Australian psychiatry.

Table 8.1. Demographics of Australian States (Australian Bureau of Statistics, September 2001)

	Population (millions)	Population in capital (millions)	Area (million km²)
New South Wales	6.55	(3.99)	0.8
Victoria	4.84	(3.37)	0.22
Queensland	3.64	(1.57)	1.7
South Australia	1.51	(1.09)	0.9
Western Australia	1.92	(1.34)	2.5
Tasmania	0.50	(0.19)	0.06
Northern Territory	0.20	(0.09)	1.35
Australian Capital Territory	0.31	(0.31)	0.002
Total	19.5		7.7

Background – the introduction of telepsychiatry

The most important driving factor in the adoption of telepsychiatry in Australia has been need. The combination of the need, and someone able to see the role of telepsychiatry, occurred first in South Australia. Although it is one of the states with a smaller population, almost all the psychiatrists live in the state capital.

With changes in the structure of psychiatric services, readily available city-based institutional beds were no longer available for rural general practitioners to send patients to for assessment and treatment. Assessment – and as far as possible treatment – had to occur locally, and whilst mental health teams were set up in rural areas, these were without a local psychiatrist.

Telepsychiatry was one of the earliest applications of telemedicine in the state, with funding from grants and government giving rise to a specific project task group and the subsequent establishment of the telemedicine unit in 1995.[2,3] The South Australian telepsychiatry service aimed to facilitate community-based care, and to demonstrate a desire to provide equity and access to the rural population. From an early stage, it provided the Northern Territory, a vast area with a small population, with psychiatric clinical and supervisory support.

A report from the South Australian unit recommended in 1996 that a National Steering committee should be established to direct the broad issues of development and implementation throughout Australia. This resulted in the National Telehealth Committee, which became the Australian and New Zealand Telehealth committee,[4] although no longer now functional.

Following this early trial, other states have installed facilities for telepsychiatry. These are summarized in Table 8.2. Government structure has affected the number of programmes rather than the geography, with Queensland and Victoria, being regionally based and having the majority.[5]

Queensland is the second largest state geographically and has 3.6 million people, 55% of whom live outside the capital. Mental health applications along with other specialties such as paediatrics, intensive care and radiology are part of the Queensland telemedicine network of over 160 sites.[6] Besides patient need, staff support was seen to be crucial because of high staff turnover at remote locations such as Mt Isa. In addition, because of the distances, cost savings were also an important consideration.[5]

Western Australia is the largest state, with a small population, three quarters of which live in the capital. It has many of the same challenges as South Australia and New South Wales, with a number of regional centres and many small outposts. A review of mental health needs prompted the Mental Health Division of the Health Department to establish telepsychiatry initiatives in 1998/9 and subsequent expansion to 35 clinical centres. The aim has been to have comprehensive regional services with decentralized assessments, and the telemedicine service also includes ophthalmological and general medical programmes.

Table 8.2. Summary of telepsychiatry services in Australia

State	Year	No. of telepsychiatry sites (total of all telemedicine sites)	Activity	Main use
New South Wales	2002	Number of mental health sites (91)	33 clinical sessions per month (from ref. 5)	Clinical
Victoria	1998	39	195 hours per month	Clinical – CAMHS
Queensland	1999	48 (160)	91 clinical sessions per month (from ref. 5)	Clinical
South Australia	1997–8	35	107 clinical sessions per month (from ref. 5)	Clinical
Western Australia	2001	35	Not available	Clinical

In New South Wales, the telemedicine initiative has been operating since 1996 with 13 trial telemedicine programmes, evaluating effectiveness and viability in a variety of clinical areas, including psychiatry. Evaluation was an integral part of the introduction, which has been ongoing (M. Osborne, D. Lyle, K. Stevens, personal communication).

In a smaller, relatively highly populated state such as Victoria, which also has a number of moderate sized regional cities with at least one psychiatrist, the requirement has been less urgent. Child psychiatrists were not available in rural settings however, and it was in child and adolescent psychiatry where Victorian telepsychiatry became established, following the initial introduction at the Royal Children's Hospital in 1995 (see Chapter 12).[7] Following this, and results of a pilot project suggesting that improved access to mental health services in rural settings was required, the Victorian Telepsychiatry Programme was established in 1996. By 1998, there were 39 sites of which 27 were in rural locations.[8] Users included regional mental health services linking primarily to central services such as child and adolescent, and smaller satellites of their own service, but also to specialist services such as the interpreter service, mental health review board and forensic services. Mental health is the predominant user, with smaller projects in other areas such as dermatology and radiology.

Tasmania, the smallest state, both geographically and in population (less than half a million), has linked to Victoria for child and adolescent psychiatry expertise,[9] and for teleradiology.

Current practice – the successes

Delivery of clinical services

South Australia, which pioneered telemedicine in Australia, has been able to develop and sustain a model of clinical service delivery that has resulted in increasing usage over time.[3] In 1995 usage ranged from 15 to 50 hours of usage per month; in 1997 this had increased to 50 to 100 hours per month, over 35 sites (Table 8.2). This activity has been principally related to clinical service delivery with 88% of clinically related sessions being direct patient assessments. Whilst not typical of all services, this relates to the needs and geographical challenges of South Australia. Hawker et al[3] noted that the service allowed patients to be seen within 48 hours of referral rather than several months if they had waited for the visiting psychiatrist or had to travel to Adelaide. This clearly represents an improvement in care options. The importance of the driving force of need was noted by Hawker et al[3] 'it was when psychiatrists working in the emergency service area of the psychiatric hospital in Adelaide started to use the service that it began to be seen as a valuable service'.

Since this report, the number of South Australian sites has increased to over 80 and has the highest number of direct clinical sessions of all the Australian telemedicine programmes.[5] An evaluation[10] highlighted some of the continued strengths of the service. Rural psychiatry in 2000 involved general practitioners, mental health workers and some 26–30 visiting rural psychiatrists, in collaboration with a telepsychiatry programme and emergency/triage service. Ninety per cent of general practitioners referred to the visiting psychiatrist; 72% were satisfied with this component of the service, 66% were satisfied with the telepsychiatry (although 59% were concerned with problems of continuity of care) and 54% were satisfied with the liaison services. Community health workers had a higher satisfaction with telepsychiatry (90% had used it; 82% satisfied) but only 34% were satisfied with the visiting psychiatric service. These findings show a high level of use and satisfaction with telepsychiatry, but also highlight some of its limitations. Kalucy et al[10] suggest that most of the dissatisfaction experienced by the workers was not related to the telepsychiatry service, but a perceived inadequacy in the frequency of visits from psychiatrists and shortage of inpatient beds, the latter being a common perception about all psychiatric services in Australia, whether rural or not. If this is indeed the case, this report supports what has been proposed as a role for telepsychiatry; that it is a useful and important adjunct but not a replacement for face-to-face contact.

Between 1997 and 2000, regular audits of the Queensland telemedicine service have found that clinical use represented about 10–20% of all activity.[11] Why there is this variation is unclear. Mental health was the main single user of the system.

Northern Queensland's heavily clinical assessment-based service includes the delivery of psychotherapy and cognitive behavioural therapy – as a result there has been a 40% reduction in transfers.[6] Acceptance by clinicians and how this affects usage is illustrated by one clinician from Queensland who had used the service there and had subsequently moved to rural Victoria. In the Victorian review of services, this single clinician was essentially responsible for the Grampians accounting for 56% of the rural utilization, averaging 8.6 sessions per month. The next largest user region accounted for only 17%.[8]

Trott[12] reported a high apparent level of community acceptance as well in Queensland, and Trott and Blignault[6] noted the advantages of not dislocating patients from their communities, and commented that this may have particular benefits for the indigenous population. Lessing and Blignault's[5] review also suggested advantages to this group.

In New South Wales, a recent (2002) trial of telepsychiatry use linked the Black Dog Institute in Sydney with Wagga, where the Institute psychiatrists provide second opinions after interview with patients via videoconferencing. This is currently being evaluated, but there has been full utilization since its operation commenced (J. Greenwood, personal communication).

In Victoria, the principal clinical service delivery has been for Child and Adolescent Mental Health Services (CAMHS). When initially introduced the primary usage was for administration, secondary consultation, supervision and teaching[7] but consultation and clinical work were the primary uses in a later review.[13] In the 1998 Victorian review CAMHS was the most frequent user of the specialist services, averaging 30 sessions per month and accounting for 52% of the specialist use. Seventy per cent of all mental health usage in this review was for clinical purposes – either primary or secondary consultation.

Cooper and Davies[9] reported on the Monash telepsychiatry programme which provides clinical service delivery to children and adolescents in specific regions of

Victoria and Tasmania. They noted that telepsychiatry could be successful for direct consultation, but only after 'careful and comprehensive preparation' and when the case manager was present with the child/adolescent. Telepsychiatry was not for a first presentation. However, secondary consultation was thought to have a valuable role in supporting and aiding the rural workers, and hypothesized to aid in satisfaction and retention.[6,9]

Despite these reports of clinical usage, the activity overall has been low. In a review of Australian telemedicine programmes, there was an average of 123 sessions per programme per year – half that reported in the USA.[5]

Education and supervision

Education has been a strong focus for all the telepsychiatry sites. This was thought to be important in reducing isolation, and improving knowledge and job satisfaction for health care staff.

One area where this goal has been achieved in all states has been supervision. Telepsychiatry has been particularly important in enabling students and junior staff to take up positions in the country, which they would have otherwise been unable to take because of lack of supervision essential to course requirements. Trainee psychiatrists and psychologists are able to access supervision through videoconferencing – thus allowing them to benefit from the rich experience of rural psychiatry, and allowing the rural service to fill positions that might otherwise have been vacant. In the Northern Territory where there are few psychiatrists, psychiatry trainees have been able to link to Adelaide in South Australia for this purpose. Video links need not be limited by state boundaries. Supervision for a variety of other courses is also possible in this manner.

Broader applications have been scarce. The Early Psychosis Prevention and Intervention Centre (EPPIC), a state-wide service in Victoria, has been able to make use of telepsychiatry in reaching rural centres to fulfil its educational role in the management of first presentation psychotic illness. This accounted for 34% of the specialist service usage.[8] In Queensland, the weekly Grand Round held at a major teaching hospital in Brisbane can be accessed by a number of centres throughout the state, allowing skill updating and exposure to case presentations and visiting speakers.

Cost savings

Cost savings from telepsychiatry have been difficult to measure and the subject has been largely avoided in service reviews. Telepsychiatry is seen by clinicians as a supplement to improve the quality of service and not as a replacement for service delivery. Most people involved in telemedicine have emphasized this point, partly to allay the concern of clinicians and patients who fear cuts to services, and also because there are limitations to telemedicine which means that it is not useful in certain circumstances for primary consultation, particularly if the patient and clinician have not met before.[3,9] Savings in time and travel costs are difficult to quantify in many of the services, and analysis is complex and requires consideration of capital costs and variable costs such as administration, training and maintenance.

Use by the mental health review board in Victoria provides an example of savings which are easier to quantify. The board, comprising psychiatrists and lawyers, must review the case of every patient who has been involuntarily detained within 6 weeks of their detention, or within 2 weeks if a protest has been lodged. This necessitated regular flights to regional cities by the team. With telepsychiatry, many of these trips can be avoided, with estimated savings of AUS$24 500 in 1998.[8]

Trott and Blignault[6] described significant savings in the northern Queensland project. Because of the establishment costs, these were less in the first year, and maintenance costs were not included, but cost savings for patient and family health travels were thought to be about AUS$85 000–113 000 per year. In addition there were cost savings to the flying doctor service of nearly AUS$100 000 per year.

Cost analysis of the Monash project was less straightforward. Although Cooper and Davies[9] established that telepsychiatry was cost-effective compared to a visiting psychiatrist, non-salary costs for the project were high. A problem in this analysis was the low activity, and the use of private psychiatrists who at the time were not refundable through health insurance for providing the service.

Current practice – the challenges

Clinician drivers

In Yellowlees's[14] description of successful telemedicine systems he outlines seven core principles. Many of these principles are discussed in reviews of services and relate closely to outcomes with respect to usage and acceptance, at least from the health professionals and service perspective. Given the relatively low reported usage, this is an important consideration.

One of these principles is the need for strong leadership. This is relevant at two levels: first at the local level, to have an advocate for service usage – someone who keeps the service in mind, harnesses opportunities and provides a role model. At a broader level, leadership is needed to ensure that appropriate implementation occurs, adequate funding is provided and future directions are set.

The setting up of a national steering group was an important initiative in Australia. However, because of the different state health departments, this alone was inadequate to substantially effect the direction and implementation of each state service. Local interest and support are also required.

The establishment of a specific telemedicine unit in South Australia – itself evidence of a strong driver – was the initial driving force of the national body and has maintained the local focus. This service elected to minimize policies and procedures, and to encourage utilization by supporting plans for equipment maintenance and fee structure for non-health care use.

In Queensland, the telemedicine network has developed more formal policies and guidelines with specified objectives and outcomes, essentially to support, improve and increase telemedicine delivery. In both of these series there has been significant development with dissemination of information, but there is still a need for more active updating and promotion.

In Victoria, child and adolescent psychiatry had strong leadership at a local level, with the early formation of a steering group,[7] which has resulted in a strong presence of this subdiscipline amongst users. Leadership at a broader level was absent at implementation. Western Australia has also been slower to develop, though issues here are also related to geographical and population challenges.

Pragmatic sites

Another of Yellowlees's[14] principles is that the choice of service location should be pragmatic rather than philosophical. The importance of accessibility to promote usage is highlighted in the review by Hawker et al[3] of the South Australian service. A steady increase in usage was noted to the 23 rural communities that it served. From the outset the service installed ISDN sockets in several rooms to aid the transfer of the telemedicine equipment, with minimum policy barriers for usage.

By contrast, Victorian usage in some centres has been slow to take off, and clinicians identified difficulties with access as one of the barriers, although overall not the most crucial.[8] Obviously, issues such as these are best addressed *before* implementation. If they are to be overcome, a significant need, strong leadership and training are important.

Support and training

Yellowlees[14] noted that although training and support is essential to promote acceptance and clinician involvement in a user-friendly system, this frequently does not occur. Lack of support and training tend to go hand in hand with implementation where there is no clinician owner of the system, or designated manager, and is likely to increase the occurrence of technological difficulties and clinician frustration and lack of usage.

In South Australia a multidisciplinary telemedicine unit was able to provide support to centres through telephone calls, videoconferencing and visits.[3] An evaluation of the effectiveness of this is not given, but is likely to be at least amongst the factors contributing to the service uptake.

Evaluation

Evaluation of telemedicine services in Australia, as elsewhere in the world, has been limited. Yellowlees[14] noted that there is an absence of methodologically sound evaluations. In particular there has been an absence of evaluations that have looked at broader issues of the role of telepsychiatry and what changes result from its introduction. Cost evaluations have also been very narrow rather than from this broader perspective. There has been little evaluation of consumer (patient) satisfaction and it has often been restricted to comfort with the technology rather than examining different models for service delivery. Evaluation of usage also been fraught with difficulties because of methods of recording what a 'clinical session' is, i.e. whether a patient is present or not.

The ANZ Telehealth committee[4] evaluated the literature with respect to evaluation of telemedicine, and also concluded that information was scant, often theoretical, with little detail of methods given and lack of validation of survey tools. They noted the difficulties with obtaining statistically valid samples and cited barriers to performing randomized control trials as the main reason for the absence of such evaluations in the literature. In addition, the committee acknowledged the complexity of economic analysis, and the rapid advances in technology, which also hamper research. From a conference held in Melbourne, a number of recommendations resulted with respect to evaluation, with support for an internationally accepted framework.[4]

They highlighted in their recommendations that evidence-based telehealth should be developed through good practice documentation and dissemination and that feedback of telehealth evaluation is critical.[4]

Technological difficulties

One of the most frequently cited barriers to usage has been technological difficulties. Such difficulties, when associated with lack of training, support and clinician ownership, appear to be the main reason for low usage in certain areas of Victoria.[8] Even in the more successful implementations, technological difficulties are cited as a significant problem – 40% in Gelber and Alexander's[13] study. In minimizing these problems the choice of the right equipment is crucial. Whilst South Australia found that videoconferencing at 128 kbit/s was adequate, they noted a preference for 384 kbit/s. Cooper and Davies[9] describe videoconferencing at 128 kbit/s as unreliable, with difficulties in conveying non-verbal emotional cues. Gelber and Alexander[13] also noted this problem, but felt that even at the improved bandwidth there were difficulties in this area.

Consumer feedback

Feedback from patients who have used the service is more limited than clinician feedback and is one area that needs further work. Work to date suggests reliability with respect to diagnostic assessment[15] and acceptability by patient and referrer, at least when introduced appropriately.[9,16] Patients and carers in the South Australian evaluation[10] were generally positive, with 67% finding telepsychiatry helpful or very helpful and 20% 'okay'. Other anecdotal reports, particularly of family members separated from young children and adolescents, appear to find some benefit.[7] The adolescents themselves appeared less enthusiastic, with the suggestion from the reviewer that for use in primary consultation, 'careful and comprehensive preparation is needed'.[9]

Medicolegal and remuneration issues

Though telepsychiatry has been used in Australia for at least 8 years, a number of medicolegal and renumeration issues remain unresolved. Many policies have emphasized the need for the clinical responsibility to remain with the rural treating team. In Cooper and Davies's[9] recommendations, the presence of the local team was thought to be crucial. By contrast, Hawker et al[3] suggested that excessive policies are cumbersome and a barrier to use.

Duty of care, medical indemnity and the need for registration across state boundaries are not as clear, and no universal service guideline has been developed. The Royal Australian and New Zealand College of Psychiatrists has developed guidelines which at least provide a starting point for this process (see Chapter 21).[17]

For the future development and promotion of telepsychiatry these issues need to be resolved, as does remuneration through medical benefits. Lack of remuneration was seen as a major barrier to the service development in South Australia, and a clear problem for the adoption of the model proposed by Cooper and Davies[9] which used private psychiatrists.

Summary

Since its introduction into psychiatric services in Australia in 1995, telepsychiatry has quickly expanded to all states. Both initially, and subsequently, usage has varied between states. Nonetheless, telepsychiatry in Australia is here to stay. We have learnt some lessons and have established directions that need to be further explored. The most critical step now is in dissemination of the knowledge we have, and of the evaluations that are done; in this way as a nation we will be able to move forward with the most effective way of reaching our rural colleagues and clients, enhancing health care and job satisfaction and improving the life of those in rural and remote areas.

References

1   National Mental Health Survey. Data supplied from *Department of Human Services*, 2002.
2   Yellowlees PM, McCoy WT. Telemedicine – a health care system to help Australians. *Medical Journal of Australia* 1993;**159**:437–438.
3   Hawker F, Kavanagh S, Yellowlees P, Kalucy RS. Telepsychiatry in South Australia. *Journal of Telemedicine and Telecare* 1998;**4**:187–194.
4   Australian and New Zealand Telehealth Committee. Available at http://www.telehealth.org.au [last checked 9 September 2002].
5   Lessing K, Blignault I. Mental health telemedicine programmes in Australia. *Journal of Telemedicine and Telecare* 2001;**7**:317–323.
6   Trott P, Blignault I. Cost evaluation of a telepsychiatry service in northern Queensland. *Journal of Telemedicine and Telecare* 1998;**4**(suppl 1):66–68.
7   Gelber H. The experience of the Royal Children's Hospital mental health service videoconferencing project. *Journal of Telemedicine and Telecare* 1998;**4**(suppl 1):71–73.
8   Buist A, Coman G, Silvas A, Burrows G. An evaluation of the telepsychiatry programme in Victoria, Australia. *Journal of Telemedicine and Telecare* 2000;**6**:216–221.
9   Cooper H, Davies J. *Psychiatry Pilot Project – The provision of child and adolescent psychiatric consultation and supervision to Gippsland and Tasmania via Telepsychiatry*. Monash Telepsychiatry Pilot Project Report. Melbourne: Southern Health Care Network, 2000.
10 Kalucy R, Hawker F, Delin J, Muenstermann I. *Evaluation of Specialist Psychiatric Services in Rural and Remote South Australia*. Adelaide: Department of Psychiatry, Flinders University and Commonwealth Department of Health and Aged Care, 2000.
11 Kennedy C, Blignault I, Hornsby D, Yellowlees P. Videoconferencing in the Queensland health service. *Journal of Telemedicine and Telecare* 2001;**7**:266–271.
12 Trott P. The Queensland Northern Regional Health Authority telemental health project. *Journal of Telemedicine and Telecare* 1996;**2**(suppl 1):98–104.
13 Gelber H, Alexander M. An evaluation of an Australian videoconferencing project for child and adolescent telepsychiatry. *Journal of Telemedicine and Telecare* 1999;**5**(suppl 1):21–23.

14   Yellowlees P. Successful development of telemedicine systems – seven care principles. *Journal of Telemedicine and Telecare* 1997;**3**:215–222.

15   Baigent MF, Lloyd CF, Kavanagh SJ, et al. Telepsychiatry : 'tele' yes, but what about the 'psychiatry'? *Journal of Telemedicine and Telecare* 1997;**3**(suppl 1):3–5.

16   Clarke PHJ. A referrer and patient evaluation of a telepsychiatry consultation-liaison service in South Australia. *Journal of Telemedicine and Telecare* 1997;**3**(suppl 1):12–14.

17   The Royal Australian and New Zealand College of Psychiatrists. Available at http://www.ranzcp.org [last checked 9 September 2002].

9

Telepsychiatry in Europe

Paul McLaren

Introduction

The digital revolution has yet to make a significant impact on the delivery of mental health care in Europe. There is free movement of labour and a common currency in most of the European Union, yet mental health care is still largely confined to national boundaries. There is no European model for the provision of mental health services and European telepsychiatry projects have developed in relative isolation within national services. European e-mental health projects are discussed elsewhere in this book by Simpson (see Chapter 13), who reviews telepsychology, Ball (see Chapter 14), who reviews telepsychiatry in old age services, and Birmingham (see Chapter 11), who reviews forensic services.

Telepsychiatry is the use of communications technology to deliver mental health care. The most often quoted driving force for telepsychiatry is to improve access to mental health services in areas of low population density, where there are economic or geographical barriers to travel. Western Europe, compared to western North America and Australia, where telepsychiatry services have developed more rapidly, has high population density, public transport and fewer problems with recruitment and retention of clinicians. Nonetheless, there are exceptions, where geographical barriers limit access and the telemedicine recipe, of low population density and an advanced telecommunications infrastructure, can be found. Island communities in Greece, Scotland, Jersey and Ireland have been subjects in telepsychiatry research. In northern Norway mental health applications were established at an early stage in the development of the extensive telemedicine network centred on Tromsø. While the shape of mental health services altered significantly during the second half of the twentieth century, technology has played little part. Telepsychiatry research in Europe has been small scale. Most of the work has been pilot projects and can be classified into those applications driven by geography, academic enquiry or to address communication challenges in complex service delivery systems.

The European context

Within the European Union there is an open market in medical services. Doctors registered in one country can register to practice in another. There have been recent attempts to move patients across borders for surgical treatment, for example from the

UK into northern France to take advantage of spare capacity and to reduce waiting lists in the UK. Such exchanges have not taken place in mental health care. Because of sensitivities about language and culture this is likely to remain the case for some time. The provision of mental health care in Europe is rendered even more diverse by the dominance of different therapeutic models in different states and a diversity of funding models and legislation. There are however increasing movements of population between the north and south, with people from the north retiring to the south. The open employment market means that in large population centres there are significant numbers of expatriots. If they develop an acute mental illness they are likely to receive emergency treatment from host services. If the illness becomes chronic or they require longer-term treatment they are likely to return home. Communications technology offers the potential to provide timely, culture- and language-sensitive care across national boundaries. Telepsychiatry will be judged on the contribution it makes to achieving these objectives.

The early development of telepsychiatry in Europe

The European Commission established a health telematics programme in the early 1990s to stimulate pan-European research in the field. This was known as AIM (Advanced Informatics in Medicine) and was a research and development programme to apply information and communication technologies to medicine and health care. Its overall goal was to enable a free flow of health information across Europe in line with the needs of its citizens, thus providing seamless care across borders. Its objectives were to increase harmony and cohesion in these areas, to improve the quality and cost effectiveness of medicine and to strengthen the competitiveness of European industry in informatics, telematics, pharmaceutical products and medical equipment through the stimulation of a market driven by the users, rather than pushed by the technology.[1] The AIM programme defined telemedicine as 'the investigation, monitoring and management of patients and education of staff and patients using systems which allow ready access to expert advice and patient information no matter where the patient or information is located'.[2] These principles are particularly relevant to mental heath care as service users may be unable to communicate their health needs clearly, or may be reluctant to state their histories.

Telepsychiatry research began at Guy's Hospital in London in the early 1990s and was funded by the European Commission through the RACE Telemed Programme. This was a multispeciality research programme to develop medical applications for broadband communications links. While the long-term aim was seamless care across national boundaries, the short-term aim was to stimulate the use of broadband communications. At about the same time telepsychiatry applications were being developed in northern Norway in response to political imperatives to support isolated communities and ensure equality of access to health care. The Norwegian health care system is publicly funded. In August 1996 Norway became the first country to implement an official telemedicine fee schedule for reimbursement, one of the barriers most often blamed for the sluggish diffusion of telemedicine.

Telepsychiatry in Norway

Uldal et al[3] surveyed telemedicine programmes active in Norway in 1999. Telemedicine research had been stimulated by the More Health for each bIT plan, published by the Norwegian Ministry of Health and Social Affairs.[4] A videoconferencing network was established for psychiatric teaching in Oppland county, and nine of the sites were operating within clinical psychology. Within psychiatry they found that distance learning applications were being used for education by psychiatry students and psychiatric nurses, and for lectures in both child and adult psychiatry.

The Centre for Telemedicine at the University of Tromsø in northern Norway has piloted telepsychiatry as part of a wide range of telemedicine applications in a region where travel is very difficult for half of the year. Gammon et al[5] surveyed the use of videoconferencing in mental health care in northern Norway after ISDN telecommunications became available in mid-1995. A questionnaire was distributed to all user institutions. The questionnaire completion rate for locations recorded as participants in videoconferencing sessions was 62%. Within 6 months, 1028 persons had participated in 140 videoconferencing sessions from 35 institutions. The purposes of videoconferencing included meetings (50%), supervision, training and teaching (31%), clinical consultations (14%) and tests or demonstrations (5%). The alternative forms of contact which videoconferencing replaced included travel (59%), no contact (25%), telephone (14%) and mail or fax (2%). No problems were reported in 55% of the sessions. In 19% there were audio problems, in 14% there were picture problems, in 5% attempts to connect failed and in 5% disconnection occurred. The majority of users (87%) reported that they were satisfied or very satisfied with the facility. The low rate of clinical videoconferencing, having nurses or psychiatrists communicating directly with service users, is striking and may reflect a reluctance of key professionals to offer services this way.

The Tromsø group[6] reported the use of videoconferencing to deliver psychotherapy supervision using 384 kbit/s ISDN links. Trainees had five face-to-face sessions, alternating weekly with videoconferencing sessions giving ten supervision sessions in total. All participants completed a semi-structured interview within 2 weeks of the end of the study. The eight subjects (six candidates and two supervisors) reported a wide range of experiences and attitudes. They concluded that the quality of supervision could be satisfactorily maintained by videoconferencing, for up to half of the 70 hours required for training. A precondition for this estimate was that the supervision dyad should meet face to face and establish a relationship characterized by mutual trust and respect if videoconferencing was to be used. The most obvious implication from this study is the potential for implementing decentralized models for recruiting and educating psychiatrists. The 70 hours of mandatory psychotherapy supervision for psychiatry residents in Norway is designed to develop insights into the therapeutic relationship and these authors attempted to define general characteristics of this process. A good working alliance, characterized by confidence, trust and mutuality of goals, is as essential in achieving the aims of psychotherapy supervision as it is in psychotherapy. The supervisor must be able to build a stable framework within which the candidate can openly seek an understanding of the complex interaction between the patient and therapist. The supervision process must encourage candidates to relate their personal experiences in their therapeutic relationships by exposing their personal emotions and reactions. The quality of these processes could be maintained when the supervisor and candidate communicated half the time with videoconferencing.

Major dislikes and concerns reported by the participants were the loss of non-verbal cues and the effects this had on spontaneity, the expression of personal emotional material, and the experience of social and emotional presence. These findings echoed Rutter's[7] 'Cluelessness' model for understanding the effects of mediated communication. This predicts that as we move through the four communication modes of face-to-face, communicating through a curtain (physical presence minus visual cues), closed circuit television and telephone, the smaller the available social cues become the more task-orientated and depersonalized the content of the interaction becomes. This in turn leads to a more deliberate non-spontaneous style of communicating, as well as particular types of outcome.

When subjects in the Norwegian study thought that the medium had not affected the supervision they qualified it by mentioning the previously established relationship. Several reported that being video-recorded compounded the effects of reduced non-verbal cues such as reduced spontaneity. Several reported an increased ability to overcome the limitations imposed by videoconferencing as experience accumulated. Several subjects reported the limitations imposed as having positive effects on verbalization, structure and self-representation. Some positive effects were related to the design of the study, such as better preparation for supervision due to a much shorter journey time of 10 minutes, not being interrupted by the supervisor's telephone and having a delineated neutral space, separate from the supervisor's office. Placing the quality of communication on the agenda stimulated potentially valuable insights into the role of communication in building relationships.

Telepsychiatry in Finland

Mielonen et al[8] reported on the use of videoconferencing in mental health care in Finland. Early telepsychiatry work in Finland was carried out at the Department of Psychiatry of the University of Oulu, where videoconferencing was used for family therapy, occupational counselling, clinical consultation and teaching. ISDN is available across Finland and this work was conducted at a bandwidth of 384 kbit/s. In 1996 videoconferencing was used for a total of 249 hours, which increased to 434 hours in 1997. During 1997, 45% of the time was used for teaching, 26% for occupational counselling, consultations and therapies, 23% for training and 6% for administration. In a survey of user responses, 37 participants rated the videoconferences on a scale from 4 (poor) to 10 (excellent). The audio quality had a mean value of 8.0 (SD 0.9), the picture quality 7.5 (SD 1.5) and the general value of the videoconference was rated at 7.5 (SD 1.0).

This project took place in Northern Ostrobothnia, a sparsely populated area with about 360 000 inhabitants. The farthest municipality from the hospital is over 200 km away. Between 1994 and 1997 the total number of consultations did not increase but a greater proportion of the consultations and discussions were performed by videoconferencing. Staff attitudes to videoconferencing became progressively more positive as experience grew. Participants in family therapy and counselling by videoconferencing generally wanted to continue with the medium.

This same group[9] reported on the use of videoconferencing for discharge planning from an inpatient mental health unit. They performed a cost analysis taking account of the fact that other speciality applications were using the equipment. They estimated that 30% of use of the videoconferencing equipment at the Department of Psychiatry and 60% at the primary care centres were psychiatry. Fourteen patients, 44 health care staff, five nursing students, 35 primary care workers, 13 social service workers and 13 relatives in the municipalities participated. All the inpatients involved suffered from psychosis. The majority of participants stated that they would prefer to have their next meeting by videoconference. The most important reason given was the reduced need for travelling, and the ease and speed of the consultations.

The economic analysis showed that at a volume of 50 care planning consultations per year the videoconferencing alternative was about FM 2340 cheaper than conventional meetings and the municipality would save about FM 117 000 by using the medium (1 FM is approx 0.17 Euro or US$ 0.17). Six hours of travelling time could be used for other purposes when the meeting was held by videoconferencing. This area of Finland suffers from a chronic shortage of psychiatrists with 20 posts out of 100 without a qualified holder in 1998–99. This makes the loss of working time through travelling particularly undesirable.

In Finland meetings with relatives and friends are held for about half of all psychiatric inpatients. This study consisted of 14 videoconferences with an intentional sample, so that its generalizability is limited. The authors noted that prejudices against videoconferencing were expressed by health care personnel, which limited the number of videoconferences that actually occurred. They stressed the need to structure the meetings to suit the medium.

Sorvaniemi and Santamaki[10] reported on the use of videoconferencing to support emergency consultations in Satakunta District Hospital on the west coast. Patients referred for emergency assessments were assessed for the first time on a video link operating over ISDN at 384 kbit/s. The link was between Harjavalta Hospital, a psychiatric institution, and the Satakunta District General Hospital 35 km away. Although there were two open psychiatric wards in Satakunta the only on-call psychiatrist was based in Harjavalta. They used a PC-based videoconferencing unit. To investigate the appropriateness of the technology, 19 consecutive patients who were referred to the ward at Satakunta were approached. None refused to participate. One patient was dissatisfied with the medium but none would have preferred to have been referred on to Harjavalta for face-to-face assessment. All patients were admitted as a result of the assessment, and follow-up judged management to have been appropriate.

Telepsychiatry in the UK

Guy's Hospital in London was the site for the earliest reported telepsychiatry research in the UK.[11,12] The mental health services at Guy's served a deprived and inner city catchment area with high levels of psychiatric morbidity. In the early 1990s a prototype low-cost digital videoconferencing system, known as the LCVC, was developed for remote diagnosis and treatment in psychiatry. This generated a monochrome picture with 64 grey levels refreshed at 12.5 frames/s or 16 grey levels at 25 frames/s. Its use was piloted using an analogue link between two acute adult psychiatric wards at Guy's Hospital.

Although this research was funded to develop an application for new communications links, responses of professional and service users were studied. Service users were in acute phases of illness and came from a wide range of ethnic backgrounds. User responses were generally positive. In a 4-month study period 44 patients were approached, eight refused or were unable to give informed consent and three refused after initial use.[11] One patient suffering with schizophrenia stopped talking in the middle of a videoconsultation and said that he felt uncomfortable with the TV. This patient had previously reported experiences of influence from television. A second acutely depressed patient froze in front of the screen and asked to stop. One senior psychiatrist refused to use the link to inform a patient, who did not want to leave, of their discharge and to give another a diagnosis of a life-threatening illness. He was concerned that he would be unable to manage the situation if these patients reacted in an unexpected way. The observations were consistent with the hypothesis that individual attitudes and user psychopathology were stronger determinants of the outcome of clinical tasks than the technical specification of the equipment.

In the final phase of the Telemed project a link was established between Guy's Hospital and the Speedwell Mental Health Centre about 10 km away (Fig. 9.1) using a 2 Mbit/s link.[13] Of 26 patients asked to participate, 11 refused. Five said that they were concerned about confidentiality and video recording, three said that they had used it before and three said that they did not understand. The views on the medium of those who participated were significantly more positive than clinicians' for every question on the satisfaction instrument. The sound quality was reported as disappointing. Users were much more likely to complain of sound problems than video problems. Sound seemed to be more critical to the consultation than the image. Clinicians rated themselves as less confident in judging the presence of symptoms via the video link. Although service-user responses to outpatient management by videoconferencing were positive, the high cost of the link at that time rendered it unsustainable.

The Guy's group went on to pilot a range of telepsychiatry applications, within the South London and Maudsley NHS Trust, using ISDN videoconferencing systems operating at 128 kbit/s. Applications have included remote psychotherapy supervision in Cognitive Analytical Therapy (CAT) for trainee psychiatrists in Belfast given by a supervisor in London.[14] The videoconferencing equipment used in this study was PC-based, cheaper and operated at a lower bandwidth (128 kbit/s vs. 384 kbit/s) than that reported in the Norwegian work. The therapeutic model was also different (CAT versus psychodynamic) and the CAT supervisor found the medium challenging and

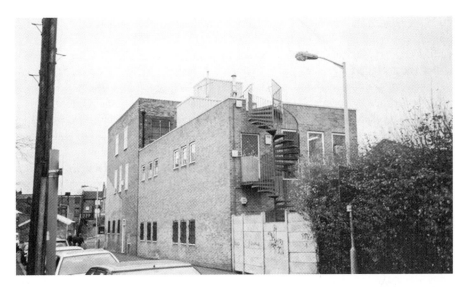

Fig. 9.1. The Speedwell Community Mental Health Centre in London, about 10 km from Guy's Hospital.

disruptive to normal therapeutic processes. She reported (M. O'Kane, personal communication) of using the video link:

> I feel de-skilled. Many of the things I am used to using are not available to me: complex body language that I am bound to read at a subliminal level. Emotional responses that I may pick up through transference and counter transference. The chance to think creatively, using a reflective space with others that has an alive quality. In discussions we looked at what de-skilled meant. ...We discussed whether what is needed is a larger than life personality (like a TV presenter) to get points across!

Manchanda and McLaren[15] reported a case study of cognitive behaviour therapy with a patient suffering from mixed anxiety and depressive disorder. This was delivered over a video link using ISDN at 128 kbit/s to connect the patient in his general practice with the therapist at Guy's. The patient reported:

> I do wonder whether the slightly more impersonal nature of the contact by videolink might have as many advantages as disadvantages for the relationship between the therapist and client. It is possible that I may have been less self-conscious, perhaps less inhibited due to the distance.

In more recent work the Guy's group have used videoconferencing to address communications problems within a community mental health service in Lewisham. Distances are modest, but travel is difficult because of traffic congestion and limited parking space. Services are dispersed, struggling to meet demands, and professionals have to spend time travelling between sites. This time represents a cost to the service.

The Lewisham Telepsychiatry Project at present has two main strands, the first to link primary care mental health teams, such as that at the Grove Medical Centre (Fig. 9.2), with secondary services and the second to improve communication between sites within the secondary service.

This work has demonstrated that there are high levels of service-user acceptance of videoconferencing when it is used to obtain specialist psychiatric help.[16] Not all users are willing to use videoconferencing in all circumstances and some service users have asked to stop using the link because they felt unable to close painful personal issues. Gathering information on refusals to use or on individuals who having used a video link then seek face-to-face treatment instead, has been a useful aspect of this urban research where the benefits to service users are more marginal and more subtle than in areas of low population density. Some service users see it as an advantage to be interviewed in their general practitioner's surgery rather than the community mental health centre. Others may feel they are 'missing out' and prefer to travel. Dropout rates were no higher for patients treated by video link than face-to-face but patients treated by video link may stay in the service longer than those seen face-to-face within the same service[16].

The other major strand in the Lewisham telepsychiatry research has been the use of videoconferencing in discharge planning.[17] A 128 kbit/s ISDN link has been used to connect set-top videoconferencing equipment in the Speedwell Community Mental Health Centre and the catchment area inpatient unit at the University Hospital in Lewisham (Fig. 9.3). It has been used by community mental health team professionals

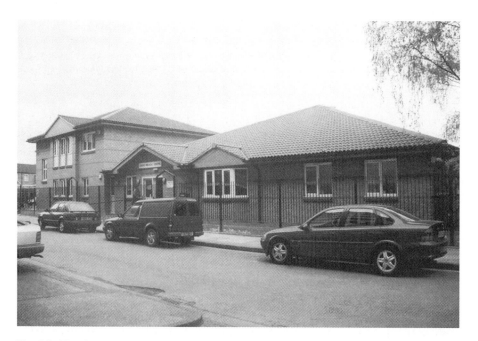

Fig. 9.2. The Grove Medical Centre.

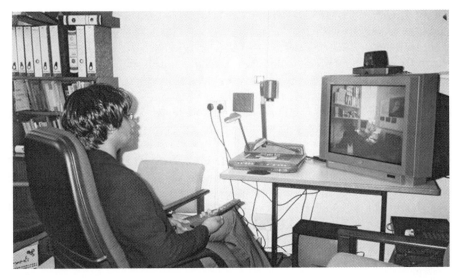

Fig. 9.3. Senior social worker using a videoconferencing system to participate in a discharge planning meeting.

to participate in discharge planning meetings without having to travel to the ward. Satisfaction results for professional and service users have been positive and an economic analysis of this work is currently underway. This application has 'taken off' and has been sustained by professional users who believe that it improves both their efficiency and job quality.

In a study looking at communication within a specialist service, Haslam and McLaren[18] reported on the use of a set-top videoconferencing system, operating at 128 kbit/s, to improve communication between a psychiatric Intensive Care Unit and a referring acute adult ward 8 km away. Images were displayed on a 63-cm monitor. More staff were able to participate in clinical communication on patient transfers between the units than would otherwise have been the case. One assessment was completed, as were two episodes of patient review from the remote ward. One patient commented:

> It was nice to know she (the keyworker) would be there (in the referring ward) when I got back

Two male patients with histories of aggression refused to use the system. One was deluded and refused, the other was found to be incapable of giving informed consent. The feasibility of this link was demonstrated but the enthusiasm of the staff was low and the equipment was subsequently withdrawn from the unit.

In Scotland Freir et al[19] described the use of videoconferencing to deliver psychology services in the Highlands, where there is a population of 210 000 at a density of 8 people per km^2, one of the lowest in the European Union. The clinical psychology service operated from 1997 and extended over a distance of 200 km between Inverness, where most of the population is situated, and Portree Hospital on the Isle of Skye, which has a population of 9000. This study used desktop videoconferencing units connected by ISDN at 128 kbit/s. They surveyed 27 adults and seven children referred to clinical psychology outpatient clinics and treated with cognitive behavioural therapy over the video link. Most complained of poor sound and picture quality but were satisfied with the medium. A third expressed a preference for face-to-face consultation. The links were used to advise parents on managing their children's behavioural problems, to consult directly with young people for phobias and depression and to treat parents.

May et al[20] established a telepsychiatry referral service in the north-west of England for patients suffering from anxiety and depression. Desk-top videophones were used connected with ISDN at 128 kbit/s. Qualitative data were collected from participants using a semistructured interview schedule. This study ran for 12 months from April 1998 and 22 patients and 13 doctors were interviewed after their video-link consultation. Tape recordings were transcribed and analysed using a conventional method of discourse analysis. Patients were interviewed within 3 days of using the system.

None of the professional subjects were active proponents of telemedicine. In most of the Guy's work they have been. Professionals stated that they did not see a need for videoconferencing where accessibility was not a problem. One psychiatrist said he found it difficult to get patients to settle over a videophone. Some patients saw the technology as having the potential to reduce stigmatizing encounters with mental health services. Patients saw it as a means of obtaining additional 'expert' advice. The general practitioners felt that the service might adversely affect the doctor–patient relationship. The most important problem identified was the extent to which communication skills needed to be adjusted to meet the demands of the medium. They concluded that patients need an induction session to facilitate communication and professionals need to learn new ways of communicating in mediated spaces.

In a further qualitative analysis of this data,[21] it was reported that the use of the videoconferencing equipment threatened professional constructs about the nature and practice of therapeutic relationships. These authors concluded that satisfaction and acceptability are complex phenomena that need to be considered in the context of the particular ecologies in which they are expressed.

Other European telepsychiatry projects

Gonçalves and Cunha[22] described a telepsychiatry component in a Portuguese telemedicine link between Lisbon and the Azores. This was designed to operate at 384 kbit/s.

Mannion et al[23] reported on a link established in 1996 between the island of Inishmore, off the west coast of Ireland, and the Department of Psychiatry in University College Hospital, Galway. There is one general practitioner on the island and admission rates are high compared with other areas within the catchment area. Two rollabout videoconferencing systems were connected using 384 kbit/s. The link was mainly used to facilitate emergency consultations between patients on the island and the duty psychiatrist, at the request of the island's general practitioner. Nine patients were referred for assessment over 8 months. Three patients had their first psychiatric contact and assessment through the video link, and were followed up as outpatients via the link to eventual resolution of the episode of illness and discharge at the outpatient clinic. They reported that the videoconferencing systems are acceptable and satisfactory for patients and staff alike.

The States of Jersey Health and Social Services have purchased tertiary mental health care from the UK mainland. Encouraging results have been reported for a videoconferencing link between the island and the South London and Maudsley NHS Trust to deliver further opinions on difficult psychiatric cases.[24] An economic analysis of this link is currently under way.

Conclusion

Telepsychiatry in Europe has developed in a piecemeal fashion despite the early recognition by the European Commission of the potential of communications technology to deliver services across borders within the European Union. Pilot studies have shown that communications technology can improve access to services at the peripheries. Work in urban settings, particularly in the UK, has revealed the complexity of user responses to mediated communication, which may not have been so apparent in areas of the world where the benefits of using the technology for service users are more obvious.

Professionals have been shown to vary widely in their willingness to use videoconferencing for clinical consultations with service users. Supervision in psychotherapy by videoconferencing has been tested in Scandinavia and the UK. While economic advantages have been demonstrated professionals have been reported to be wary of the effects the medium may have on the process.

The economics of telepsychiatry will be marginal in much of Europe but the potential of the technology to improve communications in complex service delivery systems demands closer examination. Large networks employing high bandwidth and high specification videoconferencing systems may be economically justifiable in areas of Europe with low population density but the implications of this technology for service delivery remains unclear. In urban centres communications technology is more likely to diffuse through incorporation into existing community mental health service delivery models, where it should bring efficiency gains through reducing the needs for professionals to travel between sites.

References

1   Sosa M. Telematics in Europe. *Journal of Telemedicine and Telecare* 1995;**1**:61–62.
2   Commission of the European Communities. *Advanced Informatics in Medicine (AIM). Supplement. Application of Telecommunications to Health Care Telemedicine, AI 1685*. Brussels: CEC, 1990.
3   Uldal SB. A survey of Norwegian Telemedicine. *Journal of Telemedicine and Telecare* 1999;**5**:32–37.

4   Norwegian Ministry of Health and Social Affairs. *More Health for Each bIT. Information Technology for Better Health Services in Norway.* Oslo: Norwegian Ministry of Health and Social Affairs, 1996.

5   Gammon D, Bergvik S, Bergmo T, Pedersen S. Videoconferencing in psychiatry: a survey of use in northern Norway. *Journal of Telemedicine and Telecare* 1996;**2**:192–198.

6   Gammon D, Sorlie T, Bergvik S, Hoifodt TS. Psychotherapy supervision conducted by videoconferencing: a qualitative study of users' experiences. *Journal of Telemedicine and Telecare* 1998;**4**(suppl 1):33–35.

7   Rutter DR. *Looking and Seeing: the Role of Visual Communication in Social Interaction.* Chichester: Wiley, 1984.

8   Mielonen M-L, Ohinmaa A, Moring J, Isohanni M. The use of videoconferencing for telepsychiatry in Finland. *Journal of Telemedicine and Telecare* 1998;**4**:125–131.

9   Mielonen M-L, Ohinmaa A, Moring J, Isohanni M. Psychiatric inpatient care planning via telemedicine. *Journal of Telemedicine and Telecare* 2000;**6**:152–157.

10   Sorvaniemi M, Santamaki O. Telepsychiatry in emergency consultations. *Journal of Telemedicine and Telecare* 2002;**8**:183–184.

11   McLaren PM, Ball CJ, Summerfield AB, Watson JP, Lipsedge M. An evaluation of the use of interactive television in an acute psychiatric service. *Journal of Telemedicine and Telecare* 1995;**1**:79–85.

12   Ball CJ, McLaren PM, Summerfield AB, Lipsedge MS, Watson JP. A comparison of communication modes in adult psychiatry. *Journal of Telemedicine and Telecare* 1995;**1**:22–26.

13   McLaren PM, Laws VJ, Ferreira AC, O'Flynn D, Lipsedge M, Watson JP. Telepsychiatry: outpatient psychiatry by videolink. *Journal of Telemedicine and Telecare* 1996;**2**(suppl 1):59–62.

14   McLaren P, O'Kane M. Remote psychotherapy. *Journal of Telemedicine and Telecare* 1998;**4**:122.

15   Manchanda M, McLaren P. Cognitive behaviour therapy via interactive video. *Journal of Telemedicine and Telecare* 1998;**4**(suppl 1):53–55.

16   McLaren P, Ahlbom J, Riley A, Mohammedali A, Denis M. The North Lewisham telepsychiatry project: beyond the pilot phase. *Journal of Telemedicine and Telecare* 2002, **8**(suppl 2):98–100.

17   McLaren P, Jegan S, Ahlbom J, Gallo F, Gaughran F, Forni C. Controlled trial of discharge planning by video-link in a UK urban mental health service: responses of staff and service users. *Journal of Telemedicine and Telecare* 2002;**8**(suppl 3):44–46. In press.

18   Haslam R, McLaren P. Interactive television for an urban adult mental health service: the Guy's Psychiatric Intensive Care Unit Telepsychiatry Project. *Journal of Telemedicine and Telecare* 2000;**6**(suppl 1):50–52.

19   Freir V, Kirkwood K, Peck D, Robertson S, Scott-Lodge L, Zeffert S. Telemedicine for clinical psychology in the Highlands of Scotland. *Journal of Telemedicine and Telecare* 1999;**5**:157–161.

20   May C, Gask L, Ellis N, et al. Telepsychiatry evaluation in the north-west of England: preliminary results of a qualitative study. *Journal of Telemedicine and Telecare* 2000;**6**(suppl 1):20–22.

21   May C, Gask L, Atkinson T, Ellis N, Mair F, Esmail A. Resisting and promoting new technologies in clinical practice: the case of telepsychiatry. *Social Science and Medicine* 2001;**52**:1889–1901.

22   Gonçalves L, Cunha C. Telemedicine project in the Azores Islands. *Archives d'Anatomie et de Cytologie Pathologiques* 1995;**43**:285–287.

23   Mannion L, Fahy TJ, Duffy C, Broderick M, Gethins E. Telepsychiatry: an island pilot project. *Journal of Telemedicine and Telecare* 1998;**4**(suppl 1):62–63.

24   Harley J, McLaren P, Blackwood G, Tierney K, Everett M. The use of videoconferencing to enhance tertiary mental health service provision to the island of Jersey. *Journal of Telemedicine and Telecare* 2002;**8**(suppl 2):36–38.

10

Mental Health Correctional Telemedicine

Charles Zaylor, Ashley Spaulding and David Cook

Introduction

In the USA 'correctional facilities' is the term for prisons run by the federal state and local government. Generally, local county jails typically house less than 200 inmates, but a few like Rikers Island in New York may house several thousand inmates. Inmates in a jail setting are rarely incarcerated for more than a year and may be incarcerated for only a few days. State prison inmates are often incarcerated for much longer periods of time. Most correctional facilities have some procedure for screening inmates for physical and mental illness. This could involve the correctional officers having an inmate complete a questionnaire regarding physical and mental illness. This might be the case in small jails with limited staff. State prisons have a central correctional facility where all inmates enter the correctional system. In the Kansas Department of Correction (KDOC) at the time of entry an inmate will have a physical examination to asses any physical illness or disability. The inmates also undergo a battery of psychological testing and interviews with mental health staff to determine if any mental illness is present. With this information the Department of Correction can provide any necessary health care.

In the year 2000, an estimated 191 000 inmates in state correctional facilities throughout the USA experienced mental illness.[1] The United States Department of Justice's Bureau of Justice Statistics recently reported that behavioural therapy/counselling and psychotropic medication were the most common mental health services offered among confinement facilities. Therapy/counselling accounted for 84% of the services rendered, while 83% of the total number of services offered involved medication.[1] These numbers highlight the necessity of offering mental health services to individuals during incarceration. While the initial screening process identifies a large majority of individuals with mental illness prior to placing them in correctional facilities, some inmates develop mental illness after entering the correctional environment. These illnesses can include adjustment reactions, major depression, schizophrenia and anxiety disorders.

Inmates with mental illness may sometimes not receive mental health assistance because of financial constraints or poor access to mental health care providers. This is particularly true in rural jail populations. Many correctional facilities are located in counties that have been designated as 'Health Professional Shortage Areas' for the mental health discipline,[2] which underscores the fact that being able to provide mental health services to these facilities is frequently a difficult task. Even if a psychiatrist is available, correctional psychiatry may make up only a small fraction of their clinical practice leaving relatively inexperienced clinicians providing care to this challenging population.

Telemedicine offers a solution to these problems, linking qualified mental health providers with inmates in correctional facilities to provide patient care at a distance. The technologies include videoconferencing and electronic medical records. Although providing medical care at a distance has been the focus of telemedicine, information technology such as an electronic medical record aids in the delivery of care to patients even if they are not seen at a distance.

Symptom improvement is the fundamental aim for offering mental health services via telemedicine in the correctional setting, although safety is another crucial issue. Transporting inmates to health care facilities poses a serious security risk to those involved in the transport process and to community members due to the increased potential for the inmate to escape.[3-5] Telemedicine allows inmates to receive regular, efficient care for mental health problems, which ideally enables them to be better prepared for reintegration into the community. In addition to safety, significant cost savings are possible because of money saved when correctional officer time is not needed to transport inmates and/or physician time is not used to travel to the inmate. Videoconferencing with use of an electronic medical record (EMR) allows an on-call psychiatrist to be more accessible to several correctional facilities spread out over a large geographical area. Even in an urban setting where the psychiatrist is only a few miles from a correctional setting, hours can still be spent travelling to the correctional facility and passing security check points before the psychiatrist is face to face with the patient.

Inmates benefit by having appropriate care initiated thus relieving symptoms that make them unable to function in the general inmate population. The care may be in the form of being given medication and placed in a holding cell under 24-hour observation. Whenever an inmate's disruptive behaviour can be controlled by psychiatric intervention the correctional staff are better able to manage them. At the administrative level, tele-mental health services are advantageous because of their ability to assist administrators to meet their responsibility to provide mental health services for inmates at a reasonable cost. Furthermore, administrators in correctional settings benefit from having telemedicine available in their facilities because they can use the equipment for inmate parole hearings in addition to other administrative meetings.

Mental health correctional telemedicine services – USA

As inmates continue to be identified as needing mental health services, the demand for such services is increasingly being met by offering telemedicine as a health care delivery mechanism. The Association of Telehealth Service Providers (ATSP)[6] identified nine programmes in the USA that were providing mental health telemedicine services to correctional facilities. These programmes were very diverse in terms of activity.[6] Although the ATSP report is the most comprehensive report of its kind, the information in it depends on programmes reporting their telemedicine activity to the ATSP. I believe that other individuals and organizations use videoconferencing to provide psychiatric care, but it is not reported in the literature. For example, the United States Bureau of Prisons has been operating a telepsychiatry programme since 1997 (C. Tomelleri, personal communication).

Three of the nine programmes – the California Department of Corrections (DOC) Telemedicine Services Programme, Texas Tech University Center for Telemedicine, and Mountaineer Doctor Television (MDTV) in West Virginia – report mental health consultations (i.e. in the general population) as their most active tele-medicine specialty.[6] Inmates at a California state prison have been able to benefit from being able to access mental health services via the DOC Telemedicine Services Programme – there were 3888 tele-mental health consultations in the year 2000. Texas Tech University Center for Telemedicine utilizes interactive video to manage patient conditions in addition to monitoring medications of inmates in a state prison. MDTV conducts more general telemedicine mental health consultations than any other type. Many of these consultations are conducted with inmates at a state prison for the purpose of managing mental health conditions and medications.

The Arizona Telemedicine Programme, the Center for Health and Technology in California, the University at Buffalo (SUNY) Telemedicine Services Programme and Maine Telemedicine Services all reported that tele-mental health is their second most active clinical specialty.[6] Interactive video and store and forward technologies available through the Arizona Telemedicine Programme are well utilized by health care providers offering services to inmates of the state prison. Sacramento's Center for Health and Technology also utilizes interactive video to provide tele-mental health services to inmates at a state prison as well as those at a county jail. The SUNY Telemedicine Services Programme offers telemedicine services such as referrals to specialists and continual management of patients' conditions to inmates at a state prison as well as a county jail. Reporting mental health as its second most active clinical specialty, the Maine Telemedicine Services Programme additionally provides services to inmates in these two types of facilities.

The Michigan Department of Corrections (DOC) provides clinical tele-mental health services to inmates at a state prison. The DOC reports that their main administrative use for the technique is to conduct parole hearings for correctional facility inmates. The Office of Telemedicine in Charlottesville, Virginia also reports mental health services among their active specialties. A state prison is one of the facilities receiving telemedicine services from the Virginia-based programme.

The United States Bureau of Federal Prisons began its telepsychiatry network in 1997. At present there are two primary sites. Fort Devens Federal Prison uses videoconferencing to provide psychiatric services to medium and minimum security federal prisons in their area. The other site is in Springfield Missouri, where Carlos Tomelleri is the chief of psychiatry for the United States Medical Center for Federal Prisons. He has been the leader in developing a telepsychiatry service at his facility. Their programme uses videoconferencing to provide psychiatric consultation and management for psychiatric patients in six federal prisons throughout the USA. They currently have an active caseload of 594 patients and have conducted over 2000 consultations in the past 18 months. The reason for the Federal Bureau of Prisons' interest in videoconferencing to deliver psychiatric care was to reduce the cost of care and to bring the most experienced clinicians to where they are needed.

Mental health telemedicine services – Kansas

Kansas has been an active centre in terms of tele-mental health activity and continues to augment current services as the demand for regular, efficient, timely health care services remains an important issue. It is helpful to appreciate the scope of mental health telemedicine services available in Kansas in order to understand the process by which providers began offering these services to correctional facilities in rural areas of the state.

In 1994, the Center for TeleMedicine and TeleHealth at the University of Kansas Medical Center (KUMC) initiated tele-mental health services for child psychiatry consultations. Inaugural services for routine telemedicine clinics were established in the following year when physicians from adult psychiatry at KUMC in Kansas City, Kansas were linked with a mental health centre 180 km away in Pittsburg, Kansas. A child psychiatry telemedicine clinic soon followed, with services initiated in 1996. Between 1995 and 1998, over 3200 adult and child psychiatry patient consultations and follow-up visits occurred throughout 15 different Kansas communities. These services continue today with regular weekly clinics.

Telemedicine mental health services at the University of Kansas Medical Center have grown in function and scope over the years to include schools and group homes. A school-based telemedicine programme – known as TeleKidcare – was established in 1998 in four inner city schools throughout the Kansas City, Kansas metropolitan area. At present, 26 sites throughout the state of Kansas have the capability to provide mental health services via telemedicine to school age children in their communities.

Adult and child psychiatry services were also provided to two group homes in Kansas from 1997 to 2000. Services occurred on a weekly basis using videophones over the ordinary telephone network (PSTN). Over 300 consultations occurred during the 3-year time period. To date, the University of Kansas Medical Center has conducted over 7000 mental health telemedicine consultations.

Tele-mental health in Kansas also involves behavioural health services, which are provided by psychologists. Tele-psychology services have operated as stand-alone clinics and have been blended with the mental health services as child psychiatrists and psychologists collaborate on patient care. For example, a stand-alone clinic currently connects Hays, Kansas with a child psychologist at the University of Kansas Medical Center in Kansas City on a weekly basis. In addition a psychologist has provided individual and group therapy for adults with depression via telemedicine, primarily to the western portion of the state, since the late 1990s. From 1999 to 2000, a project offered behavioural therapy for children with depression while they remained in school. To date, behavioural health specialists at KUMC have conducted over 500 consultations using telemedicine.

Figure 10.1 shows locations in Kansas where mental health telemedicine services are provided. It also shows sites that provide tele-mental health services to correctional facilities across the state.

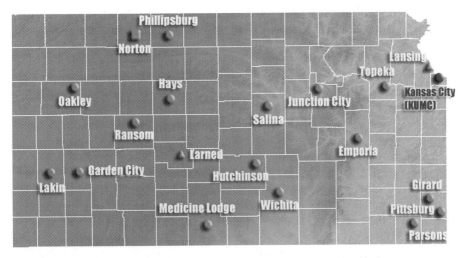

Fig. 10.1. Kansas tele-mental health sites and correctional tele-mental health sites.

Mental health correctional telemedicine services – Kansas

The Kansas Department of Corrections (DOC), in association with Prison Health Services, began its telemedicine initiative in 2000. The Kansas DOC currently oversees more than 8500 inmates at 13 correctional facilities throughout the state. Prison Health Services is a private correctional medical services company that provides health care – both medical and psychiatric – to inmates within the Kansas DOC. The telemedicine initiative at the Kansas Department of Corrections was developed as a result of the Kansas DOC identifying a need to save paper and improve continuity of care by use of an electronic medical record (EMR). Use of an EMR improves continuity of care by making the medical record readily available to clinical staff. In a correctional setting inmates are often transported from one facility to another and it is imperative that the medical records are always available to maintain continuity of care when inmates arrive at their new placement. Videoconferencing was incorporated into the delivery of patient care because of its ability to provide psychiatric care to inmates at some rural correctional facilities. An EMR not only saves paper, but also allows for a legible medical record that is accessible to all medical staff throughout the state.

Funding for the initiative was provided by the DOC's existing budget. To date, external sources such as federal grants have not been required. The fact that the programme has been funded entirely from an existing budget highlights the support that the programme has received from the Kansas DOC and certainly emphasizes the significant effect that the programme has had in correctional facilities throughout the state.

Economics of telemedicine

In a report by the United States National Institute of Justice ('Implementing telemedicine in correctional facilities', May 2002),[7] it was noted that a demonstration project ending in 1998 showed that a telemedicine consultation resulted in savings of nearly 60% when compared to a conventional (face-to-face) consultation. This demonstration project was carried out by a Joint Program Steering Group (JPSG) established by the United States Department of Justice and the United States Department of Defense. Since the time of that report the cost of videoconferencing equipment and transmission costs have decreased considerably. The present cost of videoconferencing equipment for the Kansas DOC program is under $1000 per unit. This does not include the cost of the computer because no additional computers had to be purchased for this purpose. All computers used for telemedicine are also used as work stations for accessing the EMR.

The report further states that telemedicine is most effective under the following conditions: when the cost for onsite medical specialists is high; medical specialists are not available when needed; the small number of requests for a specialist does not warrant a contract for outside services; the cost to transport patients to outside medical services is high. Other benefits noted were improved safety by avoiding transport of high-risk inmates and improved response time to inmates' medical needs. One common mistake made when starting a telemedicine programme is that more technology is provided than is actually needed. The Kansas DOC programme is not set up for multipoint videoconferencing. This was a deliberate choice because there was no need for that capability. It would add considerable cost to provide this facility. There are times when less technology is better.

Equipment

Videoconferencing was based on Intel Proshare software and an existing T1 network in Kansas. All 13 correctional facilities have taken advantage of the opportunity to connect to the central EMR. Five sites are also linked by videoconferencing, which allows the clinician to see the patient while viewing their medical record.

Technical specifications have varied across the different telemedicine mental health applications. Initial tele-mental health services in 1995 and 1996 broadcast clinics at 384 kbit/s. However, due to high telecommunications costs, services were frequently provided at 128 kbit/s. In the case of the previously mentioned group homes, services were provided over ordinary telephone lines using standard videophones. Today, the majority of telemedicine mental health services are conducted at either 128 kbit/s or 384 kbit/s (Fig. 10.2).

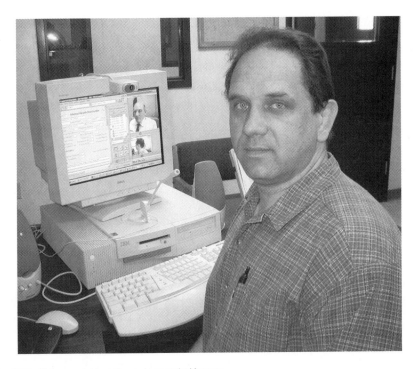

Fig. 10.2. Tele-mental health equipment in Kansas.

First telemedicine link

The Kansas DOC tele-mental health programme began with the EMR and videoconferencing was added as the need presented itself. The first telepsychiatry clinic linked Larned Correctional Mental Health Facility (LCMHF) with Lansing Correctional Facility (LCF), approximately 500 km away. The purpose of this video link was to allow a physician at LCF to chair an involuntary medication hearing (IMH) for patients at LCMHF. Prior to the video link, a psychiatrist would need to travel up to 6 hours one way to LCMHF for a meeting that might last 2–4 hours. Furthermore, situations often develop where the need for an IMH arises quickly, and it is in the best interests of the patient that the hearing is held without undue delay. Videoconferencing makes it possible to schedule IMHs quickly as no time needs to be allocated for travel. Additionally, the consulting psychiatrist does not have to leave his or her site unattended, which allows for efficient use of staff time and resources.

The protocol for the IMH is the same via telemedicine as it is in a face-to-face encounter; the only difference between the two settings being the presence of the computer and the monitor at each site. The IMH is conducted in a conference room in the medical clinic area. Those in attendance include the site psychiatrist, internist, registered nurse, unit team counsellor, clinical director and correctional officers if needed. The chairman of the hearing is present via videoconferencing and can interact with the inmate and the other members of the hearing. The inmate is present as his/her case is reviewed and the reasons for involuntary medication status discussed. After the hearing the inmate is informed of the decision of the hearing. Telemedicine has made it feasible to have patients on involuntary medication at several correctional facilities, as the need to have a physician travelling around to each site in order to participate in the IMH in person no longer exists. Involuntary medication hearings between LCMHF and LCF occur every 4–6 months, on average.

Because many of the correctional facilities are located in rural areas of Kansas, more time is often spent travelling to the facility than actually conducting consultations with patients. Consequently, two sites were identified as potential sites to provide mental health care using videoconferencing. The first link was established between Larned Correctional Mental Health Facility-West (LCMHF-West) and Lansing Correctional Facility (LCF). LCMHF-West is a minimum security facility located in Larned, Kansas, where a shortage of physician time was identified. The case load for LCMHF and LCMHF-West was determined to be one full-time equivalent. Both facilities were being staffed by a part-time psychiatrist. For this reason additional psychiatrist time was needed and telemedicine was established to address that need.

In order to facilitate telemedicine consultations, a nurse is present with the patient while the psychiatric visit takes place. The nurse's presence serves several purposes. The nurse acts as a liaison between the psychiatrist at LCF and the correctional and medical staff at LCMHF-West. In addition, the nurse provides assistance for the psychiatrist regarding procedural issues at the site where the patient is located, which may differ from those at the correctional facility where the psychiatrist is based. Furthermore, the nurse has first-hand knowledge of the information discussed between the patient and the psychiatrist, which can aid in maintaining effective follow-up.

Telemedicine and an EMR allow the psychiatrist to continue following patients as they move through the correctional system, which occurs commonly. On occasion, inmates who were seen in person at LCF were transferred to LCMHF-West, where the psychiatrist at LCF could continue to provide their care via telemedicine.

Second telemedicine link

The second tele-mental health link established was between Lansing Correctional Facility and Norton Correctional Facility (NCF) in Norton, Kansas. The connection between these two facilities was established because of the significant demand for psychiatry services in the rural town. Norton's remote location made it difficult to staff the correctional facility with health care providers. The clinic is run in an identical fashion to the clinic established through the connection of LCF and LCMHF-West. A psychologist at the NCF is present during all psychiatric visits. The psychologist serves as a liaison between the NCF and the consulting psychiatrist and also acts as an information source for the psychiatrist about the patient's psychiatric and medical history. Progress notes and orders are entered into the EMR, thus enabling the nursing staff at the NCF to take orders just as they would if the psychiatrist had consulted with the patient face to face. Communication is maintained between the psychiatrist at LCF and the nursing staff at the NCF via email, which is also linked to the medical record. The ability to link email to the EMR allows for efficient communication between staff at remote sites and consulting providers at hub sites.

Both the LCMHF-West and the NCF tele-mental health clinics are scheduled at regular intervals during the week. Sometimes a tele-mental health visit will be scheduled outside the traditional clinic time if warranted. Therefore, the remote sites essentially have access to a psychiatrist via telemedicine for 5 days a week if the need arises.

Additional consultations are initiated by the social worker at the NCF. The social worker, who has been identified as the telemedicine liaison person, calls the psychiatrist at LCF and arranges a time for NCF to call LCF to conduct the consultation. Once the videoconferencing link is established the consultation is carried out. The psychiatrist at LCF is a full-time staff member so that he/she is available to respond to needs at NCF 5 days a week. In a correctional setting it is much easier compared to a non-correctional outpatient clinic to reschedule inmates that are being seen for follow-up so that emergency consulations can be given priority.

While the Kansas Department of Corrections began tele-mental health services to prisons in 2000, KUMC began providing mental health telemedicine to a jail setting in a rural community in southeastern Kansas 2 years before that. In 1998, the Lyon County Jail located in Emporia began offering mental health services via telemedicine to inmates due to a lack of access to such services in the surrounding community.[8] Since the inception of services at the jail, over 700 consultations have been conducted with inmates.[8] While the need for mental health services in jails is consistent with the need for the same services in prisons – as highlighted by the number of consultations conducted since 1998 in Emporia – many differences exist between the two settings, which subsequently affect the delivery of health care to these facilities.

Perhaps the most notable difference in the two correctional facility settings – jails and prisons – can be found in the populations they serve. Jails typically house short-term offenders who may be incarcerated for 24 hours to 12 months. Up to 70% of inmates in jails have a diagnosis of chemical dependency and have been under the influence of some illicit drug up to the time of incarceration. For this reason many are in the process of drug withdrawal and experience physical and mental symptoms of withdrawal requiring medication management. Prisons, on the other hand, tend to accommodate individuals who have committed more serious crimes and, accordingly, have been given longer sentences ranging from 90 days to life. Consequently, jail populations are often transient in comparison to more stable prison populations. How does this population difference affect the delivery of health care services? Although both populations exhibit chronic and acute medical and psychiatric conditions, jail populations are more likely to exhibit acute psychiatric conditions because of the high level of recent substance abuse and the demands of adjusting to incarceration. These conditions dictate that medical and psychiatric services are readily available. The needs of the inmates of Lyon County Jail, for example, outweighed the services that the community mental health center in Emporia, Kansas could offer. The initiation of telemedicine services at the jail helped alleviate the burden placed on the community mental health center.

Face-to-face mental health services are provided to jails by contracting services with outside organizations. This is typically done with the local mental health centres. If the jail is large enough medical and psychiatric staff are present on site. If the jail is small contract medical staff from the outside may have to come to the jail as needed.

In addition to a difference in populations, jails and prisons also differ in their financial resources. These resources affect health care services available in the two settings. With limited operating budgets, jails may not have the resources necessary to offer health care services to inmates. Telemedicine provides a cost-effective alternative for the delivery of health care by eliminating the costs of transporting the inmates to a health care facility. Furthermore, telemedicine eliminates the cost of providing security during the transport process. The size of jails and prisons also affects the delivery of health care. In a small rural jail it may not be cost effective to have a full-time medial staff. Again, telemedicine is a potential solution.

Tele-mental health has been integrated into the delivery of health care services within Kansas's correctional facilities without adding additional infrastructure to maintain or to continue to develop applications. In essence, the process of integrating such technology has been quite seamless. Furthermore – consistent with findings from a study conducted with a prison in Ohio a few years ago[9] – the Kansas programme has been well received by inmates who have used tele-mental health services. At present, over 500 patient visits are conducted each year via telemedicine for evaluations, follow-up or involuntary medication hearings. At LCF approximately 35 of the 335 patient visits per month are provided via videoconferencing. Approximately 14% of the inmates serviced through LCF are being seen for medication management.

I believe that videoconferencing to provide psychiatric care in the correctional setting is only limited by access to the technology itself. For patients who cannot be physically restrained and brought to the videoconferencing equipment, videoconferencing equipment can be brought to them in the cell house. This is already the case at LCF. Videoconferencing equipment is used in the segregation unit so that inmates can visit, via videoconferencing, their visitors who are located at the part of the prison facility where normal face-to-face visitation occurs. Providing visitation this way decreases the security risk of transporting inmates from a high-security segregation unit to a less-secure visiting area.

Conclusion

There is a significant need for mental health services in correctional facilities. Since state prisons typically screen inmates for mental disorders prior to placing them in a facility,[1] it is imperative that these facilities – and other similar facilities – are equipped with the means to provide services to meet the behavioural health needs of those identified with such disorders. While 1394 of the 1558 state public and private adult correctional facilities in the USA offered mental health services to inmates as of June 2000,[1] telemedicine offers an additional means of providing those services in a more efficient manner. Telemedicine presents one solution to the problem of not being able to provide behavioural health care services to inmates due to geographical barriers, time constraints and health care professional shortages.

Acknowledgements

Any opinions expressed in this chapter are those of the authors and do not necessarily reflect the position or policies of the Kansas Department of Corrections. TeleKidcare is a registered trademark.

References

1 US Department of Justice. *Bureau of Justice Statistics: mental health treatment in state prisons, 2000.* Available at http://www.ojp.usdoj.gov/bjs/abstract/mhtsp00.htm [last checked 3 September 2002].
2 National Center for Health Workforce Analysis (NCHWA). *Health professional shortage areas.* Available at http://bphc.hrsa.gov/databases/newhpsa/newhpsa.cfm [last checked 3 September 2002].
3 Brecht RM, Gray CL, Peterson C, Youngblood B. The University of Texas medical branch – Texas Department of Criminal Justice telemedicine project: findings from the first year of operation. *Telemedicine Journal* 1996;**2**:25–35.
4 Zaylor C, Nelson EL, Cook DJ. Clinical outcomes in a prison telepsychiatry clinic. *Journal of Telemedicine and Telecare* 2001;**7**(suppl 1):47–49.
5 Ventetuolo A, Travisono A. Justice videoconferencing: a technology whose time has come. *Corrections Today* 1998;**60**:94–96.
6 Dahlin MP, Watcher G, Engle WM, Henderson J. *2001 Report on US Telemedicine Activity.* Portland, OR: ATSP, 2001.
7 Nacci R, Turned A, Waldron R, Broyles E. 2002. *Implementing telemedicine in correctional facilities.* National Institute of Justice. Available at http://www.ncjrs.org/pdffiles1/nij/190310.pdf [last checked 3 September 2002].
8 Zaylor C, Whitten P, Kingsley C. Telemedicine services to a county jail. *Journal of Telemedicine and Telecare* 2000;**6**(suppl 1):93–95.
9 Mekhjian H, Turner JW, Gailiun M, McCain TA. Patient satisfaction with telemedicine in a prison environment. *Journal of Telemedicine and Telecare* 1999;**5**:55–61.

11

Forensic Psychiatry in the UK

Luke Birmingham and Sarah Leonard

Introduction

Forensic psychiatry is a branch of psychiatry particularly concerned with the law, the management and treatment of mentally disordered offenders (MDOs), and providing assistance and support to the court and related agencies. It is also concerned with the prediction and, if possible, the amelioration of dangerousness, psychiatric ethics and the psychiatric contribution to criminology and penology.

Mentally disordered offender populations

The MDO population mainly comprises people with serious and enduring mental illness, such as schizophrenia and mood disorder.[1] However, many MDOs have co-morbid mental disorders such as personality disorder and substance-related disorders. Whilst their treatment needs are likely to be similar to those of general psychiatric patients, the level of diagnostic co-morbidity and their offending behaviour means that MDOs usually have more complex needs requiring input from a range of health care professionals and other services. Because they may present serious risks to others as well as to themselves they are likely to require care and treatment in a secure setting.

There are nearly 3000 MDOs detained in National Health Service (NHS) and private secure hospitals in England and Wales. This only includes the number of MDOs on restriction orders who reside in NHS/private secure care. The largest single group is those with a history of violence against the person.[2]

The current prison population in the UK is over 70 000.[3] Psychiatric morbidity in prison compared to the general population is high. A systematic review of psychiatric morbidity by Fazel et al[4] indicates that one in seven prisoners has a psychotic illness or major depression, and about one in two male prisoners and one in five female prisoners have an antisocial personality disorder.

Services for mentally disordered offenders

MDOs may have contact with several different services at any one time, including general, forensic and other specialist mental health services, social services, the police, courts, probation services, prison services, housing and voluntary sector organizations. Although these organizations may have different roles and different objectives, it is important that health, social services, criminal justice and other agencies communicate effectively when dealing with a mentally disordered offender.

Services for MDOs are present in hospital, prison and the community. Assessment and treatment in hospital is usually carried out in secure conditions, but some MDOs are managed on open wards. In England and Wales, treatment for the most dangerous MDOs takes place in conditions of maximum security in the three special hospitals, Broadmoor, Ashworth and Rampton. Beneath this are medium-security institutions, provided in NHS regional secure units and secure hospitals in the private sector. MDOs who do not require higher levels of security can be managed on locked and open psychiatric wards.

MDOs in the hospital system move through different levels of security according to the risk they pose to others. They also move in and out of prison and the community. In England and Wales, health and social services provide police liaison, court diversion and prison liaison services to divert MDOs from custody to hospital or suitable community settings where they can receive treatment.[5]

The organization of community-based services for MDOs depends on the relationship locally between general and forensic mental health services.[6] In some areas community services are delivered by dedicated forensic community teams; some forensic services work with local mental health teams to provide shared care, and the remainder hand on forensic outpatients to local services.

Health care in prison is rudimentary and inadequate.[7] Support is available from visiting NHS psychiatrists in larger prisons, but the conditions in which mentally disordered prisoners are kept are unacceptable.[8,9]

Difficulties associated with providing health care in secure settings

Providing care for MDOs in the community can be difficult due to the lack of cooperation and non-compliance on the part of the patient. However, trying to provide care in a hospital or prison also presents problems. In England and Wales, the Mental Health Act 1983 does not extend to cover prisons.[10] Therefore, prisoners with serious mental disorders who cannot be managed in prison have to be transferred to psychiatric hospitals for treatment.

Prisons and special hospitals are remote, security conscious institutions (Figs 11.1, 11.2). The emphasis they place on security can have a profound effect on the delivery of health care. Visiting clinicians have to make arrangements to see patients in advance; they have to travel there and further delays are caused by security arrangements that hinder them getting in and out again. In prison, the situation is made worse by the fact that mentally disordered inmates requiring transfer to hospital can wait a long time for a bed. Because there are very few vacancies, patients who need care in a secure hospital may have to be admitted to units in other areas of the country. This problem also affects patients who require specialist secure services, such as women, personality-disordered patients and those with learning disability.

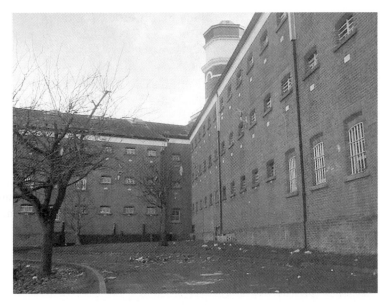

Fig. 11.1. B- and C-wings at Winchester prison (reproduced with the kind permission of the Governor of Winchester Prison).

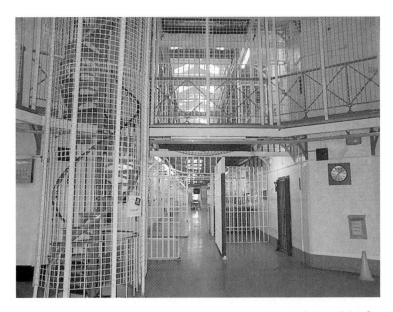

Fig. 11.2. C-wing at Winchester prison (reproduced with the kind permission of the Governor of Winchester Prison).

Health care policy relating to mentally disordered offenders

Since the 1950s, changes in mental health policy and law in England and Wales have resulted in a move away from detaining mentally disordered people in hospitals towards caring for them in the community. During the 1990s shortfalls in community care and a series of inquiries into homicides committed by psychiatric patients led to increasing concern about public safety.[11] In a subsequent policy document the Government stated unequivocally that community care had failed.[12] Proposals were put forward to develop extra beds, improve outreach and crisis intervention services and provide better access to treatment in order to make services 'safe sound and supportive'.[12] This approach was developed further with the publication of the National Service Framework for Mental Health, the intention of which was to improve quality and reduce unacceptable variations in health and social services.[13] Financial support to implement this strategy was promised by the Government in the NHS Plan.[14]

Another development is the reform of the Mental Health Act in which the Government has put forward a new legal framework to reflect the major changes that have occurred in mental health services, with more emphasis placed on public protection.[15]

Since the publication of the Butler report in 1975,[16] there has been a drive to develop regional (medium) secure services to reduce the inpatient populations of the special hospitals and provide treatment for MDOs closer to home. Even with the contribution made by the private sector, demand for medium-secure beds has outstripped supply and the very real need for longer-term secure provision was overlooked until relatively recently.[17]

The Reed report published in 1992 provided a wide-ranging review of health and social services for MDOs. The report established the policy that 'MDOs needing care and treatment should receive it from health and personal social services rather than in custodial care'.[18] The report recommended an increase in the number of secure psychiatric beds to address the shortfall. It also recommended the development of a nationwide network of court assessment and diversion schemes, bail information schemes and specialized bail accommodation.

In the last 10 years there has been an expansion in local diversion initiatives, especially those operating at the court level. However, this has not been centrally coordinated or strategically planned. As a result the network is patchy and there are a variety of different service models in operation. Bail information schemes and specialized bail information schemes have hardly developed at all.[5,19]

Recent changes in mental health policy brought about by mounting concerns over public safety are reflected in the reform of the Mental Health Act[9] and additional security measures introduced into the special hospitals as a result of the Tilt report.[20]

Prison health care in England and Wales is currently undergoing major reform. Until very recently the NHS had no statutory responsibility for prisoners, but in 2000 the NHS entered into a formal partnership with the Prison Service to improve health care in prisons. Prisoners are now entitled to have access to the same range and quality of services that everyone else receives from the NHS.[21]

Videoconferencing in forensic psychiatry

Although videoconferencing is not yet a part of routine psychiatry in the UK, it is widely used in psychiatry elsewhere in the world, including Australia, Canada and the USA.[22] Telepsychiatry has a great deal to offer in forensic settings where patients are 'hard to reach' and staff are relatively isolated from mainstream services.

Clinical

Telepsychiatry will not replace existing services or reduce the need for face-to-face contact, but it will allow a greater diversity of services to be delivered with greater efficiency.[23] Potential clinical applications in forensic psychiatry include diagnostic assessment, mental state assessment, treatment, aftercare and education. Different forms of therapy could also be delivered using videoconferencing, including psychotherapy, cognitive behavioural therapy, psychodynamic therapy and family therapy. It is also feasible to conduct case conferences and discharge planning meetings using videoconferencing.

MDOs in prison have limited access to mental health care. Despite the fact that the mental health needs of the prison population are recognized, the problem remains that these needs are not met. Telepsychiatry could provide obvious benefits for prisoners, including early intervention, improved follow-up and speeding up transfer to hospital.

MDOs placed in special hospitals and other secure units outside their own health district may find themselves many miles from home. Local general and forensic services have a responsibility to monitor these patients and contribute to discussions about their treatment and rehabilitation. Using videoconferencing to assess patients in these settings and virtual attendance at case conferences could help to improve communication between services and aid decision-making (Fig. 11.3).

Features of successful court diversion schemes include having close links with local psychiatric services and having good methods of obtaining health, social services and criminal record information.[19] Using telepsychiatry to assess MDOs in custody and gather background information could help to make some court diversion schemes function more effectively.

Supervision

Access to supervision can be difficult for some health care professionals working in the forensic field. Many professionals such as psychiatrists, nurse specialists, psychologists and therapists work in isolation. Within the Prison Service access to adequate supervision is particularly difficult. This is largely because of the structure and culture, small numbers of health professionals and isolation of health care staff.[21]

Telepsychiatry can offer opportunities for network supervision from peers or senior clinicians. Whilst it is important that all health care professionals receive support and guidance in the work that they undertake, this is especially important when working with MDOs because of the risks involved. Videoconferencing offers the possibility of real-time supervision which allows professionals to discuss complex issues.

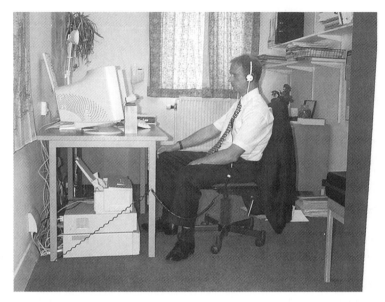

Fig. 11.3. A telepsychiatry session in progress at Ravenswood House.

Education

Teleconferencing technologies used for education purposes encompass a broad range of applications, which include one-to-one or multi-attendance sessions in which distance learning is supported. The education and training needs of health care professionals working in the field of forensic psychiatry are diverse. Many educational opportunities require significant travel time and for prisons especially it is only feasible to release a limited number of staff at any one time. Videoconferencing could facilitate access to training and educational sessions for a greater number of professionals, especially those who work in isolation. Videoconferencing also appears to be suitable for medical education in forensic psychiatry, although to date the evidence remains largely anecdotal.[24]

Assessment for legal reports

Health care professionals who work in the forensic setting are often asked to prepare medicolegal reports on MDOs. This can be a time-consuming process involving the need to travel great distances compounded by difficulties in accessing MDOs due to security orientated and institutional regimes. Videoconferencing offers the opportunity for the health care professional to carry out a real-time assessment in a time-efficient manner.

Practical, ethical and legal issues

The use of telemedicine brings with it practical, ethical and legal challenges. In forensic psychiatry, a thorough assessment requires the assessing clinician to possess appropriate skills and expertise, and to have access to adequate information about the patient and the legal background to the case. Issues relating to security, confidentiality, consent and the implications of the assessment require careful consideration. There are also a number of legal issues that merit discussion.

Practical considerations

Before a new patient is seen the forensic psychiatrist needs to know who has referred them and why. They also need to be familiar with the background to the case. It may be possible to provide some paperwork by fax, but large volumes of notes and bundles of legal papers will have to be sent by post or courier.

There are resource implications for training clinicians using telemedicine. Those who use it should be familiar with the equipment, its operation and limitations, and means of safeguarding confidentiality and security.[25,26] They should also ensure that they maintain good medical records and make suitable arrangements for storing notes. The American Psychiatric Association recommends that if the record is kept at the site where the patient is, a copy should also be kept at the site of the treating clinician for routine care and in case of emergencies.[25]

If the forensic psychiatrist is providing treatment they should have a working relationship with the prison or local mental health services where the patient is located. This should include suitable arrangements for communicating information and providing ongoing care and supervision. The need for good communication is especially important in forensic psychiatry because of the nature and severity of the risks posed by MDOs.

Videoconferencing equipment needs to be set up in a room that is suitable for conducting an interview in comfort and privacy. There must be a connection to the network used to transmit and receive information and, assuming the equipment is to be stored there, the room must be suitably secure. This can be a problem in secure hospitals and prisons where space is at a premium. The equipment has to be operated and maintained. If the equipment fails and it cannot be serviced on site it may take a long time to arrange for equipment located in a secure setting to be taken away, repaired and reinstalled. Staff are also required to supervise patients whilst they are being interviewed.[25] This has implications for confidentiality, especially if the patient is a prisoner. Low staffing levels in prison may prevent the equipment being used at all.

Videoconferencing has been used with patients suffering from mental illness,[27-29] and in America Zaylor et al[30] have reported some success using telepsychiatry in a prison setting (see Chapter 10). However, commonsense suggests that it would be unwise to try and use the equipment with a MDO or any other patient who is very disturbed, aroused and aggressive.

Ethical aspects

A small number of studies have looked at the reliability of psychiatric diagnoses and assessments of psychopathology using videoconferencing,[27-29] but more research is needed to investigate the pitfalls of assessing patients using telepsychiatry. The forensic psychiatrist who considers using videoconferencing to interview a patient must consider the potential limitations, because the conclusions they draw from their assessment, for example in relation to risk assessment, may have far-reaching implications for the patient and potential victims.

Having a third party present during the interview raises issues of confidentiality, particularly if the patient being assessed is a prisoner. Forensic psychiatrists using videoconferencing facilities to assess patients should follow standard guidance on confidentiality such as that produced by the General Medical Council[31] and the Royal College of Psychiatrists,[32] and systems should be developed to maintain security and protect confidential patient information that is transmitted.[33]

The consulting psychiatrist's role and their responsibilities must be clearly defined. At the outset of the interview the forensic psychiatrist should explain the nature and purpose of the assessment and the limits of confidentiality to the patient as they would if they were seeing them face to face. Also, an explanation of the benefits of using videoconferencing and, very importantly, the possible limitations must be provided in order to obtain the patient's consent. The patient should be assured that if they choose not to take part, care will not be withheld. However, what care they do receive may be subject to available resources.

Legal aspects

It has been suggested that in legal terms, a telemedicine consultation is deemed to have occurred where the patient is rather than where the clinician is.[34] In countries such as the USA and Australia where legislation varies from state to state, the consulting psychiatrist should ensure that they have the appropriate credentials, a suitable license and malpractice cover assessments of patients in a given state.

In the USA telepsychiatry assessments have been used for involuntary commitment[25,35] and Yellowlees[36] has described the use of telemedicine to perform assessments under the Mental Health Act in New South Wales. In England and Wales the current 1983 Mental Health Act requires that medical recommendations 'shall be given by practitioners who have personally examined the patient'.[10] There have been no reports yet of videoconferencing being used for examinations under the English Act. If this is not tested whilst the current Act remains in force it will certainly need to be considered for the new Mental Health Act.

There are other issues relating to malpractice and liability that the forensic psychiatrist should consider. There is an assumption that the foundation of the teleconsulting doctor's duty to a patient is the same as that which any conventional doctor owes to any patient. This means that the doctor may incur liability at any time after accepting responsibility for the patient.[37] In forensic psychiatry this situation is complicated by the fact that forensic psychiatrists routinely undertake work which involves a duty to others. Breaches of security and confidentiality may result in the disclosure of highly sensitive information about patients and third parties such as victims. In England and Wales general principles of the common law duty of confidentiality and the 1998 Data Protection Act apply to videoconferencing; other legislation relating to computer hacking and eavesdropping may also be relevant.[37]

In England and Wales a doctor is not guilty of malpractice if it can be shown that he or she has acted in accordance with the practice of a responsible body of professionals skilled in that art.[38] One difficulty for forensic psychiatrists is that there are relatively few examples of integrated telepsychiatry systems in operation and even fewer in the field of forensic psychiatry. So far the courts have not considered standards of care involving this technique and the extent of liability and professional negligence in telepsychiatric practice is still to be determined.[37,39]

Experience to date

A wide variety of studies concerning telemedicine in general have been conducted in different settings throughout the world. However, there are relatively few studies of telepsychiatry and these tend to focus on satisfaction and cost effectiveness.[40] Some studies have looked at the reliability of using such a method.[27,29,41–46] These studies indicate that telepsychiatry does offer the potential to extend treatments to individuals who may otherwise be neglected due to remoteness, security and at times reduced staffing levels.

Telepsychiatry in correctional facilities in the USA

In the USA the American Psychiatric Association report on the work undertaken by the Michigan Department of Corrections project indicates that significant savings have been made. The report advocates that telepsychiatry can be used in courts, prisons and other secure settings.[25]

Telepsychiatry applications have been used in the US prison service. Zaylor et al[30] established a telepsychiatry pilot between the Kansas University Medical Center and Lyon County Jail. Their main findings indicate that moderately to severely ill inmates with a broad range of psychiatric illness can be seen and treated effectively using a videoconferencing system. Further work by Zaylor et al[47] has also shown the service to be effective from both the prisoners' and the psychiatrists' perspective in terms of satisfaction. Forensic telepsychiatry services have also been reported to be a cost-effective method of health care delivery in the USA (see Chapter 10).[48]

Telepsychiatry in prisons in England and Wales

In the UK there have been few studies of the suitability of using videoconferencing equipment to deliver services to MDOs and none appear to have been published.

In June 2001 the Wessex Forensic Service established a telepsychiatry service at Parkhurst Prison on the Isle of Wight. This service supplements the weekly visiting forensic psychiatric service and is used to provide psychiatric assessment and follow-up of prisoners. In December 2001 this service was underpinned with a research study. The purpose of the study was to determine whether the videoconferencing facility provides a robust method of assessing patients' psychopathology.

The Manchester Crown Court video-link project

While this study is not strictly telepsychiatry it is relevant to MDOs. This pilot project involved the installation of a video link between Manchester Prison and Manchester

Crown Court to conduct plea and directions hearings. The purpose of the evaluation was to examine the suitability of the video link for conducting preliminary hearings in the Crown Court. The evaluation of this system involved 92 Crown Court hearings conducted over the link between September 1999 and April 2000. The following areas were investigated:

- the configuration and performance of the video link
- the effect of the video link on the relationship between advocate and client
- the arrangements for pre- and post-hearing consultations between lawyer and client
- the scheduling and length of hearings
- the effectiveness of consultation about new working practice
- the impact of the link on the prison regime
- the associated training needs.

The evaluation concluded that the use of technology could significantly enhance security, reducing the need to transport prisoners. It also found that 76% of defendants preferred to be in prison for their hearing rather than travelling to the court. Some initial difficulties with equipment and sound quality were encountered but quickly resolved, and generally the equipment was found to be reliable. Issues surrounding confidentiality were raised with concerns relating to conversations conducted between lawyer and client. The importance of joint working was highlighted and the need to maintain a strategic approach when wider implementation commences. Training of all those who participate in video-link hearings was recommended. Some cost savings were identified; it was felt that the benefits and savings would be made predominately by the prison service.[49]

Since 1999 video-link hearings between the Court and Prison Service have become more accepted as a routine service. Plans are currently under way to extend these services further. It is expected that by September 2002, 57 prisons and 156 magistrates courts will be using the new technology.

Hospital inpatient and community forensic services in England and Wales

Forensic psychiatric services in south-east London and the Maudsley hospital are embarking on a feasibility study of using videoconferencing to follow up MDOs in custodial, community and out-of-area secure hospital settings. The study will focus on the practical aspects of using the system, such as cost implications, the training needs of staff, and equipment and systems requirements. It will also examine the potential for facilitating the transfer of MDOs to hospital and discharge planning.

Conclusions

In forensic psychiatry videoconferencing offers real opportunities to help reduce the level of health care inequality experienced by MDOs. It has the potential to improve access to a better range and quality of services for a population that is hard to reach by conventional means, to substantially reduce the time it takes for assessments to be carried out, and to help improve communication between the various agencies involved. Videoconferencing also has a role in providing education, training and support to staff, which should in turn benefit patients.

English courts are now using video links to reduce the need to escort prisoners to court. Reducing the amount of time it takes to obtain psychiatric reports by making more use of videoconferencing facilities could speed the progress of MDOs through the criminal justice system. Policy-makers will no doubt support such developments because they appear to be cost effective.

Nevertheless, the use of videoconferencing in forensic psychiatry raises some very important ethical and legal questions. We do not fully understand how assessments and treatment conducted by telepsychiatry resemble conventional psychiatric practice and how it differs. Bearing in mind that the conclusions drawn from a psychiatric assessment can have significant implications for a mentally disordered offender, questions about the reliability and validity of such assessments carried out using telepsychiatry are very relevant to forensic psychiatry.

References

1   United Kingdom Central Council for Nursing. *Nursing in Secure Environments*. London: UKCC, 1999.
2   Johnson R, Taylor R, eds. *Statistics of Mentally Disordered Offenders 2000, England and Wales*. London: Home Office, Research Development and Statistics Directorate, 2001.
3   Walmsley R. *World Prison Population List*, 2nd edn. London: Home Office Research Development and Statistics Directorate, 2000.
4   Fazel S, Danesh J. Serious mental disorder in 23 000 prisoners: a systematic review of 62 surveys. *Lancet* 2002;**359**:545–550.
5   Birmingham L. Diversion from custody. *Advances in Psychiatric Treatment* 2001;**7**:198–207.
6   Snowden P, McKenna J, Jasper A. Management of conditionally discharged patients and others who pose similar risks in the community: integrated or parallel? *Journal of Forensic Psychiatry* 1999;**10**:583–596.
7   Smith R. Prisoners: an end to second class health care? *British Medical Journal* 1999;**318**:954–955.
8   Reed J, Lyne M. The quality of health care in prison: results of a year's programme of semi-structured inspections. *British Medical Journal* 1997;**315**:1420–1424.
9   Reed J, Lyne M. Inpatient care of mentally ill people in prison: results of a year's programme of semistructured inspections. *British Medical Journal* 2000;**320**:1031–1034.
10   Department of Health and Social Security. *The Mental Health Act 1983*. London: HMSO, 1983.
11   Reith M, ed. *Community Care Tragedies: a practice guide to mental health inquiries*. Birmingham: Ventura, 1998.
12   Department of Health. *Modernising Mental Health Services, Safe Sound and Supportive*. London: HMSO, 1998.
13   Department of Health. *The National Service Framework for Mental Health*. London: HMSO, 1999.
14   Department of Health. *The NHS Plan. A plan for investment a plan for reform*. London: HMSO, 2000.
15   Department of Health. *Reforming the Mental Health Act 1983*. Cm5016: I and II. London: HMSO, 2000.
16   Butler RA. *Report of the Committee on Mentally Abnormal Offenders*. London: HMSO, 1975.
17   Reed R. The need for longer-term psychiatric care in medium or low security. *Criminal Behaviour and Mental Health* 1997;**7**:201–212.
18   Department of Health and Home Office. *Review of Health and Social Services for Mentally Disordered Offenders and Others Requiring Similar Services: final summary report*. London: HMSO, 1992.
19   James D. Court diversion at 10 years: can it work, does it work and has it a future? *Journal of Forensic Psychiatry*. 1999;**10**:507–524.
20   Department of Health. *Report of the Review of Security at the High Security Hospitals*. London: HMSO, 2000.

21 Prison Service and NHS Executive Working Group. *The Future Organisation of Prison Health Care.* London: HMSO, 1999.

22 Reid D, John B, Toone H, Storey C. Video-conferencing in community mental health care: a pilot study of psychiatric assessment. *Mental Health Care* 2000;**3**:156–159.

23 Kavanagh SJ, Yellowlees PM. Telemedicine – clinical applications in mental health. *Australian Family Physician* 1995;**24**:1242–1247.

24 Baer L, Elford R, Cukor P. Telepsychiatry at forty: what have we learned? *Harvard Review Psychiatry* 1997;**5**:7–17.

25 American Psychiatric Association. *Resource Document on Telepsychiatry Via Videoconferencing.* 1998. Available at http://www.psych.org/archives/980021.pdf [last checked 16 September 2002].

26 World Medical Association Statement on Accountability, Responsibilities and Ethical Guidelines in the Practice of Telemedicine. Adopted by the 51st World Medical Assembly, Tel Aviv, Israel, October 1999. Available at http://www.wma.net/e/policy/17–36_e.html [last checked 16 September 2002].

27 Baer L, Cukor P, Jenike MA, Leahy L, O'Laughlen J, Coyle J. Pilot studies of telemedicine in psychiatric patients with obsessive-compulsive disorder. *American Journal of Psychiatry* 1995;**152**:1383–1385.

28 Ruskin PE, Reed S, Kumar R, et al. Reliability and acceptability of psychiatric diagnosis via telecommunication and audiovisual technology. *Psychiatric Services* 1998;**49**:1086–1088.

29 Zarate CA Jr, Weinstock L, Cukor P, et al. Applicability of telemedicine for assessing patients with schizophrenia; acceptance and reliability. *Journal of Clinical Psychiatry* 1997;**58**:22–25.

30 Zaylor C, Whitten P, Kingsley C. Telemedicine services to a county jail. *Journal of Telemedicine and Telecare* 2000;**6**(suppl 1):93–95.

31 General Medical Council. *Confidentiality: protecting and providing information.* London: General Medical Council, 2000.

32 Royal College of Psychiatrists. *Good Psychiatric Practice: confidentiality.* Council Report CR 85. London: Royal College of Psychiatrists, 2000.

33 Stanberry B. The legal and ethical aspects of telemedicine. 1:Confidentiality and the patient's right of access. *Journal of Telemedicine and Telecare* 1997;**3**:179–187.

34 Norwell N. Hang-on-a-minute.com. *Journal of the Medical Defence Union* 2000;**16**:6–7.

35 Bear D, Jacobson G, Aaronson S, Hanson A. Telemedicine in psychiatry – making the dream a reality. *American Journal of Psychiatry* 1997;**154**:884–885.

36 Yellowlees P. The use of telemedicine to perform psychiatric assessments under the Mental Health Act. *Journal of Telemedicine and Telecare* 1997;**3**:224–226.

37 Stanberry B. Medicolegal aspects of telemedicine. In: Wootton R, Craig J, eds. *Introduction to Telemedicine.* London: Royal Society of Medicine Press, 1999: 159–175.

38 Bolam v. Friern Hospital Management Committee [1957] 1 WLR 582.

39 Merideth P. Forensic applications of telepsychiatry. *Psychiatric Annals* 1999;**29**:429–431.

40 Mair F, Whitten P. Systematic review of studies of patient satisfaction with telemedicine. *British Medical Journal* 2000;**320**:1517–1520.

41 Ball CJ, Scott N, McLaren PM, Watson JP. Preliminary evaluation of a Low-Cost VideoConferencing (LCVC) system for remote cognitive testing of adult psychiatric patients. *British Journal of Clinical Psychology* 1993;**32**:303–307.

42 Salzman C, Orvin D, Hanson A, Kalinowski A. Patient evaluation through live video transmission. *American Journal of Psychiatry* 1996;**153**:968.

43 Baigent MF, Lloyd CJ, Kavanagh SJ, et al. Telepsychiatry 'tele' yes, but what about the 'psychiatry'? *Journal of Telemedicine and Telecare* 1997;**3**(suppl 1):3–5.

44 Elford R, White H, Bowering R, et al. A randomized, controlled trial of child psychiatric assessments conducted using videoconferencing. *Journal of Telemedicine and Telecare* 2000;**6**:73–82.

45 Brodey BB, Claypoole KH, Motto J, Arias RG, Goss R. Satisfaction of forensic psychiatric patients with a remote telepsychiatry evaluation. *Psychiatric Services* 2000;**51**:1305–1307.

46 Jones BN, Johnston D, Reboussin B, McCall WV. Reliability of telepsychiatry assessments: subjective versus observational ratings. *Journal of Geriatric Psychiatry and Neurology* 2001;**14**:66–71.

47 Zaylor C, Nelson E, Cook DJ. Clinical outcomes in a prison telepsychiatry clinic. *Journal of Telemedicine and Telecare* 2001;**7**(suppl 1):47–49.

48 Zollo S, Kienzle M, Loeffelholz P, Sebille S. Telemedicine to IOWA's correctional facilities: initial clinical experience and assessment of program costs. *Telemedicine Journal* 1999;**5**:291–301.

49 Evaluation of video link pilot project at Manchester Crown Court. Available at http://www.hmprisonservice. gov.uk/library/dynpage.asp?Page=262 [last checked 23 October 2002].

12

Telemedicine for Child and Adolescent Psychiatry

Harry Gelber and Jean Starling

Introduction

Child and adolescent psychiatry aims to alleviate serious psychiatric disturbance in children and adolescents by providing assessment and treatment services. Within the subspecialty of child and adolescent psychiatry, further specialist streams are developing. For example, infant mental health is a subspecialty developing in response to increasing knowledge about early infancy and childhood. Adolescent mental health is also a long-established subspecialty. These areas demand extra training and workers in child and adolescent psychiatry generally receive further education and ongoing supervision to enhance their specialist skills.

Child and adolescent mental health services (CAMHS) in rural regions are often unable to attract professionals who offer the range of specialist expertise needed to meet the complex needs of children, adolescents and their families. Those who do work in rural areas face difficulties due to their isolation. These difficulties include isolation from their peers, the demand that they offer services across a range of specialties, burnout and low retention rates. As a consequence, attracting and retaining specialist staff in rural locations is difficult.

Given the imbalance in resources between metropolitan and rural CAMHS, innovative strategies are needed. Videoconferencing may be useful to rural staff for a number of reasons:

▶ accessing a range of specialist advice which would not normally be available

▶ meeting case managers with whom they are working closely

▶ 'visiting' their child or adolescent during admission to inpatient units

▶ maintaining contact with case managers after the child or adolescent has returned home.

In this context the development of telepsychiatry has emerged as an important tool in enhancing service delivery in several areas of Australia. Two services are described below.

Brief literature review

There is a growing literature related to telemedicine generally and to telepsychiatry. However, most of the work on telepsychiatry concerns adults. There are relatively few reports specific to child and adolescent telepsychiatry.

One of the first CAMHS to use telepsychiatry was in Melbourne, which began a pilot project in 1995 to provide services for rural areas of Victoria.[1] Following an evaluation of the pilot, it was expanded[1,2] (see case study 1 below). Subsequently, a child and adolescent telemedicine psychological outreach service (CAPTOS) was established in Sydney. The pilot service started in 1996, from the Children's Hospital at Westmead.[3] It too, was evaluated and then expanded in 1999[4] (see case study 2 below).

In the USA, the University of Kansas Medical Center's long-established telemedicine programme has a child and adolescent telepsychiatry clinic which links the medical center and a county mental health center in rural Pittsburg, Kansas. The clinic provides 10–18 consultations per week and has been able to serve severely disturbed children and children in crisis. The quality of clinical interactions in the telepsychiatry clinic is reported to be comparable to that in face-to-face meetings.[5]

All these reports suggest that telepsychiatry works well for children and adolescents. To that extent, they are reassuring, although as an evidence base the reports are largely anecdotal. There appears to have been only one formal study of the efficacy of telepsychiatry for child and adolescent work. In Canada, Elford et al[6] set up a child and adolescent telepsychiatry project in Newfoundland. They conducted a randomized controlled trial to compare diagnoses, treatment recommendations and other outcome measures between patients seen by videoconferencing and the same patients seen face to face. There were no significant differences in outcome,[6] and the cost of telepsychiatry was less than the patients' travel costs.[7]

What do the users think? There are few reports of user satisfaction with child telepsychiatry. Dongier et al[8] found no difference in patient satisfaction between telemedicine and usual care. Blackmon[9] found that all nine children and 98% of the 46 parents surveyed reported that they were as satisfied with the telemedicine consultation as with an in-person visit. Elford et al[7] completed a comprehensive evaluation of user satisfaction with a videoconferencing system used for child psychiatry. They found that the pilot telepsychiatry service was successful in that both parents and children "liked using it".[7]

Case study 1: Melbourne

Pilot service

The Royal Children's Hospital in Melbourne established a pilot project in 1995. In the period April–August 1995, a total of 38 videoconferences took place linked with three sites.[10] This included 29 clinical secondary consultations, five primary consultations with clients and four administrative meetings.

Evaluation of the pilot

A total of 125 evaluation questionnaires were returned from videoconference participants who made use of the equipment during the trial period. The evaluation found evidence of a number of benefits to consumers and clinicians from the introduction of telepsychiatry to regional services. Not only had it enabled much more interaction between staff at distant sites, supporting remote workers who often had limited professional contact, but it also allowed for more involvement of rural-based staff in the client and family assessment and in the treatment process. Case conferences could be held regularly between metropolitan and rural facilities through videoconferencing.[10]

The evaluation of the pilot resulted in a number of recommendations to enhance the service and facilitate the integration of telepsychiatry into the mainstream service delivery system of the Royal Children's Hospital. The main recommendations included:

▷ incorporating videoconferencing into the consultation process offered to regional services, rather than offering it as a stand-alone service

▷ preparing orientation materials, including protocols and standard forms to obtain informed consent

▷ introducing an ongoing monitoring framework and process

▷ consumer representation on the monitoring body.

These recommendations are in line with some of Yellowlees' principles of successful development of telemedicine systems.[11] Their subsequent implementation may be a reason why the service has been well accepted.

New clinical applications

The main purpose of the pilot project was to test the effectiveness of telepsychiatry as an innovative clinical tool. In addition, various new clinical applications have been developed.

Pre-admission work

The use of telepsychiatry has allowed families to participate in the preliminary clinical assessment of their child or adolescent without the need to travel long distances. Where this assessment leads to the clinicians and family deciding on an admission to an inpatient unit, the family have the benefit through the telepsychiatry experience of having already met the staff who will provide treatment.

Case conferences

Telepsychiatry has enabled rural workers to be involved in the decision-making process about assessment and treatment alternatives. This is important because in the past rural workers have felt isolated through their inability to travel, thereby losing contact with their clients.

Parent and family interviews

The project team has been able to include parents in the treatment process through the use of telepsychiatry. This has meant that parents have not had to travel while remaining actively involved in the treatment of their child as an inpatient in Melbourne. A key protocol, which developed out of the pilot was the importance of the rural worker being present for any telepsychiatry session involving their clients.

Post discharge

Similar to the pre-admission work, the availability of telepsychiatry has facilitated continuity of care and enabled rural workers to have ongoing support from the Royal Children's Hospital Mental Health Service (RCHMHS) team following discharge.

Education and training

A further use of telepsychiatry has been to provide education and training to community-based rural workers. This has been popular because it is a cost-effective method of receiving expertise and training that they would not normally have received. Telepsychiatry has also strengthened links between rural CAMHS and community-based rural workers. The Royal Children's Hospital, in collaboration with the Bendigo Health Care Group division of psychiatry, have also implemented a major mental health education initiative to rural Victoria using telepsychiatry.[12]

Current status

In the 5-year period ending December 2001 a total of 587 videoconferences took place across five rural sites. The purposes were 475 clinical secondary consultations and supervisory sessions, 93 inpatient assessments and consultations, and 19 education and training sessions.

Five key features have characterized the successful development of the pilot into a routine service.

1. *Collaborative relationships and the culture of partnership.* From the outset, there was a culture of partnership between the participants in the mental health service and in the rural CAMHS.

2. *Consumer participation.* From the outset the project team spoke with service users who had difficulty in accessing the CAMHS because of the long distances they needed to travel. The project team also monitored every videoconference by inviting the participants to answer a questionnaire. In addition, a former parent user of telepsychiatry had been engaged to advise the service on how to be more consumer friendly. The development of user-friendly information and an informed consent process for parents was one example of her contribution.

3. *Broadening clinical applications.* During the pilot phase of the project the clinical applications had only begun to be used. Once the pilot was found to be successful (after September 1995) the equipment was used for a wide range of clinical activities including pre-admission work, case conferences, parent and family sessions, post-discharge interviews and education and training.

4. *Technology as a tool.* Staff at the Royal Children's Hospital and in rural areas were anxious that the technology would not replace face-to-face contact, particularly in the context of the economic pressure in Victoria for service providers to use less costly interventions.

5. *Evaluation.* There has been a commitment to continuing evaluation.

Case study 2: Sydney

Pilot service

The Child and Adolescent Psychological Telemedicine Outreach Service (CAPTOS) started as a pilot service from the Westmead Children's Hospital in Sydney to two sites (Dubbo and Burke) in New South Wales (NSW). The pilot service began in December 1996.[3] In the period to July 1997 there were 72 videoconferencing interviews and 54 patients were seen.

Evaluation of the pilot

Although only 24% of families returned the questionnaire, they reported a high level of satisfaction with the service. Rural clinicians and rural families expressed high levels of satisfaction with the services: 96% of families and 99% of rural clinicians rated the quality of service as good or excellent, were very or mostly satisfied with the services they required, and felt that they received the service that they wanted.

After the evaluation of the pilot, the NSW health department provided funds for staff and equipment so that the service could be extended from the Children's Hospital to all of remote and rural NSW (except for the southern area) (Fig. 12.1). This service was evaluated between September 1999 and September 2000 inclusive.[4] Data were collected from 136 telepsychiatry consultations.

The mean age of the young people seen was 11.9 years (SD 3.7, range 4–23 years), 65% were male and 28% had safety or at-risk issues. The most common diagnostic group seen were the behaviour disorders (37%), followed by depression (22%) and anxiety disorders (13%).

There was disagreement between rural families and clinicians at the Children's Hospital about their satisfaction with technology. Rural families found that the equipment was easy to use (97%) and interfered little with the consultation (97%). Less than half of the clinicians (48%) found the equipment easy to use, although 87% felt that it did not interfere with the consultation. Rural families felt that the sound (91%), visual (95%) and overall quality (96%) were good or excellent. By contrast, clinicians were less happy with the technology. Overall, only 26% were happy with the sound, 14% with the visual quality and 18% with the overall quality. Finally, 91% of rural families felt that telepsychiatry was as good or almost as good as a face-to-face consultation, compared to 16% of the clinicians.

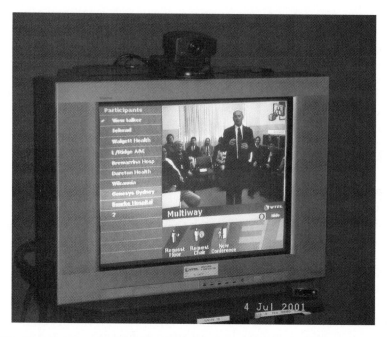

Fig. 12.1. Craig Knowles, the State Health Minister, launching the CAPTOS service to the Far West region, one of eight areas of New South Wales. The launch was held in July 2001, with a multipoint videoconference (Broken Hill, Bourke, Dareton, Lightening Ridge, Walgett, Brewarrina Wilcannia and the Children's Hospital). The minister was at Bourke.

New clinical applications

Telenursing

The CAPTOS telenursing service started in late 2001.[13] The Clinical Nurse Consultancy (CNC) Service serves a network of 27 rural wards throughout NSW. At times, all of these wards care for children or young people with mental health problems. These young people may be unsuitable for a gazetted unit because of their presenting problem, age or developmental level. There may also be no appropriate psychiatric beds available. The nurses on these wards rarely have specialized training in child and adolescent mental health. They want to support rural families in obtaining local treatment, but are concerned that they are being asked to perform tasks beyond their level of education and experience.[14] The CAPTOS telenursing initiative aims to enhance the skills of rural nurses using the Caplan model.[15] The focus of the CNC Service can be clinical supervision, patient management issues or problem solving for a specific situation. The CAPTOS CNC also offers rural site visits as well as the telemedicine consultations.

Professional skills training

Training programmes were begun when it became clear that some rural clinicians lacked the skills to implement treatment recommendations. Family therapy was the most requested clinical skill. Since 2001, three rural teams have been involved in family therapy training. A rural area forms a training group of clinicians, and a children's hospital clinician skilled in family therapy becomes the supervisor. Preliminary theoretical reading is sent out, and the group meets once face to face to plan the course, which lasts 12 months. The group then meets via videoconferencing for tutorials and case discussions. At the end of the 12-month period the group has acquired basic family therapy assessment and treatment skills. A similar model is being piloted for individual work with children and adolescents. A children's hospital psychotherapist participates in theoretical and case discussions with a group of rural clinicians via videoconferencing.

Sabbaticals for rural clinicians
Rural clinicians often have limited access to formal training, and few other ways of accessing evidence on good practice. Even Internet access is poor in some rural areas. Because of this, CAPTOS has been offering 1-week sabbaticals to rural clinicians. The rural clinicians negotiate learning goals for their visit with their child and adolescent mental health area director, and are supported by a children's hospital clinician on their visit. The goals can vary from learning a clinical skill, researching a specific topic or even writing a policy document. The visit not only helps to achieve learning goals, but also allows the rural clinician to feel part of a wider CAPTOS network.

Clinical skills workshop
In December 2001, CAPTOS coordinated a workshop for 42 clinicians from eight rural areas, with the goals of developing a collegiate network across rural areas and developing clinical skills. The event was very successful.

Current status
The CAPTOS service currently links all eight rural and remote areas of NSW. There are 25 videoconferencing units in community health or psychiatry facilities, and this number is increasing. There are also videoconferencing units in hospitals for nursing and other hospital staff to access. About eight half-day sessions per week of child psychiatry are offered across the areas and more than 300 new patients a year are seen. Extra time is allocated for telenursing and other forms of supervision and teaching.

Conclusions

The experience of the two services described above is that telepsychiatry has facilitated the development of partnerships between mental health clinicians across the region. There are now more opportunities for rural CAMHS clinicians in Victoria and NSW to access specialist mental health training opportunities via telepsychiatry than there were 5 years ago. Notwithstanding the technological advances in recent years, and the benefits that the participants have identified, one of the common themes to emerge is that the full benefit of telepsychiatry will only be realized when the equipment is more effective and participants feel comfortable with its use.

Yellowlees[16] has argued that traditional evaluations of telehealth programmes ask the wrong questions. They should be asking if the telehealth programme is useful enough to be part of clinical practice. The experience described in this chapter suggests that telepsychiatry is a useful and essential part of clinical practice in child and adolescent psychiatry.

Nonetheless, it is clear that the task of integrating the use of telepsychiatry is a continuing one for child and adolescent psychiatry services. Yellowlees' solution was to propose *nurturing, experience and success*, complemented by a national forum or association supported by the federal government.[16] By *nurturing*, Yellowlees meant 'the provision of money, ideas, education, training and innovation'. *Experience* referred to 'an integrated management process, the achievement of long and wide patterns of usage, the development of updated policies and procedures and the involvement of multiple disciplines'. *Success* referred to 'evidence of outcomes, evaluation and research and, most important, the sharing of information through scientific and popular press publications, and conferences and collaborations with internal and external groups'.

Yellowlees' recommendations could be proposed as a gold standard for all telemedicine work, not only that in the field of mental health. The child and adolescent telepsychiatry programmes described above can only claim to have achieved some of the elements of Yellowlees' vision so far. Their full realization will require appropriate structures, processes and continuing commitment to improvement and evaluation.

References

1 Gelber H, Alexander M. An evaluation of an Australian videoconferencing project for child and adolescent telepsychiatry. *Journal of Telemedicine and Telecare* 1999;**5**(suppl 1):21–23.
2 Gelber H. The experience in Victoria with telepsychiatry for the child and adolescent mental health service. *Journal of Telemedicine and Telecare* 2001;**7**(suppl 2):32–34.
3 Dossetor DR, Nunn KP, Fairley M, Eggleton D. A child and adolescent psychiatric outreach service for rural New South Wales: a telemedicine pilot study. *Journal of Paediatrics and Child Health* 1999;**35**:525–529.
4 Kopel H, Nunn K, Dossetor D. Evaluating satisfaction with a child and adolescent psychological telemedicine outreach service. *Journal of Telemedicine and Telecare* 2001;**7**(suppl 2):35–40.
5 Ermer DJ. Experience with a rural telepsychiatry clinic for children and adolescents. *Psychiatric Services* 1999;**50**:260–261.
6 Elford R, White H, Bowering R, et al. A randomized, controlled trial of child psychiatric assessments conducted using videoconferencing. *Journal of Telemedicine and Telecare* 2000;**6**:73–82.
7 Elford DR, White H, St John K, Maddigan B, Ghandi M, Bowering R. A prospective satisfaction study and cost analysis of a pilot child telepsychiatry service in Newfoundland. *Journal of Telemedicine and Telecare* 2001;**7**:73–81.
8 Dongier M, Tempier R, Lalinec-Michaud M, Meunier D. Telepsychiatry: psychiatric consultation through two-way television. A controlled study. *Canadian Journal of Psychiatry* 1986;**31**:32–34.
9 Blackmon LA, Kaak HO, Ranseen J. Consumer satisfaction with telemedicine child psychiatry consultation in rural Kentucky. *Psychiatric Services* 1997;**48**:1464–1466.
10 Blaskett B. *Personal Connections: an evaluation of the Royal Children's Hospital Mental Health Service Videoconferencing Project.* Parkville, Victoria: Social Work Department, Royal Children's Hospital, 1996.
11 Yellowlees P. Successful development of telemedicine systems – seven core principles. *Journal of Telemedicine and Telecare* 1997;**3**:215–222.
12 Fahey A, Gelber H. *Tele-education: a collaborative project in the delivery of mental health education in rural Victoria.* Victoria: Bendigo Health Care Group and Royal Children's Hospital Mental Health Service, 2001.

13   Rosina R, Starling J, Nunn K, Dossetor D, Bridgland K. CAPTOS Telenursing: clinical nurse consultancy for rural paediatric nurses. *Journal of Telemedicine and Telecare* 2002;**8**(suppl 3):48–49.

14   Hegney D, McCarthy A. Job satisfaction and nurses in rural Australia. *Journal of Nursing Administration* 2000;**30**:347–350.

15   Caplan G, ed. *The Theory and Practice of Mental Health Consultation.* London: Tavistock Publications, 1970.

16   Yellowlees P. An analysis of why telehealth systems in Australia have not always succeeded. *Journal of Telemedicine and Telecare* 2001;**7**(suppl 2):29–31.

13

The Use of Videoconferencing in Clinical Psychology

Susan Simpson

Introduction

Clinical psychology is one of the smallest health care professions, comprising only 3% of the NHS workforce in Scotland, a problem compounded by 20% of posts in the UK being vacant. Attempts to address this shortfall have included psychologists adopting a larger role in teaching and training. Supervision and consultancy to other professionals is an increasingly cost-effective way of delivering psychological treatments.

Livingstone[1] described the difficulties of recruiting psychologists to remote areas and noted that most posts are filled by new graduates, who have a greater need for supervision and support. In these areas, professional isolation and opportunities for professional development are extremely limited. In addition, rural-based psychologists are often expected to function as 'specialist generalists' and may be the most qualified mental health practitioner in the area. Geographical impediments have been addressed through letter writing,[2] the telephone,[3,4] email,[5] 'online' communications[6,7] and videoconferencing.

Videoconferencing in clinical psychology

Psychological assessments

Psychological assessments are usually accomplished through face-to-face interviews and standardized psychometric instruments. Most studies in this area have been reported by psychiatrists. Baer et al[8] assessed patients with obsessive-compulsive disorder by both videoconferencing and face to face. Inter-rater reliability was found to be high (0.97–0.99) for scores obtained by interview on the Hamilton Anxiety Rating Scale, the Hamilton Depression Rating Scale and the Yale–Brown Obsessive Compulsive Scale. Zarate et al[9] reported that patients with schizophrenia could be reliably assessed via face-to-face, low- and high-bandwidth videoconferencing systems. No significant differences were found using the Brief Psychiatric Rating Scale and the Scale for the Assessment of Positive Symptoms in all three settings. The Scale for the Assessment of Negative Symptoms produced less reliable results in the low-bandwidth condition due to it being more difficult to detect less obvious non-verbal information from patients.

Psychometric testing

Psychometric assessments detect changes in psychological functions such as those recurring after head injury or dementia. Ball et al[10] tested a group of psychiatric patients via face-to-face and low-cost videoconferencing conditions within 48 hours of each other using the Mini-Mental State Examination (MMSE). A high correlation was found between groups (r = 0.89–0.92).

A similar study by Ball and Puffett[11] examined the reliability of the CAMCOG (a subsection of the CAMDEX structured interview schedule designed to identify early cognitive impairment) via videoconferencing using a PC-based unit at 128 kbit/s. Correlations between subtests ranged from 0.10 (calculation) to 0.84 (memory), suggesting that reliability levels vary widely between subtests and that caution should be exercised when interpreting results. It was suggested that these variations were due to intermittent technical problems caused by the relocation of telecommunication lines within the hospital site.

Montani et al[12] tested 15 hospitalized elderly patients using the MMSE, and the Clock Face Test (CFT), a measure of cognitive and visuospatial ability, 8 days apart. The videoconferencing equipment consisted of a television screen, microphone and a camera which could be focused remotely by the psychologist. Correlations between face-to-face and videoconferencing assessments were high on the MMSE (r = 0.95) and lower on the CFT (r = 0.55). In a similar study Montani et al[13] found that these tests were reliable via videoconferencing for patients with dementia, but not for those without cognitive impairment. It was suggested that the quality of the sessions might have been influenced by the lack of direct eye contact and poor sound quality.

Troster et al[14] reported a neuropsychological assessment via videoconferencing in conjunction with a psychometrician at the remote site, who had been trained in test administration and scoring. The neuropsychologist received information about the patient prior to appointments and then met the patient for up to 60 minutes for a videoconferenced interview. Following this, he was able to advise the psychometrician about which tests to administer. These were then scored and returned to the neuropsychologist for interpretation. The results were then communicated to the patient and family via videoconferencing. Reliability was not reported.

Kirkwood[15] found that neuropsychological testing could be reliably administered via videoconferencing at 128 kbit/s. He assessed a group of subjects with a history of alcohol abuse using a battery of cognitive tests which measured pre-morbid and current intellectual functioning, visual and verbal memory, and concentration levels. The assessments were made face to face and via videoconferencing on the same day. To minimize practice effects, a parallel version of the tests, except the NART (National Adult Reading Test), was used at the second testing. A number of modifications were necessary to carry out testing in the videoconferencing mode, including providing materials for each test in separate envelopes, making adjustments in light and brightness, and minimizing movement to ensure the clear presentation of visual material. For the majority of outcome measures, testing was found to be equally reliable for both modes.

Testing via videoconferencing produced less performance anxiety in participants, due to the absence of the assessor in the same room. Kirkwood suggested that inconsistencies in results obtained between presentation modes for the Quick Test and the Information Processing test were caused by difficulty hearing the instructions and image clarity.

Biggins[16] supported the notion that neuropsychological testing may be conducted via videoconferencing with adaptations in the way the material was presented using a slide projector, video-recorder and document camera. Although a health worker was recruited to assist in test administration, the testing was administered by a remote neuropsychologist. Twenty-eight subjects were tested using a battery of tests in face-to-face and videoconferencing modes. These included the National Adult Reading Test (Revised), the Weschler Adult Intelligence Test (Revised), the Rey–Auditory Verbal Learning Test, the Rey–Oesterriech Complex Figure Test, the Benton Visual Retention Test, the Boston Naming Test (short-form), the Controlled Oral Word Association Test and the Trail Making Test (forms A and B). No significant differences were found between test scores presented via face to face or videoconferencing, except on the Trail Making Test (form B) which is a measure of concentration, attention, information processing and executive functioning. In the videoconferencing mode the time delay may have affected performance of the test. The authors recommended that test instructions be kept clear and brief.

Rather than trying to adapt tests for videoconferencing use, it would be better to use tests specifically designed for administration by computer in the first instance. Some tests have already been developed for computerized administration, such as the Cambridge Neuropsychological Test Automated Battery (CANTAB), which covers a range of neuropsychological functions, and is administered on a computer with a touch-sensitive screen.[17]

The use of videoconferencing for psychological therapies

Most studies of remote psychological therapy have used a hybrid form of delivery with a face-to-face assessment followed by videoconferenced treatment. The earliest such report is from the University of Nebraska Medical Centre and provided training, education and psychiatric treatment via video link.[18] A group of clients were placed in one room facing a TV monitor, which displayed their therapist, while the therapist was in another room viewing the group on another monitor. Group psychotherapy was conducted in this way with four groups over six sessions. These were compared with four face-to-face groups. The diagnostic categories of the clients and the therapeutic model employed were not described. The presence of the TV monitor did not influence the therapists' or clients' views about treatment. The results showed that the choice of therapist and group members had more impact on the effectiveness of therapy and therapeutic alliance than the presence of the videoconferencing technology. However, data supporting these conclusions were not provided.

Acceptability to clients

The majority of studies published on this subject have reported that clients rate high levels of satisfaction with videoconferencing as a means of therapy delivery and in many cases would choose this modality over face to face. Simpson et al[19] found that nine out of ten clients from Shetland were satisfied with low-cost videotherapy sessions using a rollabout system at the hospital site, and a PC-based system at the remote site. Videoconferencing was conducted at a bandwidth of 128 kbit/s. Client satisfaction was shown to increase with experience and familiarity with the technology. It was also found to be adversely affected by sound and picture difficulties and by the complexity of their psychological difficulties. In another study by Simpson et al,[20] 10 out of 11 clients were satisfied with a single session of video-hypnosis and all indicated that they would like to have further video-hypnosis sessions in the future. This study used a set-top videoconferencing system at the hospital site and a rollabout system at the remote site connected at 384 kbit/s. Freir et al[21] reported on a sample of 27 adults and seven children (or their parents) in the Highlands of Scotland who were treated using a cognitive behavioural approach via low-cost videoconferencing units with a document imager. The majority indicated that they would accept further treatment via videoconferencing in the future. However, one third of participants rated a preference for face-to-face sessions. No reasons were given for this, but a number of technical problems with sound and picture were encountered.

In these Scottish studies, clients did not have the opportunity to experience both modes of treatment delivery and their 'preferences' may simply reflect a tendency to be satisfied with whatever was available. Clients included in these samples were self-selected and had indicated a desire to use video-therapy. This limits the generalizability of these results. In each of the studies by the author, there was one client who refused to take part. The client who dropped out of video-therapy was fearful that her sessions might have been watched or recorded without her knowledge. Her paranoid and avoidant personality traits may have made it more difficult to trust the therapist and technology. The client who did not participate in the video-hypnosis study was more concerned by the hypnosis than videoconferencing, as he believed that this would conflict with his Christian beliefs. Further studies are needed to establish whether personality characteristics or psychological issues are more suited to mediated or face-to-face treatment.

Results from these studies suggest that given the choice, a number of clients may prefer video-therapy sessions to face-to-face sessions.[19,20] Reasons given include video-therapy sessions being less 'threatening', 'intimidating' and 'unnerving', particularly with sexual or body-image issues when clients may feel ashamed or anticipate disapproval. The perceived distance afforded by video-therapy seems to allow clients the space to feel more comfortable and less 'scrutinized'. They do not feel as pressurized to respond quickly as they might in a face-to-face setting. It takes place in 'neutral territory' and gives the client a greater sense of power and control than might be the case in a face-to-face setting. This was also reported by Omodei and McClennan,[22] who added that clients expressed greater levels of satisfaction when they were able to control the video camera. Other clients felt more protected by the confidentiality of discussing their private issues via video-therapy sessions (Fig. 13.1). This may be particularly relevant for small communities on remote islands or in rural areas, where privacy is difficult to sustain.[19]

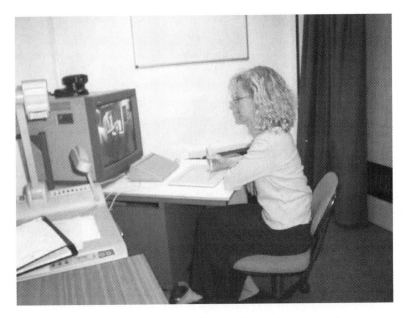

Fig. 13.1. Video-therapy in progress, using a rollabout videoconferencing unit.

Acceptability to psychologists

Feedback from psychologists suggests that this is a challenging but satisfactory means of providing therapy to remote areas. When using systems where the picture size, resolution and frame rate are limited, it can be difficult to read clients' facial expressions and to detect tearfulness (e.g. Simpson et al[19]). Some studies have reported reluctance on the part of therapists to participate in video-therapy. Omodei and McLennan[22] compared counselling across face-to-face, videoconferencing and telephone modes, reporting that counsellors perceived that video-therapy sessions were cognitively biased, with a loss of emotive content and 'social presence', the level at which it is possible for the presence of individual participants to be conveyed within any interactive setting. They also expressed dissatisfaction with the loss of non-verbal cues such as reduced eye contact and gesturing. This contrasts with the views of Hodges (unpublished work), who found that videoconferencing was an ideal means of communicating non-verbal information, citing as an example the extensive use of videoconferencing by Australian aboriginals, whose language includes a sophisticated range of non-verbal gestures. Such differences are more likely to be due to individual preferences and experience than technical differences in equipment and quality of calls. Schneider[23] suggested that media richness and presence are complex concepts which are influenced by a range of factors, including verbal and non-verbal cues, the communication setting, and the ability of the therapist to use the modes available to them in developing a therapeutic relationship with the patient.

Therapeutic alliance

A number of recent studies have examined whether it is possible to develop a positive therapeutic alliance in video-therapy. Therapeutic alliance is a strong predictor of clinical effectiveness across a range of psychotherapy models.[24] Therapeutic alliance is comparable in face-to-face and video-therapy, and personality characteristics of clients and therapists influence attitudes to therapy more than the technology. Ghosh et al[25] found that when using a psycho-educational and eclectic model of therapy, a working alliance was developed via videoconferencing. Although some non-verbal cues were lost and there was a slight sound delay due to the use of a lower bandwidth (128 kbit/s), these were easily accommodated. Both therapists and clients felt sufficiently comfortable to discuss personal issues freely and openly. Simpson[26] found similar results in a study in which 10 clients rated therapeutic alliance using the Penn Helping Alliance Questionnaire[27] over an average of 12 sessions. When compared with a similar group studied in a face-to-face setting, clients' ratings of therapeutic alliance were found to be equivalent. These results were based on small sample sizes limiting generalizability.

Clinical effectiveness of psychological therapy by video link

There have been few studies of the clinical efficacy of video-therapy. The largest study to date was conducted by Schneider[23] on the delivery of brief cognitive behavioural psychotherapy via videoconferencing. A sample of 80 clients made contact with the clinic by telephone and were randomly assigned to one of three treatment groups: face-to-face, two-way audio, two-way video or a waiting list control group. Client demographic details were recorded. Therapists had master's degrees in clinical or counselling psychology, and were supervised by a doctoral level psychologist. A closed circuit television system was used, with two 50-cm television sets used to simulate a high-quality two-way video delivery. The same system was used without a picture to simulate a two-way audio system. All sessions were video-recorded. A range of outcome measures was used to assess general personality characteristics and satisfaction levels, as well as more specific problem inventories. No significant differences were found between treatment groups across outcome measures, although all three groups were significantly superior to the no-treatment group. Although drop-out rates were low for all modes, both the audio and video groups had higher rates than the face-to-face group. Clients from the audio and video groups became more comfortable with their therapy mode over time, suggesting a tendency to adapt to the medium in question. Individual factors such as problems, comfort level and personality may be important in matching clients to the best therapy mode.

Simpson et al[19] compared pre and post scores from two questionnaires measuring clinical improvement (the General Health Questionnaire[28] and the CORE[29]). Results suggested that all clients but one improved over the course of therapy. Positive outcome results were also found in the video-hypnosis study (S. Simpson et al, unpublished work). Nine of the 11 clients indicated that following their session they had increased confidence in their ability to cope with their problem. The remaining two rated no change. In addition, 10 of the 11 clients rated an increase in their relaxation levels from pre to during and post video-hypnosis. Case vignettes from both of these studies are described in Boxes 13.1 and 13.2.

Harvey-Berino[30] compared a 12-week behavioural weight-control programme for clients with obesity via videoconferencing and face to face. Details of the videoconferencing equipment used and bandwidth of calls were not described. Both

---

Box 13.1.

Mr S was referred for help with recurrent depression and sexual difficulties. He was a 55-year-old man who had lived in the Outer Hebrides for many years, and had been unable to access specialist psychological treatment locally (Fig. 13.2). He had been prescribed antidepressant medication. As he was a health professional on the island, he had felt unable to consult with local health professionals about his sexual difficulties due to fears about confidentiality. Following a face-to-face assessment, he was offered 12 sessions of cognitive behavioural therapy via videoconferencing, using a set-top videoconferencing unit at the hospital site and a PC-based system at the remote site at a bandwidth of 128 kbit/s. A manual-based approach was used to treat his depression. He was required to fill out thought and mood diaries on a weekly basis and these were then examined together with the use of the document imager. Handouts and information sheets were faxed or posted to him regularly in order to help him to learn to manage his difficulties more effectively. His sexual problems were addressed using a behavioural approach and email was used in between sessions to monitor his progress. Mr S commented that although he had initially felt anxious at the prospect of discussing such personal problems with a younger female psychologist, he actually found that videoconferencing made this easier than anticipated. He felt more able to discuss his problems without feeling scrutinized or judged. The distance made him feel less self-conscious.

Box 13.2.

Miss F was a 25-year-old woman living on a remote island, who was referred for difficulties associated with generalized worry, anxiety and insomnia. She was offered a course of video-therapy sessions to address her generalized anxiety, followed by a single session of video-hypnosis to address her insomnia. The client used a set-top videoconferencing unit at the remote site, and the psychologist used a rollabout system. Sessions took place at a bandwidth of 384 kbit/s. The video-hypnosis session began with her sitting in a large comfortable chair, with the camera closely focused on her face and upper body. The psychologist was able to move the camera at the remote site, which facilitated close monitoring of the patient's breathing, facial expressions and body posture throughout the procedure. A 'deepening' script was used to induce a state of relaxation and this was timed with Miss F's own breathing pattern. The session focused on helping her learn to reduce tension through a series of relaxation techniques, including diaphragmatic breathing and visualizing herself in a situation where she felt comfortable, safe and able to let go of negative or unhelpful thoughts. She was then able to utilize these techniques when going to bed at night. Miss F commented that the videoconferencing gave her a sense of 'space', which reduced any self-consciousness. She suggested that her attendance at previous video-therapy sessions enabled her to relax more fully during video-hypnosis in that she had already established a 'video-rapport' with the psychologist. Her ratings showed that she was substantially more relaxed following the video-hypnosis and more confident in her ability to fall asleep at night.

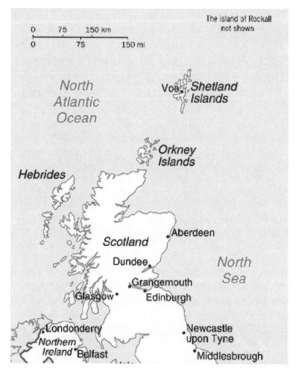

Fig. 13.2. The Outer Hebrides are about 100 km west of the Scottish mainland.

treatment modalities led to significant and comparable levels of weight loss and improvements in eating and exercise behaviours. Attrition rates were similar for both groups. A cost-effectiveness analysis found that the video condition was more expensive, partly because site facilitators were provided at all remote clinics. Bakke et al[31] described the treatment of two women with bulimia nervosa using manual-based cognitive behavioural therapy via videoconferencing. Videoconferencing systems with 48-cm screens were used, at a bandwidth of 128 kbit/s. Both subjects abstained from binge eating and purging for the last 4 weeks of treatment and continued to be abstinent at 1 month follow-up.

Supervision via videoconferencing

A few studies have examined the feasibility of providing clinical supervision over videoconferencing. Gammon et al[32] examined the use of psychotherapy supervision via videoconferencing for psychiatric trainees in Norway. Six trainees met individually with one of two supervisors for 10 supervision sessions, alternating between videoconferencing (at 384 kbit/s) and face-to-face modes from week to week. Rollabout videoconferencing units were used. The results of this study suggested that supervision for up to half of the sessions could be satisfactorily carried out by videoconferencing, but that rapport-building should take place on a face-to-face basis in order to establish mutual trust prior to embarking on video-supervision. Observing the adaptations participants made in communication via videoconferencing facilitated the overall quality of supervision.

A similar study by Sorlie et al[33] examined six supervisor/supervisee pairs for the quality of contact and working alliance as measured by an independent rater. The two conditions did not differ on ratings of quality of communication and alliance for supervisors, but supervisees preferred the face-to-face condition, in particular when it came to discussing unpleasant or difficult issues. Analysis of sessions revealed that there were no differences between conditions in relation to gesturing, turn-taking, listener-response and note-taking. It was concluded that individual differences should be taken into account and that whereas younger and less experienced supervisees may in general benefit from beginning the supervision process on a face-to-face basis, video-supervision may become more acceptable to them as they become more familiar with the process and relationship. In addition, those who are more likely to intellectualize and avoid emotional engagement may be less suited to a video-supervision setting. Similarly, supervisors who are anxious about using videoconferencing may not be suitable for this mode of working. Supervisors should be aware of the effects of videoconferencing throughout the supervision process. Openly reflecting on these issues can stimulate learning in supervision.

As in video-therapy, it is important for future studies to ascertain which modes of communication suit which participants.

Recommendations for future research

Larger-scale randomized controlled trials are lacking. The undertaking of more robust evaluation trials is likely to require collaboration between sites, which should be facilitated through the use of existing videoconferencing facilities.

There is a need for an appropriate evaluation paradigm. Wide variation exists in the clinical and technical details provided by studies conducted to date. Few give full descriptions of the clinical samples used, the diagnostic groups included or details of the videoconferencing equipment. Sampling procedures are of particular importance, with implications as to the generalizability of findings in the wider population. Future studies should provide diagnostic details, including how this was ascertained. The model of intervention (e.g. cognitive behavioural, psychodynamic) and number of sessions should also be detailed. In addition, adherence to the therapeutic model specified (treatment integrity) needs to be checked. Researchers should specify whether clinicians are qualified and experienced in this model, and their adherence to the model can be checked through filling out ongoing rating forms and/or by an independent observer. Outcome measures should also be specified.

Potential areas for investigation include clinical effectiveness, drop-out rates, DNA (did not attend) and cancellation rates. It will also be of value to ascertain whether certain patients become more or less comfortable with video-consultations with familiarity, experience with technology, and how this is influenced by factors such as therapeutic rapport, the presence of equipment-related technical problems, and patient and psychologist personality factors. Schneider[23] suggested that certain clients may have an aptitude or higher level of comfort for one mode over another. It may also be useful to explore whether clinical effectiveness and therapeutic rapport are influenced by conducting sessions exclusively via videoconferencing, face to face or a combination. Nickelson[34] highlighted the importance of carrying out research into conditions which enhance or impede privacy and confidentiality and so influence patients' decisions to engage in treatment via videoconferencing. Other factors worthy of consideration include cost effectiveness, and structural aspects of conversation conducted via videoconferencing as compared with other modes including turn lengths, pauses, interruptions, feasibility and user satisfaction.

Legal and ethical issues

As videoconferencing becomes a more popular medium for providing psychological services, it will be essential to establish the ethical and legal implications of offering services across states and countries that have differing regulations for registration. Capner[35] suggested that if clients give their agreement then all services are considered to take place at the psychologist's place of work. This may provide some protection from litigation. However she cautioned that if psychologists choose to collaborate with local psychologists at remote sites, it is essential that the boundaries are clarified as to who is responsible and who is qualified to carry out which tasks. It is particularly important, in this early stage of developing videoconferencing psychology services, that psychologists retain their professional standards and are conscious of upholding their duty of care to patients.

Psychologists should be involved in the development of guidelines and protocols to direct the expansion of mental health services through the use of videoconferencing. This will allow working more flexibly across a range of settings, whilst putting procedures in place to ensure that patients are aware of their rights and are able to protect themselves in this novel environment.

Conclusions

Early studies on the use of videoconferencing in clinical psychology show great potential. In the absence of robust randomized controlled trials, preliminary work has shown that therapy via videoconferencing may be effective and in many cases acceptable to both patients and psychologists. In some cases, patients have been shown to prefer videoconferencing to face-to-face sessions due to greater perceived confidentiality, personal control and a reduced sense of intimidation. This may be particularly relevant for those with body-image distortion or other shame-based disorders, although further research is needed to verify which client groups are most suited to which modes.

Initial studies which have examined the use of videoconferencing in conducting psychometric and neuropsychological assessments have also shown good levels of reliability, with some adaptations necessary to ensure that loss of image is kept to a minimum. With the availability of additional equipment such as document imagers and video recorders, even the most complex material can be effectively transmitted to the far site and when necessary local aides may be recruited to assist in test presentation.

Videoconferencing is a way forward for people living in remote areas or traffic-congested cities to access psychological services. As the cost of equipment and calls decreases, videoconferencing will become an increasingly attractive option. It will soon be technically possible to deliver services into the home. This will greatly reduce the isolation associated with living in remote areas and make access to health care more equitable.

As supervision and training roles are further developed via videoconferencing, it will also become more attractive for clinical psychologists to live, work and train in remote areas, in the knowledge that they will have access to the support and supervision they require.

Acknowledgements

I thank Stephen Bell and Emma Morrow for their helpful comments.

References

1   Livingstone A. *Professional supervision and support in rural and remote psychology: telemedicine and other approaches.* Paper presented at South Australian State Psychology Conference. Adelaide: Australia, September 1999.

2   Davidson H, Birmingham CL. Letter writing as a therapeutic tool. *Eating and Weight Disorders* 2001;**6**:40–44.

3   Lester D. Counseling by telephone: advantages and problems. *Crisis Intervention* 1995;**2**:57–69.

4   Rosenfield M. *Counselling by Telephone.* London: Sage, 1997.

5   Robinson PH, Serfaty MA. The use of e-mail in the identification of bulimia nervosa and its treatment. *European Eating Disorders Review* 2001;**9**:182–193.

6   Castelnuovo G, Gaggioli A, Riva G. Cyberpsychology meets clinical psychology: the emergence of e-therapy in mental health care. In: Riva G, Galimberti C, eds. *Towards Cyberpsychology: mind cognition and society in the Internet age.* Amsterdam: IOS Press, 2001:229–252.

7   Lange A, van de Ven JP, Schrieken BA, Bredeweg B, Emmelkamp PM. Internet-mediated, protocol-driven treatment of psychological dysfunction. *Journal of Telemedicine and Telecare* 2000;**6**:15–21.

8   Baer L, Cukor P, Jenike MA, Leahy L, O'Laughlen J, Coyle JT. Pilot studies of telemedicine for clients with obsessive-compulsive disorder. *American Journal of Psychiatry* 1995;**152**:1383–1385.

9   Zarate CA, Weinstock L, Cukor P, et al. Applicability of telemedicine for assessing clients with schizophrenia: acceptance and reliability. *Journal of Clinical Psychiatry* 1997;**58**:22–25.

10 Ball CJ, Scott N, McClaren PM, Watson JP. Preliminary evaluation of a Low-Cost VideoConferencing (LCVC) system for remote cognitive testing of adult psychiatric patients. *British Journal of Psychology* 1993;**32**:303–307.

11 Ball C, Puffett A. The assessment of cognitive function in the elderly using videoconferencing. *Journal of Telemedicine and Telecare* 1998;**4**(suppl 1):36–38.

12   Montani C, Billaud N, Tyrrell J, et al. Psychological impact of a remote psychometric consultation with hospitalized elderly people. *Journal of Telemedicine and Telecare* 1997;**3**:140–145.

13   Montani C, Klientovsky K, Tyrrell J, Ploton L, Couturier P, Franco A. Feasibility of psychological consultation with elderly demented patients. *Journal of Telemedicine and Telecare* 1998;**4**(suppl 1):111.

14   Troster AI, Paolo AM, Glatt SL, et al. "Interactive video conferencing" in the provision of neuropsychological services to rural areas. *Journal of Community Psychology* 1995;**23**:85–88.

15   Kirkwood K. *The Validity of Cognitive Assessments via Telecommunications Links.* University of Edinburgh: PhD Thesis, 1998.

16   Biggins N. *'Virtual Reality' or 'Virtual Unreality'? A 'face-to-face' vs 'teleconferencing' comparison of neuropsychological assessment.* Flinders University of South Australia: PhD Thesis, 1998.

17   Morris RG, Evenden JL, Sahakian BJ, Robbins TW. Computer-aided assessment of dementia: comparative studies of neuropsychological deficits in Alzheimer-type dementia and Parkinson's disease. In: Stahl SM, Iversen SD, Goodman EC, eds. *Cognitive Neurochemistry.* Oxford: Oxford University Press, 1987:21–36.

18   Wittson CI, Benschoter R. Two-way television: helping the medical center reach out. *American Journal of Psychiatry* 1972;**129**:624–627.

19   Simpson S, Deans G, Brebner E. The delivery of a tele-psychology service to Shetland. *Clinical Psychology and Psychotherapy* 2001;**8**:130–135.

20   Simpson S, Morrow E, Jones M, Ferguson J, Brebner E. Video-hypnosis – the provision of specialised therapy via videoconferencing. *Journal of Telemedicine and Telecare* 2002;**8**(suppl 2):78–79.

21   Freir V, Kirkwood K, Peck D, Robertson S, Scott-Lodge L, Zeffert S. Telemedicine for clinical psychology in the Highlands of Scotland. *Journal of Telemedicine and Telecare* 1999;**5**:157–161.

22   Omodei M, McClennan J. 'The more I see you?' Face-to-face, video and telephone counselling compared. A programme of research investigating the emerging technology of videophone for counselling. *Australian Journal of Psychology* 1998;**50**(suppl):109.

23   Schneider PL. Psychotherapy using distance technology: a comparison of outcomes. 1999, August. In: Glueckauf RL (Chair). *Using Distance Technologies to Deliver Health Care Services: Empirical Comparisons.* Symposium conducted at the Annual Meeting of the American Psychological Association, Boston, MA.

24   Horvath AO, Luborsky L. The role of the therapeutic alliance in psychotherapy. *Journal of Consulting and Clinical Psychology* 1993;**64**:561–573.

25   Ghosh GJ, McLaren PM, Watson JP. Evaluating the alliance in videolink teletherapy. *Journal of Telemedicine and Telecare* 1997;**3**(suppl 1):33–35.

26   Simpson S. The provision of a telepsychology service to Shetland: client and therapist satisfaction and the ability to develop a therapeutic alliance. *Journal of Telemedicine and Telecare* 2001;**7**(suppl 1):34–36.

27   Alexander LB, Luborsky L. The Penn Helping Alliance Scales. In: Greenberg L, Pinsof W, eds. *The Psychotherapy Process: a research handbook.* New York: Guildford Press, 1986:325–366.

28   Goldberg DP. *The Detection of Psychiatric Illness by Questionnaire.* London: Oxford University Press, 1972.

29   Core System Group. *Core System (Information Management) Handbook.* Leeds: Core System Group, 1998.

30   Harvey-Berino J. Changing health behavior via telecommunications technology: using interactive television to treat obesity. *Behavior Therapy* 1998;**29**:505–519.

31   Bakke B, Mitchell J, Wonderlich S, Erickson R. Administering cognitive behavioral therapy for bulimia nervosa via telemedicine in rural settings. *International Journal of Eating Disorders* 2001;**30**:454–457.

32   Gammon D, Sorlie T, Bergvik S, Hoifodt TS. Psychotherapy supervision conducted by videoconferencing: a qualitative study of user's experiences. *Journal of Telemedicine and Telecare* 1998;**4**(suppl 1):33–35.

33   Sorlie T, Gammon D, Bergvik S, Sexton H. Psychotherapy supervision face-to-face and by videoconferencing: a comparative study. *British Journal of Psychotherapy* 1999;**15**:452–462.

34   Nickelson DW. Telehealth and the evolving health care system: strategic opportunities for professional psychology. *Professional Psychology: Research and Practice* 1998;**29**:527–535.

35   Capner M. Videoconferencing in the provision of psychological services at a distance. *Journal of Telemedicine and Telecare* 2000;**6**:311–319.

14

Telemedicine and Old Age Psychiatry

Chris Ball

Introduction

The world's population is growing at approximately 1.7% per year. It has been calculated that in the 25 years between 1975 and 2000 there was an increase of 54% in the number of cases of dementia in the industrialized world and 123% in the less well developed parts of the globe.[1] A recent UK study of 1083 elderly people enrolled in a hypertension study 9–12 years earlier was able to identify almost 90% of the cohort: 40% had died; all but 10.3% remained in their original practice area.[2]

In old age people are frequently afflicted by more than one condition. The problems are often of a chronic nature requiring repeated monitoring and making travelling difficult (e.g. arthritis, diabetes).[3]

The majority of elderly people in the UK have telephones – 96% of those referred to a service for mental health in older adults possessed a telephone (A.J.D. Macdonald, personal communication). Just under 10% of frail elderly people are reported to have problems using their telephones but remedial action is frequently possible.[4] The elderly are not reluctant to accept new technologies (Fig. 14.1); 58% of community alarm users owned a microwave or a video, 68% were interested in 'lifestyle monitoring' and 46% in videoconferencing.[5]

It is surprising therefore that searching the literature for telemedicine studies targeted at the elderly is a relatively fruitless task. Many studies have been small, have lacked controls and have not progressed beyond the feasibility or pilot phase. Studies of mental health problems in the elderly are even rarer. Unearthing references to psychiatric or psychological features in 'home nursing' studies, for example 'disclosing intimate information'[6] or 'feelings',[7] is not a challenge I have risen too. Nor, largely, is the other task of extrapolating from work undertaken with working-age adult subjects, unless the gains seem particularly pertinent. Few descriptions of telepsychiatry projects from around the world have directly concerned the elderly (e.g. Gammon et al[8]).

This review looks at the literature in which the mental health problems of older adults are specifically addressed or which have a particularly pertinent part to play in the management of those suffering from mental health problems in later life.

Assessing cognitive impairment and diagnosing dementia

The development of mental health in older adults (MHOA) services has come about from the recognition that the needs of those who develop dementing illnesses in later

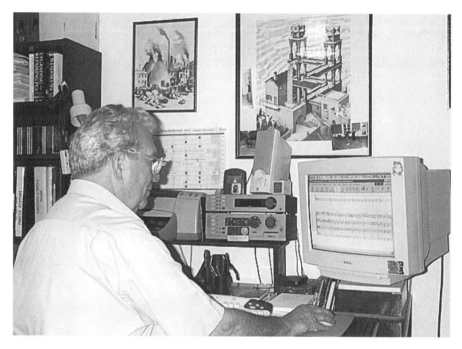

Fig. 14.1. Using new technology is no preserve of the young.

life have been largely ignored. The creation of Alzheimer's disease as a major public health issue has been the spur for an increasing research and service effort.[9] Assessing the cognitive abilities of a subject is a core activity for those in MHOA teams.

The search for a reliable telemedicine assessment of cognitive function began in the late 1980s with long batteries of tests performed via the telephone.[10,11] This required the sending of packages to the subjects' home before testing could be undertaken. Despite good correlation between face-to-face and telephone testing in younger adults, concerns about cheating and the length of the tests led the authors to conclude that this method was not suitable for assessing those who might have a dementing illness.

This led to attempts to use shorter instruments to assess cognitive function in the elderly. The Short Portable Mental Status Questionnaire and the Information Orientation and Memory Test proved adaptable for use via the telephone, as all the questions are spoken and only verbal responses are required.[12-14] The specificity of these very short tests is unfortunately rather low for routine clinical use or screening.[15] In the search for better tests the adaptability to telephone use has proved to be the crucial issue.

Possibly the most widely used brief assessment of cognitive function is the Mini-Mental State Examination (MMSE).[16] Although heavily language based it does ask the subjects to respond to visual material and to undertake tasks that the assessor has to see (e.g. to copy pentagrams and to obey a written command). One approach to such problems is merely to omit the visual parts of the test. Because of the heavy language bias there is a reasonable correlation with the full MMSE, for example the Telephone Assessed Mental State (TAMS) $(r = 0.81, P < 0.001)$.[17] However, this strategy weakens the number of cognitive domains that can be tested, especially if dysphasia is prominent, for example after stroke.

In order to fill the gaps left by omitting the visual tasks some have attempted to replace the tasks with something similar. Such tasks include naming, 'What is the name of the thing you are speaking into now?' (telephone version of the MMSE),[18] or the three-part command, 'Tap the receiver five times'.[19] It is not always clear that these substitutions represent items of equal cognitive difficulty or even if they represent tasks in similar cognitive domains. Nevertheless they have some face validity.

To substitute for these deficiencies others have chosen to extend the tasks that are undertaken as part of the test, for example to general knowledge 'Who is the President?'[18] or opposites.[20] There is no doubt that the range of tests is extended but whether this adds greatly to the sensitivity or specificity of the tool or its ability to measure change in cognitive functioning is not clear. A third option has been to engage a caregiver to score the task and report back to the investigator.[21]

Perhaps the most successful of the MMSE adaptations is the telephone interview for cognitive status (TICS)[19] and its later modification TICS-m.[20,22] This substitutes a 10-item delayed word recall for the usual 3-item recall, asks for opposites, name, age and telephone number as well as a general knowledge question. Omitting a question on orientation helps to eliminate those questions that cannot be verified by the interviewer (particularly with the advent of mobile phones, making the orientation-to-place question something of a lottery). The TICS has been used in a number of research studies aimed at identifying cognitive impairment,[23–25] whilst the TICS-m has been used as screening in a population of 12 709 individuals. The sensitivity was estimated to be more than 99% and the specificity to be 86% at a cut-off score of 27/28. Creatively the TICS was suggested as a substitute for the MMSE where the subjects being tested are blind.[26] The MMSE has been translated into many languages and the process has now begun with telephone versions.[27,28] The expanded and modified MMSE (3Ms)[29] has also had an outing in telephone form[30] but the results show no big advantages over other versions (Table 14.1).

A number of other researchers have brought together tests that they felt would be useful to test cognitive status via the telephone. Often these have been from disparate sources, for example the Telephone Screening Questionnaire (TELE)[32] and the Telephone Cognitive Assessment Battery.[33] Sometimes these have been tied in with more detailed questioning. The Structured Telephone Interview for Dementia Assessment (STIDA)[34] is also able to generate a score for the subscales for the Clinical Dementia Rating Scale.[35]

The STIDA includes a second innovation because it includes an informant interview. Taking a history from an informant is vital in establishing that cognitive impairment is part of a progressive picture, i.e. part of a dementing illness.[36] However, it is not always clear that informant interviews for the identification of cognitive impairment have been validated for use on the telephone. Mintzer et al[37] interviewed carers over the telephone and validated the interview against in-person assessment of

Table 14.1. The Mini-Mental State and its variants for telephone. (Adapted from Ball & McLaren.[31])

Mini-Mental State Examination (MMSE)[16]	Telephone Interview for Cognitive Status (TICS)[19]	Telephone Interview for Cognitive Status modified (TICS-m)[20]	Telephone version of the MMSE[18]	Telephone Assessed Mental State (TAMS)[17]
Orientation in time	Orientation in time	Orientation in time	Orientation in time	Orientation in time
Orientation in place	Orientation in place	Orientation in place	Orientation in place	Orientation in place
Concentration Serial 7's or spell WORLD backwards	Serial 7's and count from 20 down to 1	Serial 7's and count from 20 down to 1	Concentration Serial 7's or spell WORLD backwards	Spell HOUSE backwards
Delayed recall of three objects	Delayed recall from a list of 10 items	Delayed recall from a list of 10 items	Delayed recall of three objects	Delayed recall of three objects
Naming (pen and watch)	Responsive naming (What do people use to cut paper?)	Responsive naming (What animal does wool come from?)	Naming (What is the thing you are speaking into called?)	—
Read and obey a written command (Close your eyes)	Obey a verbal command (Tap five times on the part of the phone you speak into)	Obey a verbal command (Tap five times on the part of the phone you speak into)	—	—
Three-part command (Take a paper in your right hand fold it in half and put it on the floor)	—	—	—	—
Write a sentence	State full name	State full name	—	—
Copy a design	Opposites (What is the opposite of west?)	Opposites (What is the opposite of west?)	—	—
—	—	State age and telephone number.	—	—
—	General knowledge (Who is the president of the USA? Who is the vice-president?)	General knowledge (Who is the president of the USA? Who is the vice-president?)	—	—

the subjects. Gallo et al[25] used the telephone dementia questionnaire when their subjects scored poorly on the TICS and validated this against a sample which scored highly. A number of interviews exist for the identification of cognitive impairment through informant interview (e.g. Informant Questionnaire for Cognitive Decline in the Elderly (IQCODE)[38]), but these have not been validated by correlating face-to-face with telephone interviewing.

Mundt et al[39] developed the informant interview (using the Symptoms of Dementia Screen) by asking the informant to respond using a touch-tone telephone. This was then extended to test the subjects using an interactive voice response system. The average length of the call was 12 minutes 27 seconds. Sixteen of 89 cognitively impaired subjects were unable to complete the task. Although there were problems with the technique the authors concluded that this could be a cost-effective screening method for cognitive impairment. Informant and subject interviews are required for the completion of staging tests for dementia. Monteiro et al[40] undertook a number of different tests (Global Deterioration Scale (GDS), Functional Assessment Staging (FAST), Behavioural Pathology in Alzheimer's Disease Rating Scale (BEHAVE-AD) and Brief Cognitive Rating Scale (BCRS)) in a relatively small sample (n = 30). The authors concluded that telephone administration of these tests was able to distinguish those with normal cognition from those suffering with dementia, measure the severity of the dementia and identify behavioural problems. The authors raise some doubt as to whether the telephone interview can substitute for a face-to-face interview in the diagnostic phase.

The four problems with telephone assessment of cognitive state identified by Desmond et al[23] were:

1. inability to assess writing and drawing

2. subjects who were testable in the presence of a physician, might not be testable by telephone (it was not considered that the reverse might be true!)

3. the problems associated with reduced auditory acuity

4. the ability to refer to external sources of information.

These problems could be addressed by the use of videoconferencing.

Assessing cognitive function using videoconferencing is less well developed than telephone assessment. Problems using standard tests, such as the MMSE, were identified early[41] in younger adults and the methods of overcoming the presentation and scoring of visual material are not always well described.[42] Nevertheless, a good correlation between face-to-face and videoconferencing assessments has been reported in younger adults (r = 0.89).[41] Grob et al[43] undertook MMSE assessment with elderly nursing home residents and demonstrated good inter-rater reliability between assessments made remotely and in person (0.95 vs. 0.85). Montani et al[42] undertook the MMSE and the Clock Drawing test,[44] and reported a small but significant decline in the performance of the tests performed using videoconferencing. The changes were ascribed to poor hearing and manipulation of equipment but may also have been the result of fluctuations in cognitive state between interviews as delirium was not excluded.

The problems of presenting complex visual stimuli and assessing the results of material produced by patients have been highlighted in two studies. Ball and Puffett[45] undertook the CAMCOG examination of the Cambridge Assessment of Mental Disorders in the Elderly[46] and found that the correlation between face-to-face and videoconferencing assessment items was poorer when complex visual stimuli were required. Scoring patients' written material from the MMSE was less reliable when the results were seen via videoconferencing than after faxing them or seeing the results in person.[47]

With the development of anticholinesterase inhibitors for treating Alzheimer's disease[48] and the shortage of physicians, psychiatrists and psychologists to deliver the assessments required, the development of a validated videoconferencing cognitive assessment could be used to bridge an important gap in services.

Other assessments

Although MHOA services deal with a wide range of mental disorders in their day-to-day practice, depression is perhaps the commonest disorder after dementia.

The Geriatric Depression Scale (GDS)[49] is one of the most frequently used tools for identifying cases of depression in older adults and is sometimes used as (although not clearly validated as) a measure of severity. It is a self-report instrument requiring the subject to answer 'yes' or 'no' to closed questions. Burke et al[50] evaluated the 30-item GDS in a population of elderly outpatient clinic attendees. Although individual items varied in their concordance between two telephone interviews conducted about a week apart and also between the face-to-face and telephone interviews, the overall concordance was reasonable (kappa = 0.52 in both cases). Using the traditional cut-off point of 14 as defining 'a case', the telephone version had a sensitivity of 52% and a specificity of 79%. Morishita et al[51] conducted a similar exercise with a small sample size (n = 26) and found that the correlation between in-person and telephone interview was high (0.9, $P < 0.001$). Only one subject in the sample would have been wrongly classified as depressed when the two methods of interview were compared. An informant version of the GDS has also been investigated,[52] the authors concluding that it maintains its validity when used via the telephone. In a small sample of nursing home residents (n = 27) Grob et al[43] found that the GDS could be assessed reliably when assessed over a videoconferencing link. Given the nature of the scale it is unsurprising that it transfers well to the telephone and videoconferencing.

Dorfmann et al[53] have reported using the Rand Mental Health Inventory and the Centre for Epidemiological Studies Depression Scale allowed social workers to efficiently identify depressed elders by telephone, many of whom had not previously been noted to be experiencing mental health problems.

Some problems in assessing depression in younger adults using distance technology have been identified,[54,55] but in each case these have been put down to the instrument used, the Diagnostic Interview Schedule (DIS), rather than the technology itself. The Hamilton Depression Rating Scale (HAM-D)[56] has proved robust in a small telephone study (n = 30) but not in older adults.[57] An automated telephone version of the Zung

Depression Scale[58] proved successful in younger adults, as has an interactive voice response technology version of the HAM-D but with a wider age range (18–79 years).[59] B.N. Jones et al (personal communication) reported a high level of agreement between a face-to-face observer and a telemedicine interviewer when assessing depressive symptoms in older psychiatric inpatients. Using an instrument that only required yes/no answers, concerns were raised that video images would not be adequate for clinical assessment requiring observation.

The Brief Psychiatric Rating Scale (BPRS)[60] is a global scale applicable to any disorder, although traditionally used in psychotic illnesses. It consists of two parts; one of which relies on the report of the subject and the second that relies on the observations of the observer. In several studies, three with younger adults[61–63] and a fourth with elderly people,[64] the BPRS has been conducted using videoconferencing systems and face-to-face. In each case it was found that it could be reliably undertaken using videoconferencing but in two studies[61,64] the items depending on patient report were more reliable than those requiring observation.

There is little evidence that comprehensive instruments aimed at making a diagnosis except that of dementia have been employed using communication technology in the elderly population. Tunstall et al[65] took the Depression Diagnostic Scale, Dementia Diagnostic Scale and Organic Brain Syndrome from the SHORT-CARE and assessed elders from a day hospital via the telephone and face to face. They concluded that the instrument was 'broadly reliable' when administered by telephone.

A wide range of other mental health assessments have been undertaken using the telephone and videoconferencing equipment, both diagnostically and condition specific but few of these have included elderly subjects as their principal focus.[66–69] Much needs to be done to identify those formal assessments that offer most to distance providers of care to mentally ill elders. It is perhaps reassuring to note that a number of related assessments pertinent to MHOA services, for example Activities of Daily Living (ADL),[70,71] visual acuity,[72] neurological examination,[73] vascular risk factors,[74] orthopaedic assessment[75] and the diagnosis of delirium,[76] have been undertaken successfully using a variety of media.

Providing services

The principal use of the telephone in providing MHOA services has been support to carers. The telephone is a vital tool for any community team, but little formal assessment of its use has been made (when investigating a complaint about my own service, I counted 123 telephone calls to carers documented in a single set of notes over an 18-month period). Many carers express a wish for telephone support from either professionals (45%) or a fellow carer (41%).[77]

Skipwith[78] identified the principal advantages of telephone interventions with carers as being:

▶ the lack of travelling

▶ no need to arrange alternative care

▶ the ability to reach isolated and rural carers

▶ cost- and time-efficiencies

▶ cultural acceptability.

A number of descriptive studies and formal evaluations of care support systems have been made. The models employed have become increasingly complex with the availability of technology (e.g. Mahoney et al[79]). For example Goodman and Pynoos[80] found that listening to mini-lectures over the telephone led to an increase in knowledge and more emotional support from family and friends, whilst those in support networks of four or five talking on the telephone found less support from family and friends. There was no effect on carer burden, distress at relative's problems or carer's mental health. The telecomputing system developed by the Alzheimer's Disease Support Center in Cleveland Ohio[81,82] provided carers with information, decision-making assistance and communication to other carers of people with Alzheimer's disease. Despite improvements in decision making there seemed to be no reduction in the carers' sense of social isolation.

Mahoney et al[79] used an interactive voice response (IVR) system integrated with voicemail to support carers. The IVR had four components: monitoring and counselling; an in-home support group; 'ask the expert'; and a respite conversation. During a 16-month period the average usage was 55 minutes (range 1–318 minutes). The 'adopters' of the system tended to be older and more highly educated and had a greater sense of management of the situation than those who did not adopt the system.

Counselling and Diagnosis in Dementia (CANDID) offered a telemedicine (email and telephone) support service to younger people with dementia and their carers (professional and lay). They received 1121 calls during their first 2 years of operation. About half of the enquiries were for clinical advice, with other calls falling into the categories of general information and 'social issues'.[83]

It is not clear that any single model of support significantly decreases carer burden, decreases service use or delays institutionalization. Technology represents one arm of a number of possible interventions that must be tailored to the individual.[79]

A number of attempts have been made to support elders by telephone at difficult times. Discharge from hospital is a particular time of difficulty. Berkman et al[84] demonstrated that social workers were better at providing telephone support at this time than their 'secretarial staff' which is, perhaps, reassuring. Support following the death of a family member from cancer has been offered by telephone and largely received positively.[85] Problems arose when the calls did not get to their intended recipient. Stress in this study was laid on the individual nature of the support given by a nurse with whom the family member already had a relationship.

The results of telephone intervention are not always so positive. Telephoning patients after discharge from hospital has been found to make little difference in their perceived health status, service usage or death rate. It merely became an additional service.[86] Walker[87] found that using the telephone as an aid to the management of hypertension made no difference to outcomes. There may be benefits for those discharged directly from accident and emergency departments but it is not clear that there are benefits to the mental health of the elderly.[88,89]

The telephone has also been used to improve attendance at outpatient clinics, improving the attendance rate but also increasing the cancellation rate.[90,91] Danoff and Kemper[92] found that using a telephone reminder system improved attendance at a paediatric clinic in those with telephones but drew attention to the important issue of the exclusion from studies of those without telephones. There are also suggestions that concordance might be improved by using telephone reminders,[93] but this has not been demonstrated where it might be most important in dementia.

Improving concordance is perhaps one of the major effects of telephone support to depressed people. In a number of studies improvements in outcome (caseness, depressive symptoms, days lost to sickness) have been noted where telephone interventions have been part of quality improvement programmes.[94–96] These studies with working-age adults leave some doubts about the cost effectiveness of the interventions, and it is far from clear whether the results would be comparable in elderly people with depressive illnesses. A recent review of studies examining interventions to improve concordance in depressive illnesses made no mention of telemedicine interventions.[97]

The telephone has also been shown to provide more information on referral to an MHOA community team.[98] Comparing the information provided by general practitioners in their written submissions to the team and an interview on the telephone by trained administration staff showed that significantly more information was gleaned on the telephone.

Perhaps the most notable demonstration of the effectiveness of the telephone in delivering services is the reduction in suicide rate amongst 12 135 elderly subjects connected to a 'Tele-Help/Tele-Check' Service.[99] The system was portable and offered active contact to clients by trained staff who provided information, support and rapid intervention in the event of physical or psychological emergencies. Over a 4-year period only one suicide occurred in the study group. The expected number was 7.4 (standardized mortality ratio = 13%).

The use of videoconferencing services for elderly people with mental health problems is probably more common than reviewing the literature would suggest. The website of the Telemedicine Information Exchange (TIE)[100] lists many projects that appear to have a component of elderly care and perhaps even more specifically elderly mental health care. Relatively few services have produced either descriptive or randomized studies that have been published in the literature. This might be because they are not contentious in many areas where this is the only way to deliver services. It may also reflect service pressures, the funding structures or perhaps the publishing bias of the medical press.

Most studies have concentrated on delivering services to places where older persons are gathered together, usually nursing homes.[75,101]

Tang and colleagues reported using a videoconferencing system between the hospital base and a Care and Attention (C&A) home some 3 km away.[102] The team provided regular reviews and emergency consultations to the home. Forty-five of the 198 residents were seen, 30 of the 45 had dementia and seven had depression. Over a 10-month period 149 consultations were provided, of which five were urgent. During this period only one resident required an on-site visit and two were transferred to the hospital. Those patients able to express a view were largely positive, as were the C&A staff. The authors conclude that the average cost of a consultation was 13% lower by videoconferencing than an on-site visit.

Lee et al[103] developed a more extensive service, although many of their patients were in nursing homes. The service provided telemedicine, tele-education and telecounselling to two recipient sites, concentrating on those with dementing illness. They reported high consistency rates for their assessment process (76–89%) and 'a considerable proportion' (46%) of patients showing clinical improvement.

Other studies have reported the efficacy of low-cost systems linking specialist MHOA services with remote long-term care facilities with the effect of reducing admissions to the acute facilities[104] (but increasing the length of stay (17.4 days prior to telemedicine and 23.5 days after)), or to a rural hospital with skilled nursing beds.[105]

Many other mental health interventions have been described in the literature for different conditions, for example psychotherapy,[106] obsessive compulsive disorder[107] and alcohol abuse,[108] but none have concentrated on the delivery of psychotherapies to the elderly, which represents a much neglected area.

Conclusions

There are increasing numbers of elderly people in the world who experience relatively high rates of mental health problems. Provision of mental health services to these people remains patchy around the world and is almost universally inadequate. Telemedicine techniques represent an opportunity to provide services where they are lacking, to educate, to support and empower local carers to offer a flexible and knowledgeable service.

Technical issues (bandwidth, camera quality, compression algorithms, ergonomics) are important but beyond the scope of this review.[109,110] Developing the technical specification that allows not only the health care workers to do their job but also elderly people to get the most out of the system remains to be done. Financial considerations are important for all services, but the economic case for services delivered via telemedicine in different settings still needs to be made convincingly. In some situations, issues such as reimbursement to health care workers is a major issue.[111]

To date the evidence base for the assessment and delivery of services to elderly people remains underdeveloped and under-researched. What the ultimate place of telemedicine is in the assessment and management of mental health services to elders remains to be seen. There is great potential.

References

1   Mann A. Epidemiology. In: Jacoby R. Oppenheiner C, eds. *Psychiatry in the Elderly*. Oxford: Oxford University Press, 1997.
2   Cervilla JA, Prince M, Joels S, et al. Long-term predictors of cognitive outcomes in a cohort of older people with hypertension. *British Journal of Psychiatry* 2000;**177**:66–71.

3   Bennett GCJ, Ebrahim S. *The Essentials of Health Care in Old Age*, 2nd edn. London: Edward Arnold, 1995.

4   Mann WC, Hurren D, Charvat B, Tomita M. The use of phones by elders with disabilities: problems, interventions, costs. *Assistive Technology* 1996;**8**:23–33.

5   Brownsell SJ, Bradley DA, Bragg R, Catlin P, Carlier J. Do community alarm users want telecare? *Journal of Telemedicine and Telecare* 2000;**6**:199–204.

6   Agrell H, Dahlberg S, Jerant AF. Patients' perceptions regarding home telecare. *Telemedicine Journal and E-Health* 2000;**6**:409–415.

7   Arnaert A, Delesie L. Telenursing for the elderly. The case for care via video-telephony. *Journal of Telemedicine and Telecare* 2001;**7**:311–316.

8   Gammon D, Bergvik S, Bergmo T, Pedersen S. Videoconferencing in psychiatry: a survey of use in northern Norway. *Journal of Telemedicine and Telecare* 1996;**2**:192–198.

9   Holliday SG, Ancill RJ, Myrinuk L. The cognitization of dementia. In: Ancill RJ, Holliday SG, Mithani AH, eds. *Therapeutics in Geriatric Neuropsychiatry*. Chichester: John Wiley, 1997.

10 Kent J, Plomin R. Testing specific cognitive abilities by telephone and mail. *Intelligence* 1997;**11**:391–400.

11 Nesselroade JR, Pedersen NL, McClearn GE, Plomin R, Bergeman CS. Factorial and criterion validities of telephone-assessed cognitive ability measures. *Research on Aging* 1988;**10**:220–234.

12 Roccaforte WH, Burke WJ, Bayer BL, Wengel SP. Reliability and validity of the Short Portable Mental Status Questionnaire administered by telephone. *Journal of Geriatric Psychiatry and Neurology* 1994;**7**:33–38.

13 Morrison A, Kawas C. Telephone screening for dementia using the Blessed IMC test. *Neurology* 1993;**43**(suppl):A172.

14 Dellasega CA, Lacko L, Singer H, Salerno F. Telephone screening of older adults using the Orientation-Memory-Concentration test. *Geriatric Nursing* 2001;**22**:253–257.

15 Burns A, Lawlor B, Craig S, eds. *Assessment Scales in Old Age Psychiatry*. London: Martin Dunitz, 1999.

16 Folstein MF, Folstein SE, McHugh PR. 'Mini-Mental State'. A practical method for grading the cognitive state of patients for the clinician. *Journal of Psychiatric Research* 1975;**12**:189–198.

17 Lanska DJ, Schmitt FA, Stewart JM, Howe JN. Telephone-Assessed Mental State. *Dementia* 1993;**4**:117–119.

18 Roccaforte WH, Burke WJ, Bayer BL, Wengel SP. Validation of a telephone version of the mini-mental state examination. *Journal of the American Geriatrics Society* 1992;**40**:697–702.

19 Brandt J, Spencer M, Folstein M. The telephone interview for cognitive status. *Neuropsychiatry, Neuropsychology and Behavioural Neurology* 1988;**1**:111–117.

20 Welsh KA, Breitner JC, Magruder-Habib KM. Detection of dementia in the elderly using telephone screening of cognitive status. *Neuropsychiatry, Neuropsychology and Behavioural Neurology* 1993;**6**:103–110.

21 Plassman BL, Newman T, Welsh KA, et al. Properties of the telephone interview for cognitive status: application in epidemiological and longitudinal studies. *Neuropsychiatry, Neuropsychology and Behavioural Neurology* 1994;**7**:235–241.

22 Breitner JCS, Welsh KA, Magruder-Habib KM, et al. Alzheimer's disease in the National Academy of Sciences Registry of Aging Twin Veterans. *Dementia* 1990;**1**:297–303.

23 Desmond DW, Tatemichi TK, Tanzawa L. The Telephone Interview for Cognitive Status (TICS): reliability and validity in a stroke sample. *International Journal of Geriatric Psychiatry* 1994;**9**:803–807.

24 Grodstein F, Chen J, Wilson RS, Manson JE. Type 2 diabetes and cognitive function in community-dwelling elderly women. *Diabetes Care* 2001;**24**:1060–1065.

25 Gallo JJ, Breitner JC. Alzheimer's disease in the NAS-NRC Registry of aging twin veterans, IV. Performance characteristics of a two-stage telephone screening procedure for Alzheimer's dementia. *Psychological Medicine* 1995;**25**:1211–1219.

26 Ferrucci L, Del Lungo I, Guralnik JM, et al. Is the telephone interview for cognitive status a valid alternative in persons who cannot be evaluated by the Mini Mental State Examination? *Aging (Milano)* 1998;**10**:332–338.

27 Metitieri T, Geroldi C, Pezzini A, Frisoni GB, Bianchetti A, Trabucchi M. The Itel-MMSE: an Italian telephone version of the Mini-Mental State Examination. *International Journal of Geriatric Psychiatry* 2001;**16**:166–167.

28 Gude Ruiz R, Calvo Mauri JF, Carrasco Lopez FJ. Spanish version and pilot study of telephonic test of cognitive status to evaluate and detect oversights in the assessment and follow up of dementia. *Attencion Primaria* 1994;**13**:61–66.

29 Teng E, Chiu C. The Modified Mini-Mental State (3MS) examination. *Journal of Clinical Psychiatry* 1987;**48**:314–318.

30 Norton MC, Tschanz JA, Fan X, et al. Telephone adaptation of the Modified Mini-Mental State Exam (3MS). The Cache County Study. *Neuropsychiatry, Neuropsychology, and Behavioural Neurology* 1999;**12**:270–276.

31 Ball C J, McLaren PM. Tele-assessment of cognitive state. *Journal of Telemedicine and Telecare* 1997;**3**:126–131.

32 Gatz M, Reynolds C, Nikolic J, Lowe B, Karel M, Pedersen N. An empirical test of telephone screening to identify potential dementia cases. International *Psychogeriatrics* 1995;**7**:429–438.

33 Debanne SM, Patterson MB, Dick R, Riedel TM, Schnell A, Rowland DY. Validation of a Telephone Cognitive Assessment Battery. *Journal of the American Geriatrics Society* 1997;**45**:1352–1359.

34 Go RC, Duke LW, Harrell LE, et al. Development and validation of a Structured Telephone Interview for Dementia Assessment (STIDA): the NIMH Genetics Initiative. *Journal of Geriatric Psychiatry and Neurology* 1997;**10**:161–167.

35 Hughes CP, Berg L, Danziger WL, Coben LA, Martin RL. A new clinical scale for the staging of dementia. *British Journal of Psychiatry* 1982;**140**:566–572.

36 Ball CJ. Old age psychiatry. In: Rees L, Lipsedge MS, Ball CJ, eds. *Textbook of Psychiatry.* London: Edward Arnold, 1998. 196–210.

37 Mintzner J, Nietert P, Costa K, Rust P, Hoernig K. Identifying persons with dementia by use of a caregiver telephone interview. *American Journal of Geriatric Psychiatry* 1998;**6**:176–179.

38 Jorm AF, Jacomb PA. An Informant Questionnaire on Cognitive Decline in the Elderly (IQCODE): socio-demographic correlates, reliability, validity and some norms. *Psychological Medicine* 1989;**19**:1015–1022.

39 Mundt JC, Ferber KL, Rizzo H, Greist JH. Computer-automated dementia screening using a touch-tone telephone. *Archives of Internal Medicine* 2001;**161**:2481–2487.

40 Monteiro IM, Boksay I, Auer SR, Torossian C, Sinaiko E, Reisberg B. Reliability of routine clinical instruments for the assessment of Alzheimer's disease administered by telephone. *Journal of Geriatric Psychiatry and Neurology* 1998;**11**:18–24.

41 Ball CJ, Scott N, McLaren PM, et al. Preliminary evaluation of a Low-Cost VideoConferencing (LCVC) system for remote cognitive testing in adult psychiatric patients. *British Journal of Clinical Psychology* 1993;**23**:303–307.

42 Montani C, Billaud N, Couturier P, et al. 'Telepsychometry' a remote psychometry consultation in clinical gerontology. *Telemedicine Journal* 1996;**2**:145–149.

43 Grob P, Weintraub D, Sayles D, Raskin A, Ruskin PE. Psychiatric assessment of a nursing home population using audiovisual telecommunication. *Journal of Geriatric Psychiatry and Neurology* 2001;**14**:63–65.

44 Broadaty H, Moore CM. The Clock Drawing Test for dementia of the Alzheimer's Type: a comparison of three scoring methods in a memory disorders clinic. *International Journal of Geriatric Psychiatry* 1997;**12**:619–627.

45 Ball CJ, Puffett A. The assessment of cognitive function in the elderly using videoconferencing. *Journal of Telemedicine and Telecare* 1998;**4**(suppl 1):36–38.

46 Roth M, Tym E, Mountjoy CQ, et al. CAMDEX. A standardised instrument for the diagnosis of mental disorder in the elderly with special reference to the early detection of dementia. *British Journal of Psychiatry* 1986;**149**:698–709.

47 Ball C, Tyrrell J, Long C. Scoring written material from the Mini-Mental State Examination: a comparison of face-to-face, fax and video-linked scoring. *Journal of Telemedicine and Telecare* 1999;**5**:253–256.

48 Gauthier S, Lovestone S, eds. *Management of Dementia.* London: Martin Dunitz, 1999.

49 Yesavage JA, Brink TL, Rose TL, et al. Development and validation of a geriatric depression screening scale: a preliminary report. *Journal of Psychiatric Research* 1982–3;**17**:37–49.

50 Burke WJ, Roccaforte WH, Wengel SP, Conley DM, Potter JF. The reliability and validity of the Geriatric Depression Rating Scale administered by telephone. *Journal of the American Geriatrics Society* 1995;**43**:674–679.

51 Morishita L, Boult C, Ebbitt B, Rambel M, Fallstrom K, Gooden T. Concurrent validity of administering the Geriatric Depression Scale and the physical functioning dimension of the SIP by telephone. *Journal of the American Geriatrics Society* 1995;**43**:680–683.

52 Burke WJ, Rangwani S, Roccaforte WH, Wengel SP, Conley DM. The reliability and validity of the collateral source version of the Geriatric Depression Rating Scale administered by telephone. *International Journal of Geriatric Psychiatry* 1997;**12**:288–294.

53 Dorfman RA, Lubben JE, Mayer-Oakes A, et al. Screening for depression among a well elderly population. *Social Work* 1995;**40**:295–304.

54 Watson CG, Anderson PED, Thomas D, Nyberg K. Comparability of telephone and face to face diagnostic interview schedules. *Journal of Nervous and Mental Disease* 1992;**180**:534–535.

55 Wells KB, Burnam MA, Leake B, Robins LN. Agreement between face-to-face and telephone-administered version of the depression section of the NIMH Diagnostic Interview Schedule. *Journal of Psychiatric Research* 1988;**22**:207–220.

56 Hamilton M. A rating scale for depression. *Journal of Neurology, Neurosurgery and Psychiatry* 1960;**23**:56–61.

57 Simon GE, Revicki D, VonKorff M. Telephone assessment of depression severity. *Journal of Psychiatric Research* 1993;**27**:247–252.

58 Baer L, Jacobs DG, Cukor P, O'Laughlen J, Coyle JT, Magruder KM. Automated telephone screening survey for depression. *Journal of the American Medical Association* 1995;**273**:1943–1944.

59 Mundt JC, Kobak KA, Taylor LV, et al. Administration of the Hamilton Depression Rating Scale using interactive voice response technology. MD Computing: *Computers in Medical Practice* 1998;**15**:31–39.

60 Overall JE, Gorham DR. The Brief Psychiatric Rating Scale. *Psychological Reports* 1962;**10**:799–812.

61 Ball C J, McLaren PM. Comparability of face-to-face and videolink administration of the Brief Psychiatric Rating Scale. American *Journal of Psychiatry* 1995;**152**:958–959.

62 Chae YM, Park HJ, Cho JG, Hong GD, Cheon KA. The reliability and acceptability of telemedicine for patients with schizophrenia in Korea. *Journal of Telemedicine and Telecare* 2000;**6**:83–90.

63 Zarate CA Jr, Weinstock L, Cukor P, et al. Applicability of telemedicine for assessing patients with schizophrenia: acceptance and reliability. *Journal of Clinical Psychiatry* 1997;**58**:22–25.

64 Jones BN 3rd, Johnston D, Reboussin B, McCall WV. Reliability of telepsychiatry assessments: subjective versus observational ratings. *Journal of Geriatric Psychiatry and Neurology* 2001;**14**:66–71.

65 Tunstall N, Prince M, Mann A. Concurrent validity of a telephone-administered version of the Gospel Oak instrument (including the SHORT-CARE). International *Journal of Geriatric Psychiatry* 1997;**12**:1035–1038.

66 Cacciola JS, Alterman AI, Rutherford MJ, McKay JR, May DJ. Comparability of telephone and in-person structured clinical interview for DSM-III-R (SCID) diagnoses. *Assessment* 1999;**6**:235–242.

67 Kobak KA, Taylor LH, Dottl SL, et al. A computer-administered telephone interview to identify mental disorders. *Journal of the American Medical Association* 1997;**278**:905–910.

68 Fournier L, Lesage AD, Toupin J, Cyr M. Telephone surveys as an alternative for estimating prevalence of mental disorders and service utilization: a Montreal catchment area study. *Canadian Journal of Psychiatry* 1997;**42**:737–743.

69 Ruskin PE, Reed S, Kumar R, et al. Reliability and acceptability of psychiatric diagnosis via telecommunication and audiovisual technology. *Psychiatric Services* 1998;**49**:1086–1088.

70 Korner-Bitensky N, Wood-Dauphinee S. Barthel Index information elicited over the telephone. Is it reliable? *American Journal of Physical Medicine and Rehabilitation* 1995;**74**:9–18.

71 Ciesla JR, Shi L, Stoskopf CH, Samuels ME. Reliability of Katz's Activities of Daily Living Scale when used in telephone interviews. *Evaluation and the Health Professions* 1993;**16**:190–203.

72 DeiCas R, Street DA, Javitt JC. Assessment of visual acuity via a telephone interview. *Archives of Ophthalmology* 1992;**110**:1279–1282.

73 Craig JJ, McConville JP, Patterson VH, Wootton R. Neurological examination is possible using telemedicine. *Journal of Telemedicine and Telecare* 1999;**5**:177–181.

74 Kargman DE, Sacco RL, Boden-Albala B, Paik MC, Hauser WA, Shea S. Validity of telephone interview data for vascular disease risk factors in a racially mixed urban community: the Northern Manhattan Stroke Study. *Neuroepidemiology* 1999;**18**:174–184.

75 Franco A, Frossard M, Montani C. *Telemedicine en Gerontologie.* Paris: Serdi edition, 2000.

76 Marcantonio ER, Michaels M, Resnick NM. Diagnosing delirium by telephone. *Journal of General Internal Medicine* 1998;**13**:621–623.

77 Colantonio A, Cohen C, Pon M. Assessing support needs of caregivers of persons with dementia: who wants what? *Community Mental Health Journal* 2001;**37**:231–243.

78 Skipwith DH. Telephone counseling interventions with caregivers of elders. *Journal of Psychosocial Nursing and Mental Health Services* 1994;**32**:7–12.

79 Mahoney DM, Tarlow B, Jones RN, Tennstedt S, Kasten L. Factors affecting the use of a telephone-based intervention for caregivers of people with Alzheimer's disease. *Journal of Telemedicine and Telecare* 2001;**7**:139–148.

80 Goodman CC, Pynoos J. A model telephone information and support program for caregivers of Alzheimer's patients. *Gerontologist* 1990;**30**:399–404.

81 Smyth KA, Harris PB. Using telecomputing to provide information and support to caregivers of persons with dementia. *Gerontologist* 1993;**3**:123–127.

82 Brennan PF, Moore SM, Smyth KA. The effects of a special computer network on caregivers of persons with Alzheimer's disease. *Nursing Research* 1995;**44**:166–172.

83 Harvey RJ, Roques PK, Fox NC, Rosser MN. CANDID – Counselling and Diagnosis in Dementia: a national telemedicine service supporting the care of younger patients with dementia. *International Journal of Geriatric Psychiatry* 1998;**13**:381–388.

84 Berkman P, Heinik J, Rosenthal M, Burke M. Supportive telephone outreach as an interventional strategy for elderly patients in a period of crisis. *Social Work in Health Care* 1999;**28**:63–76.

85 Kaunonen M, Tarkka MT, Laippala P, Paunonen-Ilmonen M. The impact of supportive telephone call intervention on grief after the death of a family member. *Cancer Nursing* 2000;**23**:483–491.

86 Welch HG, Johnson DJ, Edson R. Telephone care as an adjunct to routine medical follow-up. A negative randomized trial. *Effective Clinical Practice* 2000;**3**:123–130.

87 Walker CC. An educational intervention for hypertension management in older African Americans. *Ethnicity and Disease* 2000;**10**:165–174.

88 Allen D. Telephone follow up for older people discharged from A&E. *Nursing Standard* 1997;**11**:34–37.

89 Poncia HD, Ryan J, Carver M. Next day telephone follow up of the elderly: a needs assessment and critical incident monitoring tool for the accident and emergency department. *Journal of Accident and Emergency Medicine* 2000;**17**:337–340.

90 Hashim MJ, Franks P, Fiscella K. Effectiveness of telephone reminders in improving rate of appointments kept at an outpatient clinic: a randomized controlled trial. *Journal of the American Board of Family Practice* 2001;**14**:193–196.

91 MacDonald J, Brown N, Ellis P. Using telephone prompts to improve initial attendance at a community mental health center. *Psychiatric Services* 2000;**51**:812–814.

92 Danoff NL, Kemper KJ. Does excluding patients without telephones affect the results of telephone reminder studies? *Western Journal of Medicine* 1993;**158**:44–46.

93 Fulmer TT, Feldman PH, Kim TS, et al. An intervention study to enhance medication compliance in community-dwelling elderly individuals. *Journal of Gerontological Nursing* 1999;**25**:6–14.

94 Tutty S, Simon G, Ludman E. Telephone counselling as an adjunct to antidepressant treatment in the primary care system. A pilot study. *Effective Clinical Practice* 2000;**3**:170–178.

95 Schoenbaum M, Unutzer J, Sherbourne C, et al. Cost-effectiveness of practice initiated quality improvement for depression: results of a randomised control trial. *Journal of the American Medical Association* 2001;**286**:1325–1330.

96 Hunkeler EM, Meresman JF, Hargreaves WA, et al. Efficacy of a nurse telehealth care and peer support in augmenting treatment of depression in primary care. *Archives of Family Medicine* 2000;**9**:700–708.

97 Pampallona S, Bollini P, Tibaldi G, Kupelnick B, Munizza C. Patient adherence in the treatment of depression. *British Journal of Psychiatry* 2002;**180**:104–109.

98 Ball C, Box O. General practice referrals to a community team for mental health in the elderly: information and the mode of referral. *British Journal of General Practice* 1997;**47**:503–504.

99 De Leo D, Carollo G, Dello Buono M. Lower suicide rates associated with a Tele-Help/Tele-Check service for the elderly at home. *American Journal of Psychiatry* 1995;**152**:632–634.

100 Telemedicine Information Exchange. Available at http://tie2.telemed.org [last checked 11 September 2002].

101 Chan WM, Woo J, Hui E, Hjelm NM. The role of telenursing in the provision of geriatric outreach services to residential homes in Hong Kong. *Journal of Telemedicine and Telecare* 2001;**7**:38–46.

102 Tang WK, Chiu H, Woo J, Hjelm M, Hui E. Telepsychiatry in psychogeriatric service: a pilot study. *International Journal of Geriatric Psychiatry* 2001;**16**:88–93.

103 Lee JH, Kim JH, Jhoo JH, et al. A telemedicine system as a care modality for dementia patients in Korea. *Alzheimer Disease and Associated Disorders* 2000;**14**:94–101.

104 Lyketsos CG, Roques C, Hovanec L, Jones BN 3rd. Telemedicine use and the reduction of psychiatric admissions from a long-term care facility. *Journal of Geriatric Psychiatry and Neurology* 2001;**14**:76–79.

105 Johnston D, Jones BN 3rd. Telepsychiatry consultations to a rural nursing facility: a two-year experience. *Journal of Geriatric Psychiatry and Neurology* 2001;**14**:72–75.

106 Kaplan EH. Telepsychotherapy. Psychotherapy by telephone, videotelephone and computer video conferencing. *Journal of Psychotherapy Practice and Research* 1997;**6**:227–237.

107 Baer L, Cukor P, Jenike MA, Leahy J, O'Laughlen J, Coyle JT. Pilot studies of telemedicine for patients with obsessive-compulsive disorder. *American Journal of Psychiatry* 1995;**152**:1383–1385.

108 Heather N, Kissoon-Singh J, Fenton GW. Assisted natural recovery from alcohol problems: effects of a self-help manual with and without supplementary telephone support. *British Journal of Addiction* 1990;**85**:1177–1185.

109 Jones BN 3rd, Ruskin PE. Telemedicine and geriatric psychiatry: directions for future research and policy. *Journal of Geriatric Psychiatry and Neurology* 2001;**14**:59–62.

110 Tyrell J, Couturier P, Montani C, Franco A. Teleconsultation in psychology: the use of videolinks for interviewing and assessing elderly patients. *Age and Ageing* 2001;**30**:191–195.

111 Jones BN III. Telepsychiatry and geriatric care. *Current Psychiatry Reports* 2001;**3**:29–36.

Section 3: E-mental Health and the Internet – diagnosis and patient management, and self-help

15

Online Mental Health Information

Helen Christensen, Kathleen M. Griffiths and Chloe Groves

Introduction

The number of current web users across the globe has been estimated as 513 million with the expectation of a billion users by the end of 2004.[1] At present there are nearly 100 million US adults using the Internet[2] and 25 million in the UK.[3] Recent Australian Bureau of Statistics figures[4] indicate that over half (56%) of all Australian homes have a computer, and the number with access to the Internet has risen to 2.7 million (37% of all homes). The Internet has been recognized as the fastest growing technology ever.

Recent data also suggest that health is one of the most common reasons for using the Internet.[5] It has also been recognized that the Internet allows individuals to take control of their own health. Eysenbach noted that 'empowerment of consumers and patients is possible by making the knowledge bases of medicine and personal electronic records accessible to consumers over the Internet'. He reported 'e health opens new avenues for patient centered medicine, and enables evidence-based patient choice'.[6]

There is also growing evidence that self-help is of major importance in western countries. There is evidence that 'more Americans try to change their health behaviors through self help than through all other forms of professionally designed programs'.[7] These same authors report that the 12-month prevalence of self-help is approximately 3–4% of the American population. In a review of online activity these authors examined for 2 weeks all postings on two online domains (America OnLine and the Internet) for 20 disease conditions. Thirty-seven virtual support groups were identified from AOL, and 40 000 newsgroups from the Internet. The third highest rate of postings on AOL was found for depression (after multiple sclerosis and diabetes). The highest for the broader Internet were chronic fatigue, diabetes and breast cancer followed by depression in fourth place. Another research report, the Harris Poll, suggested that depression is the most frequently sought topic for health information.[8] The use of the Internet for self-help may be particularly important given the evidence that only a minority of people with mental health problems in the community seek professional health.[9]

Recent research also suggests that support groups and discussion forums may be effective in relieving symptoms. Professionally mediated support groups are popular, may be effective, and are used more by individuals with stigmatizing illnesses, such as depression, than by individuals with other less stigmatizing disorders.[7,10–12]

There is growing recognition of the importance of the Internet as a means of disseminating public health and prevention messages. The sophistication and potential effectiveness of health promotion and prevention information on the Internet far exceeds that of other media. For example, the Internet is capable of supporting individually tailored prevention programmes (where individual messages are tailored to a participant's risk profile) and the information may be accessed anonymously. Research suggests that individuals prefer tailored health information.[13] The Internet can support databases that allow information about users to be collected and analysed conveniently. Research into consumer uptake and interest in medical information directly through computers and telecommunications systems is a rapidly expanding area of research.[14] The growth of the Internet has enormous potential for facilitating the development of mental health literacy in the community and for providing mental health programs that may be accessible to many who do not seek or cannot access professional treatment.

Finally, the Internet is a powerful medium for providing information about mental health issues to all the community, not just to those with mental health problems. In particular, its capacity to provide widely accessible information makes it a potentially powerful force in the destigmatization of mental health problems.

Definition of mental health information

In this chapter we use the e-Health Ethics Initiative[15] in defining health information as:

> information for staying well, preventing and managing disease, and making other decisions related to health and health care. It includes information for making decisions about health products and health services. It may be in the form of data, text, audio, and /or video. It may involve enhancements through programming and interactivity.

This definition may be broader than that commonly used in the context of patient education. However, it is a useful definition because it accurately reflects the type of information that is available to users when they seek mental health information on the Internet. Our emphasis in this chapter is on health information available to Internet users. We have not specifically examined the information provided for the medical profession (see Chapter 16). Where appropriate, we discuss briefly information provided by sites which offer support groups (see Chapter 17) and also information on sites that offer self-treatment (see Chapter 20).

There are three major issues which concern mental health information on websites:

▶ the nature of mental health information on the Internet

▶ the quality of mental health website information

▶ the potential of the Internet to deliver prevention information.

The nature of mental health information on the Internet

It is an enormous task to describe and classify the nature of mental health information available on the Internet. Sites can be described in terms of their scope (e.g. whether they are portal sites, sites specific to depression or anxiety, or whether they fulfil a clearinghouse function), ownership characteristics, the extent of their coverage (e.g. whether they cover all aspects of mental health disorders, such as prevalence, incidence, risk factors, nature and type of treatments, etc.) and specific directions (news provision, published articles, products and resources, etc). However, these classifications give little insight into the diversity of health sites available to the Internet user.

A number of additional distinctions provide a framework for discussion about websites using the Internet, and the criteria by which Internet sites might be grouped (Box 15.1).

Websites can be described in terms of their intervention type. Although most depression websites provide information about depression, particularly about its treatment, other sites aim to prevent depression, to offer early intervention or long-term rehabilitation.

Box 15.1. Useful distinctions for mental health delivery using the Internet

Type of mental health intervention
Promotion
Prevention
Early intervention
Treatment
Relapse prevention
Rehabilitation

Volume and cost structure for these sorts of delivery services
Prevention and promotion
Community care
Primary care
Specialist care
Hospital care

Type of interaction
Consumer–professional: interactions using email, web counselling
Consumer–consumer: interactions using email, chat groups, bulletin boards
Consumer–other: advice from non-professionals
Professional–professional: interactions for peer review, specialist consultation
Consumer–information: the download of information from the Internet
Consumer–interactive technology: interactions with a computer program/system
Professional–information: information targeted at professionals
Professional–interactive technology: training/continuing education using interactive systems

Type of service
Interventions initiated by doctors/other mental health professionals for patients/clients (web counselling and email)
Interventions designed by organizations to help people manage and improve health through self-help
Information sites designed by governments, universities, non-government organizations and private individuals and bodies to provide information about mental disorders and their treatment
Sites developed to provide support to those in need

A second distinction concerns the target audience for the information. Most sites are directed at users or consumers or their carers, but some are directed at primary care or specialist audiences, and yet others are aimed at hospital care administrators. Most of these sites are available to the Internet user seeking health information.

A third distinction, overlapping to some extent with the first two, is based on the type of interaction between communicators, whether this is between consumer and health care provider (e.g. doctor, psychologist, social worker) or between consumers and consumers or between health care provider and health care provider (e.g. the general practitioner and specialists). Most sites do not promote a high level of interaction but other sites invite online communication with professionals or with others who may suffer or have suffered from depression. Clearly, many more subdistinctions can be made within these categories. For example, a further distinction for the type of interaction undertaken via the Internet has been clearly articulated by the International Society for Mental Health Online,[16] which lists the types of professional interventions that are possible using the Internet.

In addition, sites can be specified by the types of services they provide. These vary widely from direct interventions initiated by doctors and health professionals, to sites designed to provide support to those with depression or other mental health problems. Information sites are designed by governments, universities, non-government organizations and private individuals to provide information about their treatments. These sites are designed largely for consumers and carers, but, particularly in the case of clearinghouse sites, may be of use to students for training and professionals for continuing education. A new class of site is one where interventions are designed to help people manage and improve their health through self-help. These initiatives do not entail direct contact between health professionals and consumers. Rather these self-help technologies involve systematically developed programs that provide interactive services to individuals, and may include Internet, email, Web or video downloading. Examples of these programs overseas for general health include One Health Plan[17] and the PA Web.[18] Most of these programs aim to prevent disorders and intervene broadly. Finally there are sites that offer support through email, counselling and chat groups. The Internet has seen a proliferation of bulletin boards and chat rooms targeted specifically at health consumers and resulting in increased facilitation of informal communication between health consumers. This development of a worldwide patient-to-patient network may lead to more effective health advocacy groups and may inform health professionals more effectively about the public's perceptions of illness.

To our knowledge there has been no major audit of the type of information provided on mental health sites. In this section of the chapter we briefly describe several health portal sites as well as a number of specific sites which cover the mental health issue of depression. To examine the depression sites we used the dmoz directory.[19] dmoz is a comprehensive human edited directory of the Internet, which has been put together by volunteer editors. dmoz is an important directory because it 'powers core directory services for the most popular portals and search engines on the Web, including AOL Search, Netscape Search, Google, Lycos, DirectHit, and HotBot, and hundreds of others. Categories that are employed on the major search engines use those already created by dmoz.

Major mental health portals on the Internet

There are a number of major mental health portal sites listed in the dmoz directory (Box 15.2). These major portal sites provide a range of information and services to users and they record high levels of Internet traffic.

Box 15.2. Examples of mental health portal sites

Mental Help Net[50]
Mental Help Net is a large mental health portal which was established in late 1995. It is now said to include 15 000 pages of information and 6000 reviewed links to resources and to have 500 000 visitors each month. The site offers information about symptoms and treatments and includes links, and support board forums and chat rooms, news and book reviews, and mental health videos for different mental disorders. It also offers several online mood and ADHD assessment tools, an online book on psychological self-help, information about medication, and bulletin boards focusing on particular medications.

Psych Central: Dr John Grohol's Mental Health Page[51]
Established in 1992, Psych Central contains a large, annotated directory of mental health resources, information about symptoms and treatments for different mental disorders, a weekly online chat group with mental health website pioneer Dr Grohol, community support forums, online tools for assessing different mental disorders, and book reviews and news items.

Internet mental health[52]
This Canadian site provides diagnostic and treatment information and resources for over 50 different mental health disorders. The site has message boards for bipolar disorder, depression and schizophrenia, as well as chat rooms, information about psychiatric medications and links to web resources. The site links to a sister site[53] which offers online diagnosis for 37 different conditions but access to this facility is available only to paid subscribers.

NIMH (National Institute of Mental Health) for the public[53]
This is a subsite of the National Institute of Mental Health, the principal mental health research agency of the US government. The 'For the public' section of the site provides educational information and links about the symptoms, diagnosis and treatment of mental disorders.

The Mental Health Foundation[54]
This is the website of the Mental Health Association of the UK. It provides educational material about different mental health disorders, information about where to seek help and links to other mental health resources. The site contains a link to its sister site,[55] which lists more than 4000 resources including information about organizations, events, websites and news. Visitors to Connect can personalize the information they receive to match their particular interests (e.g. according to the disorder of interest, country of origin).

Specific mental disorders on the Web

At the time of writing (June 2002) there were 5514 mental health sites listed in dmoz, of which 3468 were listed as sites concerned with specific mental health disorders. The category with the most sites was listed as neurodevelopmental (652), followed by child and adolescent (650). The next most common was mood (477), followed by anxiety (418), sleep (301) and impulse control (226). Schizophrenia had 101 sites listed. Substance-related sites were relatively poorly represented with 28 specific sites.

Depression-specific sites on the Internet

In dmoz, depression is categorized under mental health conditions/disorders/mood/ bipolar or depression. At the time of review (June 2002), there were 475 mood disorders sites, some of which covered bipolar disorder and some of which covered depression. Within the depression category, 15 sites were listed as involving childhood disorders and 18 as focused on seasonal affective disorder. In addition, 37 sites were categorized as containing articles and research, 22 sites as providing direct links to books, 18 sites as providing chats and forums, 54 sites as containing personal pages, 30 sites as providing products/services and there were 33 specific links to support groups. As well as these categories, there were an additional 104 sites which were not classified within these subcategories. These sites formed the basis of the present review.

To provide more detailed information about these 104 depression sites we systematically reviewed the content of the first 60. The data are displayed in Table 15.1. Three of the sixty sites were excluded because they could not be located on the day of the search, and one site was a duplicate. Appendix 15.1 outlines the specific coding criteria. As expected, most of the websites in this sample were specific to depression, with approximately 70% being single topic or 'stand-alone' sites, 14% being pages that belonged to a site with broader scope (not confined to mental health) and 16% consisting primarily of links to other sites. Mental health professionals individually, or as part of an organization, owned approximately 30% of the sites. Consumers and consumer organizations owned 25% of the sites and media companies, pharmaceutical companies and other profit-making organizations owned 35%. Fifty-three per cent of sites promoted services or products for use in depression on the site itself. Of the 56 sites reviewed, approximately 40% had health professional involvement, either through ownership or editorial functions.

Predominantly sites were concerned with the treatment and support of individuals with depression. There were few sites concerned with depression promotion or prevention. Sites targeted individuals rather than general practitioners or specialists. Most sites provided information about depression organized into various topics on the web pages. Other sites provided little information directly but aimed to provide the mechanism through which consumers could exchange information with each other (e.g. bulletin boards). Professionals (psychiatrists and psychologists) offered services including medically informed interactive feedback, invitations to seek professional consultation, research information or vetted information about other sites.

Table 15.1 clearly shows that the most frequent goal of the website was to provide emotional support to those with depression. Only two sites (3.6%) offered specific professional help through traditional or email intervention. Two sites offered interactive self-help programmes: http://www.wellmed.com/wellmed/intro/ ConditionDepression.htm[20] (owned by a US health communication company) and http://www.copewithlife.com.[21] The Wellmed site provided tailored information to users online. It specifically asked the user to provide depression information and it

Table 15.1. Characteristics of specific depression Internet sites in the DMOZ directory

Variable	% of sites
Primary ownership	
Individual psychiatrist	5.4
Individual psychologist	7.1
Professional organization	1.8
Individual with depression	19.6
Consumer organizations	5.4
University/other non-profit organization	5.4
Pharmaceutical company	7.1
Media company	16.1
Other for-profit organization	12.5
Unknown	19.6
Setting target	
Community	89.3
Primary care	7.1
Combination	3.6
Interaction type	
Professional service to consumer	14.3
Consumer to consumer (support)	21.4
Professional to professional	3.6
Consumer information	44.6
More than one of the above	9.0
Other	3.6
Unknown	3.6
Primary aim of website	
Interventions initiated by doctors or professionals for patients	3.6
Interventions designed by organizations to help people manage and improve health through self-help	3.6
Sites provided by government and universities to give information	7.1
Sites provided by commercial groups to give information or inform of services	23.2
Sites designed for consumers to provide emotional support	46.4
Other	7.2
Missing	8.9
Information	
Symptoms and diagnosis	60.7
Self-assessments and screening	28.6
Treatment	69.6
Prevention	5.4
Risk and causes	37.5
Incidence and prevalence	37.5
Specific groups (young and older)	17.9
Help resources	41.1
Recommended reading list	23.2
Stigma reduction	
Stigma reduction	25
Features	
Bulletin board	30.4
Chatroom	16.1
Online counselling	1.8

Table 15.1. – *continued*

Variable	% of sites
Audio tapes to download	12.5
e-books	10.7
Mailing list	21.4
Newsletter	25
News	12.5
Send card facility	3.6
Radio show	3.6
Visitor/guest book	16.1
Poem posting	8.9
Host email	5.4
Web pages technology	3.6

Note: With the exception of online counselling, only features recorded for more than two sites are shown above.

provided individual feedback. http://www.copewithlife.com promoted a voice-operated psychotherapy service (COPE) which can be purchased by individual consumers and which was illustrated online. COPE is designed to have the user manage their own psychological treatment.

A number of university sites provided evidence-based information for the treatment of depression, including the site we have developed – http://bluepages.anu.edu.au[22] (Fig. 15.1). Bluepages provides evidence-based information for medical, psychological and alternative depression treatments and at the time of review was

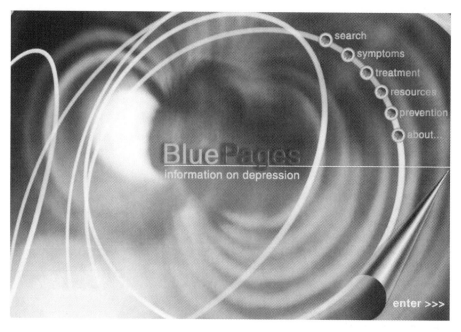

Fig. 15.1. The Bluepages site offers information on symptoms, treatment, resources and prevention. It also contains a depression-site specific search capacity.

ranked highest of all listed sites using the Google PageRank. This rating is designed to reflect the extent to which Internet sites are linked, and hence their 'quality'.[23]

Only approximately 25% of sites were rated as providing messages that might reduce stigma. To be rated as providing such information sites were required to provide messages such as 'depression does not mean that you have a weak character', 'you deserve treatment' or to describe successful individuals who had experienced or overcome mental health problems.

The resources provided by the sites in the dmoz directory are outlined in Table 15.1. The most common features on the sites were the use of bulletin boards and the availability of chat room facilities.

Table 15.2. Major quality initiatives[45]

Code of conduct/ethics	Third party certification or rating	Tool based
eHealth code of Ethics http://www.ihealthcoalition.org/ ethics/ehcode.html	URAC Health Web Site Accreditation program http://www.urac.org/ websiteaccreditation.htm	DISCERN http://www.discern.org.uk
Health Internet Ethics (Hi-Ethics) http://www.hiethics.com/Principles/ index.asp	MedPICS Certification and Rating of Trustworthy and Assessed Health Information on the Net (MedCERTAIN) http://www.medcertain.org	The Health Summit Working Group-Criteria for Assessing the Quality of Health Information on the Internet: IQ tool (HSWG IQ Tool) http://hitiweb.mitretek.org/iq/ default.asp
HON Code http://www.hon.ch/HONcode/ Conduct.html		
European Comunity Quality Criteria for Health-related Websites http://europa.eu.int/information_ society/eeurope/ehealth/quality/ index_en.htm	TNO Quality Medical Information and Communication (QMIC) http://www.health.tno.nl/homepage_ pg_en.html	
American Medical Association (AMA): Guidelines for Medical and Health Information Sites on the Internet: Principles Governing AMA Publications Web Sites http://pubs.ama-assn.org/ama_ web.html	Organizing Medical Networked Information (OMNI) http://omni.ac.uk	
British Health Care Internet Association (BHIR): Quality Standards for Medical Publishing on the Web http://www.bhia.org/reference/ documents/recommend_webquality. htm		
The International Federation of Pharmaceutical Manufacturers Associations (IFPMA) Code of Marketing http://www.ifpma.org/		

We conducted a series of analyses to see if there was a relationship between features of the site, such as site ownership, scope, resource type, PageRank, type of service provided, and whether a health professional was involved. We found that sites produced by individuals compared to organizations were more likely to provide treatment information but less likely to provide information about the risks or causes of depression, information about prevalence of depression or help resources (such as lists of contact organizations, direct help lines). However, sites owned by individuals were more likely than sites owned by organizations to provide stigma reduction messages. Individuals were more likely to offer bulletin boards, chat rooms and reading lists, but less likely to offer mailing lists and news updates. Sites with health professional involvement were more likely to describe depression symptoms and to provide self-help depression screening tests.

There were differences as a function of type of site (Box 15.1). After collapsing the categories into larger groupings, the data suggested that sites which offered professional services to consumers were more likely to provide screening tests. Sites which aimed to provide information were also more likely to include online screening tests. Bulletin boards were more likely to appear on consumer-to-consumer interaction sites, not an unexpected finding.

Higher Google PageRank was associated with the existence of an editorial board on the site ($F = 7.4$, $P = 0.03$) and with health professional involvement ($F = 10.4$, $P = 0.01$) but with no other indicators.

The information available to Internet users varies across sites. However, most sites provide information about symptoms and diagnosis and to some extent risk factors and causes. We found few sites that addressed the specific issues of depression in young people or discussed issues concerning prevention. We developed a measure of the scope of the site by counting the number of areas which were mentioned by each site and then examined it with respect to other site features. Greater scope was associated with the presence of a disclaimer on the site, the existence of a privacy policy and a professionally designed site, but not with other characteristics of the site such as site ownership or Google PageRank. The sites which provided the broadest coverage in this sample were http://www.beyondblue.org.au/site,[24] http://www.wellmed.com/wellmed/intro/ConditionDepression.htm[20] and http://bluepages.anu.edu.au.[22]

Quality of mental health information websites

It is clear that the Internet is a popular source of information on mental health and that a large number of websites provide information on mental health. But how good is this information?

The most important indication of the quality of a health website is whether it results in better health outcomes. To date there have been no studies of the effect of mental health information sites on consumer mental health or consumer mental health literacy. However, there is some evidence that health information websites can improve consumer health outcomes for other conditions.[25]

Arguably, the next most important indicator of website quality relates to the accuracy and comprehensiveness of its content. There have been at least four published studies of the quality of the content of mental health sites on the Internet.[26-29] Each of these studies has been concerned with depression and three have employed evidence-based guidelines or systematic reviews to evaluate content quality. All concluded that on average, the quality (accuracy, comprehensiveness or both) of depression information on the Internet was poor, a result which is consistent with study findings for non-mental health sites.[26,27,30] Nevertheless, most sites did have important positive features such as emphasizing that depression can be treated and encouraging help-seeking.[26,27] In addition, it is clear that there is considerable variability in the quality of sites and that there are high-quality mental health sites on the Internet.

Many other criteria have been used in evaluating the quality of health websites.[30,31] Of these, readability is clearly very important. Material may be accurate but if the reader is unable to understand it, at best it will be unhelpful and at worst misleading. A study of depression and other health websites[28] concluded that the average reading grade level of the material on the sites was 13.2 years (equivalent to US College level). This is considerably above the recommended reading level for consumer health information. The treatment information on our own site, http://bluepages.anu.edu.au, was designed to be read at year 8 reading level.

Other potentially important features of sites that have been investigated for mental health, and which we have analysed for the dmoz depression sites, include the use of disclaimers, the presence of an editorial board, the promotion of products/services, specification of a privacy policy and the availability of a feedback mechanism. Only 18% of the dmoz sites we reviewed had an editorial board, a result that is consistent with our previous findings that few depression sites have an editorial board.[26,27] However, the majority of the dmoz depression sites (75%) did have a feedback mechanism such as an email link, so that users can provide input to the webmaster. We have previously reported that most Australian depression sites use disclaimers.[27] Similarly two thirds of the dmoz sites we reviewed included disclaimers. This contrasts with the findings of another group,[32] which reported that websites concerned with eating disorders typically did not provide 'health disclaimers, caveats, and other health-related alerts'. Half of the dmoz depression sites did not include a privacy policy and 40% of Australian depression sites[27] fail to include a privacy policy on their site. Given that trust is likely to be an important factor for users who access mental health sites, this would appear to be a significant limitation of depression websites. Finally, 43% of the dmoz depression sites promoted drugs, specific services or books and one third of Australian depression sites promoted products.[27]

After content, the most frequently cited criteria for evaluating health-related websites is the design and aesthetics of the site.[31] Such a measure is clearly irrelevant if more important criteria (such as accuracy of content, readability, disclaimers) are not satisfied. Moreover, there is some evidence that aesthetics does not discriminate well between sites of high and low content quality.[33] Nevertheless, design and aesthetics may influence the degree to which a site engages and maintains the attention of a visitor. In the small number of studies of the aesthetics of non-mental health sites, few of the reviewed sites were judged seriously insufficient.[30] However, in our view, only a minority of the sites in the dmoz depression category could be classified as aesthetic (18%).

The next most commonly used set of criteria for website quality include accountability criteria (authorship, attribution of sources and references, disclosure of ownership and sponsorship; indication of when the site was created and modified), proposed by Silberg and his collaborators.[34] In a previous review we found that the majority of depression sites disclosed the authors of the content and their credentials and affiliations, the ownership of the sites and when they were created and modified. However, sites typically did not provide the sources underlying their recommendations and few attached hierarchy of evidence information to their recommendations.[26]

It has frequently been assumed that accountability criteria are indicators of the overall quality of the site. However, we failed to find a significant correlation between the Silberg criteria and content quality as assessed by evidence-based guidelines or global subjective measures of site quality.[26] A subsequent, larger study of breast cancer sites found that the Silberg accountability did correlate with accuracy of content, but content was assessed using expert ratings rather than evidence-based guidelines.[35]

More recently, focus has shifted to DISCERN, an instrument designed to measure the quality of health information. This instrument comprises 15 questions and one global item. Items include clarity of aims, relevance and currency of material, evidence of bias, inclusion of sources of information, benefits, risks and treatment choices as well as other items. In the only study to investigate the possible validity of this scale as a measure of the accuracy of health information quality, we found high correlations between the DISCERN score and content quality as measured by evidence-based information. If this result can be replicated, it may have important implications for those concerned with identifying high-quality sites. Whether such measures can or would be used by consumers is unclear.[36]

Health initiatives

Currently, the majority of people who search for information on the Internet use a search engine. Most do not look past the first 10 results returned by the search engine.[37] However, there is no guarantee that sites retrieved in the first 10 contain high-quality information. We found no correlation between the order of search engine retrieval of Australian depression sites and content quality.[27] Another group reported that website popularity as measured by the site's page rank on the popular search engine Google was not associated with quality of content.[35]

How then can a consumer access high-quality sites? There has been considerable interest in the issue over the past years and a number of major initiatives have been proposed or established to address the problem. The major Internet quality initiatives have recently been reviewed in the Journal of Medical Internet Research. The reviewers listed three means for governing quality on websites. These were: codes of conduct or ethics (self-regulation through adherence to a code of conduct); third-party certification; and tool-based evaluation.[38] However, they noted that each of these initiatives had disadvantages. These included the burden they place on health information producers, users and certifiers, the problems posed by the need to maintain the initiatives particularly in the context of unreliable funding, the difficulty in establishing 'a critical mass of acceptance' of an initiative and the problem of user indifference and the absence of meaningful enforcement mechanisms. They cautioned that quality initiatives should not be left to develop in a 'haphazard, uncoordinated way', and argued that there is a need for global leadership in the development of quality standards for Internet health, and suggested that the World Health Organization was well placed to play a leading role in the process.

The potential of the Internet to deliver prevention information and self-help

A final area to consider is the extent to which current interventions in mental health deliver public health promotion and prevention messages. Arguably, the Internet has distinct advantages as a medium for the dissemination of prevention information.

The qualities of the Internet that have led to its potential for prevention work include its capacity to reach an audience, with widely available, easily modifiable access to information, its likely cost effectiveness, and its capacity to support software applications that can be tailored to individual needs. This is particularly important, given the recognition of the importance of individually tuned messages in effective prevention. In areas other than mental health, a wide range of prevention programs have been implemented in the last two decades at workplaces and schools, and within the general community, to change risk factors such as smoking and high-fat diet consumption and thus prevent diseases such as cardiovascular disease and cancer. After reviewing the outcomes of these community intervention trials, Sorenson et al[39] noted that the 'next generation of community-based intervention' should be tailored to the needs of individuals, and involve the community in the planning process. In addiction research, Prochaska et al[40] demonstrated that successful interventions require that messages be customized to a person's motivational stage. Prochaska's transtheoretical model, which incorporates five stages of change – pre-contemplation, contemplation, preparation, action and maintenance – is now widely incorporated into studies of health treatment and prevention.[41]

The Internet has been used for the effective prevention of obesity and in exercise[18] and dietary interventions, including the prevention of eating disorders which supports its potential in mental health prevention. Moreover, there is evidence that Internet delivery may be as effective as classroom delivery for these interventions. A controlled trial comparing the effects of an Internet- and a classroom-delivered psychoeducation program for eating disorders reported no differences between these interventions, but greater effects for both treatments compared to a waitlist control condition.[42]

Highly sophisticated behavioural change programs offering tailored interventions are feasible. For example, Internet-based tailored behavioural change programs directed at exercise and nutrition have been developed, although they await full evaluation. Prochaska and his collaborators have developed PACE+ (Patient-centered

Assessment and Counseling for Exercise plus Nutrition), which is an interactive health communication techniques designed to promote physical activity and improved health nutrition in adolescents and adults.[43] The existence of these programs points to the feasibility of developing comparable programs for Internet-based mental health prevention.

All these findings indicate the potential of the Internet in the development of mental health literacy and health promotion. The question that we need to ask is whether the potential for tailored delivery of mental health prevention programs has yet been realized. Data from our searches of dmoz indicate that tailored information systems are already available. As noted above, WellMed[20] is a depression site that provides tailored messages in response to the user's symptom level. We have also developed a tailored, interactive website which offers cognitive behavioural therapy-based prevention for depression (Fig. 15.2). This site, Moodgym,[44] delivers cognitive behavioural therapy to young people. Outcome data on the use and popularity of the site are now available.[45]

The availability of these tailored information and interactive sites is an exciting development. Even more interesting are the developments which will allow material to be presented in response to the user's direct enquiry through the use of artificial intelligence. Such sites currently exist on the Internet and have been modified to sell goods and services or to provide conversation (see for example, http://www.alicebot.org[46] or http://www.maiw.com/main.html[47]).

Possible limitations to public health interventions using the Internet

In Australia, research suggests that access to the Internet is increasing more rapidly than the uptake of any other technology, but that there are inequities in its use.[48,49] In addition, higher income families, families with children and people living in cities rather than rural areas are more likely to have computer and Internet access. Internet usage was much less frequent in those aged over 55 years. Similarly, in New Zealand and the USA, studies show that the digital divide affects the less well educated, older and minority groups. Although access may be generally lower in these groups, Internet consultation may bring significant benefits to sections of the community that are disadvantaged in traditional medical health care.[49]

The future

There is a great diversity and range of mental health and depression information sites on the Internet. Websites differ in scope, aims and the provision of services. Although we need to be cautious in generalizing from our survey of depression-specific sites to those for other specific mental health conditions, our data suggest that the majority of sites may be designed with the aim of providing emotional support to people with mental health disorders. The next most common purpose

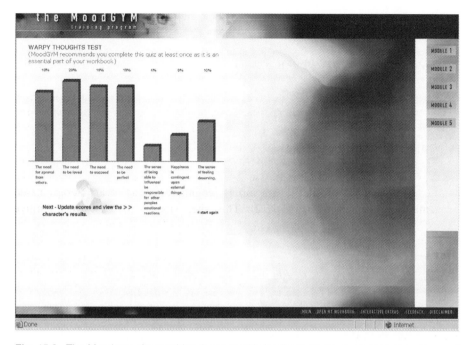

Fig. 15.2. The Moodgym site provides the user with feedback about psychological profiles and then recommends specific web pages.

seems to be the provision of advice or information about services by for-profit organizations or professionals. Interventions provided by government, not-for-profit organizations and universities are relatively uncommon. Interventions initiated by doctors or other professionals online are relatively rarely listed in the dmoz web directory. Finally, despite the potential of the Internet for supporting sophisticated tailored programs, few health communication systems are listed.

Available reviews of website quality have generally concluded that the quality of website information when compared to information from clinical practice guidelines is poor. However, there are now a number of initiatives which may increase the quality of mental health sites and assist consumers to locate high-quality information. Further research is likely to reveal how these initiatives fare.

To date the advantages of the Internet as a health promotion medium have not been realized, although there are a number of tailored and interactive sites in mental health. We believe that over the next few years there may be a disproportionate growth in consumer-driven Internet interventions such as chat groups, web counselling and self-help sites targeting consumer needs. These sectors are largely unregulated due to the relatively standard-free and egalitarian nature of the Internet. While this lack of regulation has many advantages, there is a need to develop guidelines that will facilitate safe and useful developments on the Internet.

References

1   Reuters News. November 20 2001. Available at http://www.zdnet.com/zdnn/stories/news/ [last checked 23 August 2002].

2   Risk A, Petersen C. Health information on the internet: quality issues and international initiatives. *Journal of the American Medical Association* 2002;**287**:2713–2715.

3   NetRatings Inc. Nielsen//NetRatings. Internet usage statistics for the month of December 2001 (United Kingdom). Available at http://epm.netratings.com/uk/web/NRpublicreports.usagemonthly [last checked 26 August 2002].

4   Australian Bureau of Statistics (ABS). *Use of the Internet by Householders, Australia.* November 2000. Cat No 8147.0. Canberra: ABS, 2001.

5   Powell J, Clarke A. The WWW of the World Wide Web: Who, What, and Why? *Journal of Medical Internet Research* 2002;**4**:E4.

6   Eysenbach G. What is e-Health? *Journal of Medical Internet Research* 2001;**3**:E20.

7   Davison KP, Pennebaker JW, Dickerson SS. Who talks? The social psychology of illness support groups. *American Psychologist* 2000;**55**:205–217.

8   Taylor H. *Explosive growth of 'cyberchondriacs' continues.* [The Harris Poll Number 47.] 5 August, 1999. Available at http://www.harrisinteractive.com/harris_poll/index.asp?PiD=117. [last checked 26 August 2002].

9   Andrews G, Henderson AS, eds. *Unmet Need in Psychiatry: problems, resources, responses.* Cambridge: Cambridge University Press, 2000.

10 Zrebiec JF, Jacobson AM. What attracts patients with diabetes to an internet support group? A 21-month longitudinal website study. *Diabetic Medicine* 2001;**18**:154–158.

11 Witt RT. Comparison of self-help computer-mediated communication groups: a CTF analysis. *Dissertation Abstracts International* 2000;**60**:5842.

12 Muncer S, Loader B, Burrows R, Pleace N, Nettleton S. Form and structure of newsgroups giving social support: a network approach. *CyberPsychology and Behavior* 2000;**3**:1017–1029.

13 De Nooijer J, Lechner L, de Vries H. Tailored versus general information on early detection of cancer: a comparison of the reactions of Dutch adults and the impact on attitudes and behaviours. *Health Education Research* 2002;**17**:239–252.

14 Eysenbach G. Consumer health informatics. *British Medical Journal* 2000;**320**:1713–1716.

15 Rippen H, Risk A. E-health code of ethics. *Journal of Medical Internet Research* 2000;**2**:E9.

16 International Society for Mental Health Online. Available at http://ismho.org [last checked 26 August 2002].

17 Gomaa WH, Morrow T, Muntendam P. Technology-based disease management: a low-cost, high-value solution for the management of chronic disease. *Disease Management and Health Outcomes* 2001;**9**:577–588.

18 Fotheringham MJ, Owen N. Interactive health communication in preventive medicine. *American Journal of Preventive Medicine* 2000;**19**:111–120.

19 dmoz open directory project. Available at http://www.dmoz.org [last checked 26 August 2002].

20 WellMed Depression Condition Center. Available at http://www.wellmed.com/wellmed/intro/Condition Depression.htm [last checked 16 September 2002].

21 CopeWithLife. Available at www.copewithlife.com [last checked 26 August 2002].

22 BluePages information on depression. Available at http://bluepages.anu.edu.au [last checked 26 August 2002].

23 Google PageRank. http://www.google.com/technology/index.html [last checked 26 August 2002].

24 Beyondblue. The national depression initiative. Available at http://www.beyondblue.org.au/site/ [last checked 16 September 2002].

25 Lewis D, Behana K. The Internet as a resource for consumer healthcare. *Disease Management and Health Outcomes* 2001;**9**:241–247.

26 Griffiths KM, Christensen H. Quality of web based information on treatment of depression: cross sectional survey. *British Medical Journal* 2000;**321**:1511–1515.

27 Griffiths KM, Christensen H. The quality of Australian depression web sites. *Medical Journal of Australia* 2002;**176**(suppl):97–104.

28 Berland GK, Elliott MN, Morales LS, et al. Health information on the Internet: accessibility, quality, and readability in English and Spanish. *Journal of the American Medical Association* 2001;**285**:2612–2621.

29 Lissman TL, Boehnlein JK. A critical review of Internet information about depression. *Psychiatric Services* 2001;**52**:1046–1050.

30 Eysenbach G, Powell J, Kuss O, Sa ER. Empirical studies assessing the quality of health information for consumers on the world wide web: a systematic review. *Journal of the American Medical Association* 2002;**287**:2691–2700.

31   Kim P, Eng TR, Deering MJ, Maxfield A. Published criteria for evaluating health related web sites: review. *British Medical Journal* 1999;**318**:647–649.

32   Tu F, Zimmerman NP. It is not just a matter of ethics: a survey of the provision of health disclaimers, caveats, and other heath-related alerts in consumer health information on eating disorders on the Internet. *International Information and Library Review* 2000;**32**:325–339.

33   Abbott CP. Web page quality: can we measure it and what do we find? A report of exploratory findings. *Journal of Public Health Medicine* 2000;**22**:191–197.

34   Silberg WM, Lundberg GD, Musacchio RA. Assessing, controlling and assuring the quality of medical information on the Internet. *Journal of the American Medical Association* 1997;**277**:1244–1245.

35   Meric F, Bernstam EV, Mirza NQ, et al. Breast cancer on the world wide web: cross sectional survey of quality of information and popularity of websites. *British Medical Journal* 2002;**324**:577–581.

36   Griffiths KM, Christensen H, Evans K. Pharmaceutical company websites as sources of information for consumers. How appropriate and informative are they? *Disease Management and Health Outcomes* 2002;**10**:205–214.

37   Silverstein C, Henzinger M, Marais H, Moricz M. *Analysis of a Very Large Alta Vista Query Log*. SRC Technical Note 1998-014. California: Digital Systems Research Centre, 1998.

38   Risk A, Dzenowagis J. Review of internet health information quality initiatives. *Journal of Medical Internet Research* 2001;**3**:E28.

39   Sorensen G, Emmons K, Hunt MK, Johnston D. Implications of the results of community intervention trials. *Annual Review of Public Health* 1998;**19**:379–416.

40   Prochaska JO, DiClemente CC, Norcross JC. In search of how people change. Applications to addictive behaviours. *American Psychologist* 1992;**47**:1102–1114.

41   Rosen CS. Is the sequencing of change processes by stage consistent across health problems? A meta-analysis. *Health Psychology* 2000;**19**:593–604.

42   Celio AA, Winzelberg AJ, Wilfley DE, et al. Reducing risk factors for eating disorders: comparison of an Internet and a classroom-delivered psychoeducation program. *Journal of Consulting and Clinical Psychology* 2000;**68**:650–657.

43   Prochaska JJ, Zabinski MF, Calfas KJ, Sallis JF, Patrick K. PACE+: interactive communication technology for behavior change in clinical settings. *American Journal of Preventative Medicine* 2000;**19**:127–131.

44   The Mood Gym *Training program*. Available at http://moodgym.anu.edu.au [last checked 27 August 2002].

45   Christensen H, Griffiths KM, Korten AE. Web-based cognitive behaviour therapy: analysis of site usage and changes in depression and anxiety scores. *Journal of Medical Internet Research* 2002;**4**:e3.

46   A.L.I.C.E. *AI Foundation*. Available at http://www.alicebot.org [last checked 27 August 2002].

47   Overcoming Depression. *The new computer cognitive treatment*. Available at http://www.maiw.com/main.html [last checked 27 August 2002].

48   Parent F, Coppieters Y, Parent M. Information technologies, health and globalization: anyone excluded? *Journal of Medical Internet Research* 2001;**3**:E11.

49   Bernhardt JM. Health education and the digital divide: building bridges and filling chasms. *Health Education Research* 2000, **15**:527–531.

50   Mental Health Net. Available at http://mentalhelp.net/ [last checked 26 August 2002].

51   Psych Central. Available at http://psychcentral.com/ [last checked 26 August 2002].

52   Internet Mental Health. Available at http://www.mentalhealth.com/ [last checked 26 August 2002].

53   National Institute of Mental Health. Available at http://www.nimh.nih.gov/publicat/index.cfm [last checked 26 August 2002].

54   The Mental Health Foundation. Available at http://www.mentalhealth.org.uk/ [last checked 26 August 2002].

Appendix 15.1.

A site was defined as the URL of a site listed in the dmoz directory. Links from the site to other standalone sites were not followed if these extended beyond the original URL. On some occasions it was difficult to determine the limits of the site, particularly for sites which were part of larger health or mental health sites (see below). Of the 60 sites, three were no longer available, one was a duplicate and one could not be accessed, leaving 56 sites that were examined in detail.

In addition to the characteristics noted in Table 15.1, we examined the characteristics of the site, such as its nature (standard/stand-alone, broad scope or clearinghouse site), whether it was owned by an individual or an organization, whether it included an editorial board, or had health professional involvement.

We examined its openness and attention to standards, recording whether it promoted books, products or services on a commercial basis, and whether it included a disclaimer, a privacy policy, a mechanism for feedback, collected personal information or required registration to enter the site. Often sites required registration for mailing lists and newsletters, but the registration feature was only recorded if registration was required to access the content information on the site itself.

We also reviewed the appearance of the site. In particular, we noted whether it appeared to be professionally designed (a 'yes' rating required a high degree of quality), whether it used art images that were 'goth like', or fantasy based, and whether it looked attractive (a yes rating required a high degree of quality). As noted in Table 15.1, we coded the scope of the site (whether it covered the following sorts of information: symptoms/diagnosis, treatment, prevention, risk (causes), incidence/prevalence, help resources, specific groups) in addition to stigma reduction, presence of a bulletin board, chat room, online counselling, audio tapes, music, visitor/guestbooks, mailing lists and about 30 other site features. Each of these features was examined separately. In addition, we created a variable 'scope' which provided a summary score for whether it covered the following: symptoms/diagnosis, treatment, prevention, risk (causes), incidence/prevalence, help resources and specific groups. We also sought PageRanks for each of the 56 sites.

16

Use of the Internet in Psychiatry and Clinical Psychology

Catherine Ebenezer

Introduction

The World Wide Web offers a powerful communication and delivery medium for professional and consumer health information of many kinds. In the last few years the availability of Web-based information resources, and the relative ease of access to them, has begun to effect radical changes in the practice of mental health, as with other clinical specialities. Established vehicles of professional communication have appeared in Web versions (e.g. journals, textbooks, official publications, clinical guidelines), and new Internet-only communication formats (e.g. email, newsgroups, discussion boards, weblogs, portals) have emerged. A truly vast amount of material is available.

Ready access to consumer health information on mental health subjects has also begun to affect the nature of professional–patient relationships. It is important that professionals working in these areas have some knowledge of the Web, that they are aware of ethical and quality issues relating to health information and self-help resources on the Internet and that they are able to recommend suitable sites to refer to. More generally they need to be mindful of the possible effects of the World Wide Web on their clients (e.g. Internet addiction, chatrooms, effects of exposure to pornographic or racist material).

The Web provides the advantage of being a rapid, convenient means of information delivery. Hypertext linking provides for easy cross-referencing within and between resources. The user's experience can be enriched by the use of graphical or multimedia formats. Publishing on the Internet, at least in its most basic form, is rapid and relatively cheap. Web-based sources may be readily amended and updated. Present-day Web technologies provide for a high level of interactivity, for example via forms, polls, surveys, discussion forums and rapid responses to articles. The Web also has a number of serious disadvantages. It is of vast, unmanageable size and continues to grow rapidly. It is difficult using existing search tools and technologies to locate appropriate sources within it. There is a significant problem of ascertaining the quality of material that may be retrieved using search tools, which is often highly variable. Also, Web publishing by its very nature has an ephemeral character, so there is a problem in ensuring permanent access to archival material.

Internet resources aimed at professionals in psychiatry, psychology and other mental health disciplines should ideally be discussed and evaluated within a framework of what is known of information needs and information use within them.

Very few studies exist of the information behaviour of mental health professionals, so one is required to extrapolate from studies of other groups.

At present there is a wide variation in Internet skills among mental health professionals. While members of some professional groups, particularly clinical psychologists and psychotherapists, seem to place a high priority on access to the knowledge base and are avid 'consumers' of the professional literature, workplace access to computers, despite national targets, is generally poorer than in other areas of clinical practice. Palmer,[1] for instance, in her survey of community mental health staff in Bournemouth, found that none of her respondents had access to the Internet at their team base; 15% of them had access at home, but only 9% had used it. While this group had a highly positive view of the Internet, they reported a deficiency of computer skills in general as a barrier to information seeking. Bawden and Robinson,[2] in their comparative study of information seeking by psychiatric nurses and midwives, found that the psychiatric nurses (i) demonstrated a relatively low level of information awareness and computer use, and (ii) needed access to a very wide range of information, including material on social services. These researchers considered that information resources in psychiatric nursing, both primary and secondary, were relatively poorly developed. Fakhoury and Wright's study[3] of the information and communication needs of community mental health nurses in the UK failed to mention published information sources at all. Library staff who serve mental health workers frequently mention in conversation problems of technophobia and of a lack of clear mental maps of the information resources available within their discipline.

Studies of clinicians in other specialities have discovered clear patterns and attitudes in Internet information seeking which are likely to be applicable in mental health. Obst[4] found that German medical professionals and students tended to use a relatively small number of preferred sites. This 'anchor strategy', of making regular use of a few sites which are perceived as authoritative, has also been observed in studies of primary care physicians by Westberg and Miller[5] and by Moffat et al.[6] The most recent Health On The Net Foundation[7] survey of health professionals' attitudes to Internet searching found that over 80% were concerned about the accuracy and trustworthiness of health information on the Internet, 76% were concerned about the availability of information, and 72% about the difficulty of navigating the information space and locating appropriate information. Respondents reported the following problems in using the Web: lack of time (60%), dissatisfaction with information quality (26%), inadequacy of search tools (24%) and deficient IT skills (29%).

To a large extent, practitioners' concerns about information on the Internet parallel those relating to the availability and usability of clinical evidence generally. Sources of knowledge in health care are disorganized and diffuse. For a psychiatrist, for instance, they can include the medical and popular media, recommendations and requirements of professional, political, regulatory and legal bodies, reports from charities and pressure groups; the output from educational campaigns and programmes, and marketing material from commercial sectors, primarily the pharmaceutical industry.[8] There is an additional complication with mental health, which is a multidisciplinary subject with a wide scatter of literature.[9–11] Smith,[12] in his important 1996 review of studies of the clinical information needs and wants of doctors, established that many clinical questions go unanswered and, furthermore, that particular motivational factors are significant in clinical information seeking. He refers to the 1994 study of Gorman et al,[13] which found that, of the possible factors motivating doctors to seek answers to clinical questions during consultations, only two were statistically significant: the doctor's belief that a definitive answer existed, and the perceived urgency of the patient's problem. Smith concluded that 'the ideal information source will be directly relevant, contain valid information, and be accessed with a minimum amount of work'.

In addressing the difficulties of using Internet-based health care information, Jadad[14] suggests that a three-pronged approach is required on the part of system and resource developers, health information professionals and users:

1. better coding of the information on the Internet (using metadata schemes), and development of more powerful and effective retrieval systems

2. developing predigested or 'distilled' sources of high-quality information which save clinicians' time

3. efforts to increase information literacy and to develop critical appraisal skills, among both practitioners themselves and their clients.[14]

Smith's criteria of relevance, validity and ease of use, somewhat elaborated, can serve as a basic framework for evaluating Internet-based information services for health professionals. Numerous standards for evaluating health websites have been proposed; those of Nesbitt et al[15] are concise and may serve as an example (Box 16.1). Hsiung[16] provided links to many of the major articles on Internet health information quality and an extensive bibliography on the subject is available at the University of Michigan library website: http://www.lib.umich.edu/megasite/bibl.html.

While the Internet can add vastly to a clinician's information overload, it has a major role to play in getting research evidence into practice. It provides a means of making available high-quality clinical information (such as evidence summaries, structured abstracts of key articles, clinical guidelines) at the point of care, tools for patient assessment, and a platform for professional networking in the generation of evidence-based resources.[17]

Box 16.1.   Quality criteria for websites

Accessibility – Can the site be found using common search engines?
Attribution – Are references and sources for all content provided?
Authorship – Are authors and their affiliations and credentials provided?
Content – Is the information provided valid (critically appraise using the same methods as for printed resources)? Are linked sites valid?
Currency – Are the dates of posting and last update provided?
Disclosure – Is the 'ownership' of the website clear? Are advertising, underwriting and other conflicts of interest made explicit?
Ease of use – Is the site easy to navigate? Does it load quickly? Do features work properly?
Innovation – Is the information delivered in a way that exploits the potential of multimedia without 'overdoing it'?
Readability – What is the reading age level?

Mental health care, as already stated, is very much a multidisciplinary affair. Correspondingly, professional information for mental health on the Internet is frequently cross-disciplinary in relevance, although it may be aimed at one particular group, such as clinical psychologists or psychiatric nurses. There is frequently valuable coverage of mental health within general resources in medicine, psychology and nursing as well as in specialist ones. Increasingly, mental health and social services are integrated, enhancing the importance of access to social care information (Fig. 16.1).

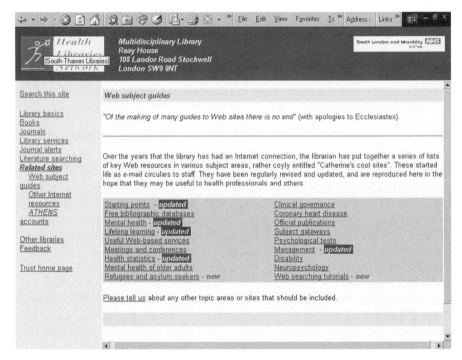

Fig. 16.1. Screen shot of the South London and Maudsley NHS Trust Library website (list of website guides).

The following offers an overview of major Internet resources for mental health care. The emphasis is on material of relevance to or developed within the UK and which is freely available. It is possible to establish a rough correspondence of professional activities with information needs, information sources and finding aids (Box 16.1). The reader should bear in mind the typology of information sources – primary, secondary, finding aids – within each category of Internet resource. I have adopted the following categories:

1. search engines and directories

2. subject gateways and portals, general and specialist

3. bibliographic databases

4. full text databases: drug information, guidelines, other clinical references

5. e-journals, directories of e-journals, table of contents (TOC) services

6. e-books

7. organizational sites

8. mailing lists.

Search engines and directories

The term 'search engine' generally refers to a system in which the database of searchable links is built automatically by a search robot or spider. In a 'directory', by contrast, the resources are selected and indexed by human agency. Search engines may be divided into primary and 'meta' engines; meta-search engines accumulate, select and display the results of a search run concurrently on several primary search tools. Primary search engines vary widely in functionality and in type of coverage.

The best general search engines, by virtue of their sophisticated searching algorithms and high level of functionality, are powerful search tools where something specific is required, such as contact information for a particular author, information about an assessment instrument, the full text of policy guidance or legislation. Google is currently perhaps the best known and most powerful; however professional searchers also hold AllTheWeb in high estimation. Both offer the ability to search PDF files. AltaVista, Lycos and HotBot are well established (Box 16.2). Teoma, while it does not have its own database, provides the facility to refine a search or go to specialized collections of links on a subject. Among the meta-search engines, the

---

Box 16.2.   Search engines

Google
   http://www.google.com   Uses PageRank search algorithm. Searches PDF and Word
                               files as well as HTML. Can limit to UK sources at
                               http://www.google.co.uk

AllTheWeb
   http://www.alltheweb.com   Comprehensive results. Searches PDF files

Teoma
   http://www.teoma.com

Lycos
   http://www.lycos.com

HotBot
   http://www.hotbot.com

AltaVista
   http://www.altvista.com   Offers search refinement feature which maps search
                               statements to subject categories

---

recently launched Vivísimo offers powerful automatic classification features which improve relevance and ease of use. Other powerful meta-search engines are Dogpile, IxQuick, SurfWax and ProFusion (Box 16.3).

For anyone who is interested in pursuing the subject in more detail, the Search Engine Showdown website provides a chart of search engine features, reviews and statistics. The CJBSJU library website has useful links to the main search engine evaluation sites, a directory of specialist search tools, search strategy guides, etc. (Box 16.4).

The databases of Web directories are much smaller than those of search engines, but have the advantage for the user of much greater precision (specificity) in the results they retrieve. Of the general directories (also known as webliographies), Yahoo!, the Open Directory (DMOZ) and WWW Virtual Library are the best known. All are US-based. A smaller, UK-based, more academically focused directory is BUBL LINK, which has a comprehensive list of links covering medical and health subjects (Box 16.5).

Box 16.3.   Metasearch engines

Vivísimo
   http://www.vivisimo.com   Powerful document clustering features. Uses Yahoo and MSN databases

DogPile
   http://www.dogpile.com

ProFusion
   http://www.profusion.com   Incorporates alerting service when sites change

Ixquick
   http://www.ixquick.com   Powerful search functionality, relevance ranking

SurfWax
   http://www.surfwax.com

Box 16.4.   Search engine evaluations

Search Engine Showdown   http://notess.com/search

CJBSJU Library search engines page   http://www.csbsju.edu/library/insearch/guides.html

---

Box 16.5.   Directories

Yahoo!
   http://www.yahoo.com   Large, comprehensive

Open Directory
   http://www.dmoz.org   Run by volunteers. Coverage is uneven

WWW Virtual Library
   http://www.vlib.org   Good psychology page; does not cover psychiatry or mental disorders as such

BUBL
   http://bubl.ac.uk   UK-based, comprehensive

Subject gateways and portals

General

Of the general health sciences and related subject gateways, BIOME (http://www.biome.ac.uk), Health on the Net (HON) (http://www.hon.ch), CliniWeb (http://www.ohsu.edu/cliniweb/), MedWeb Plus (http://www.medwebplus.com), MedWeb (http://http://www.medweb.emory.edu/MedWeb/) and the Social Sciences Information Gateway (http://www.sosig.ac.uk) are likely to be found the most useful. BIOME is a UK site which incorporates two health subject gateways with overlapping content: OMNI (Organized Medical Networked Information) and NMAP (Information for Nursing and Professions Allied to Medicine). Both use UMLS (the Unified Medical Language System) for navigation. All resources are indexed. SOSIG is a similar subject gateway for social sciences, offering access to a considerable amount of social welfare information. The Health on the Net site offers powerful mapping features using MeSH headings, and can conduct parallel searches in MEDLINE alongside searches for web resources. Hardin MD (http://www.lib.uiowa.edu/hardin/md/index.html) is an excellent resource: it has large, medium and small subject lists for each medical speciality.

Healthcare Information Resources (http://www-hsl.mcmaster.ca/tomflem/top.html), maintained by the library at McMaster University, the Karolinska Institute Library database of Diseases, Disorders and Related Topics (http://http://www.mic.ki.se/Diseases/index.html) and UK Health Centre (http://www.healthcentre.org.uk) all provide well-organized lists of links to information for patients as well as professionals. The National electronic Library for Health (NeLH) (http://www.nelh.nhs.uk) is a gateway of increasing importance for workers within the British National Health Service, providing access to a wide range of evidence-based and reference sources, news evaluations and subject briefings. Its content may be accessed via professional portals or via Virtual Branch Libraries (which include mental health and learning disabilities). It also has a reference section organized by topic: knowledge management, clinical governance and so on. Some of the material is available only to NHS staff connected to the NHS network. However, the Cochrane Library, which includes the full text of the Cochrane systematic reviews, has recently been made freely accessible to IP addresses within the UK (http://www.nelh.nhs.uk/cochrane.asp). The Electronic Library for Social Care (http://www.elsc.org.uk), while smaller and less elaborate than the NeLH, aims at providing something equivalent for social work. Finally it is worth mentioning the TRIP database, which aims to bring together all the evidence-based health care information available as full text, including guidelines, systematic reviews and material from peer-reviewed journals (http://www.tripdatabase.com). It is searchable by keyword; recent updates in a range of clinical specialities are browsable. The site offers the facility to set up automatic alerts based on customized searches.

The last few years have also seen the emergence of commercial health and medical 'one-stop' services, or portals. These provide a degree of customizability, access to a wide range of the resources that might be required in the course of professional practice, and additional facilities such as email, news and access to CME material, discussion forums, reference sources and clinical tools. Medic8.com (http://www.medic8.com), Doctor's Guide (http://www.docguide.com) and OnMedica.Net (http://www.onmedica.net) are notable examples. Doctors.net.uk (http://www.doctors.net.uk) offers comprehensive facilities, but is only available to registered medical practitioners. PharmWeb (http://www.pharmweb.net/), maintained at the University of Manchester since 1994, is an excellent pharmacy information resource.

Specialist

Many of the major general resources in mental health are of US or Canadian origin. Internet Mental Health (http://www.mentalhealth.com) is maintained and funded by a Canadian psychiatrist, Dr Philip Long. It includes information about and comprehensive lists of resources on diagnosis, therapies and research for the most common mental disorders. Mental Help Net (http://www.mentalhelp.net) is a comprehensive US-based source of mental health information for patients and professionals. Professional information includes diagnostic criteria, medication information, cognitive behavioural therapy, neuropsychology, patient assessment, links to organizations, news services and book reviews. The Online Dictionary of Mental Health (http://www.human-nature.com/odmh/), put together by the Sheffield University Department of Psychotherapeutic Studies, is in fact not a dictionary offering definitions, but an extensive list of links to resources, arranged alphabetically by topic.

Pulier's Personal Psychiatry and Behavioral Healthcare Resources for Mental Health Professionals (http://www.umdnj.edu/~pulierml/home.html) is compiled by a professor of psychiatry; it is quirky in presentation but rich in content, with particularly good listings of educational meetings, and of mental health organizations throughout the world. Dr John Grohol's site PsychCentral (psychcentral.com) claims to be the oldest-established directory of mental health resources on the Internet (see Chapter 25). Its main emphasis is on consumer mental health information, but it includes some professional resources such as guidelines and book reviews. Neuroguide.com (http://www.genetics.gla.ac.uk/neil/) is a searchable and browsable index of neuroscience resources available on the Internet: neurobiology, neurology, neurosurgery, psychiatry, psychology, cognitive science sites and information on human neurological diseases.

Some university departments and mental health libraries have well-organized collections of links and other resources: the Institute of Psychiatry (http://www.iop.kcl.ac.uk), the University of Pittsburgh (http://www.hsls.pitt.edu/index_html) and University of Adelaide (http://library.adelaide.edu.au/guide/med/menthealth/) are among the best examples. The library of the South London and Maudsley NHS Trust maintains a site that includes lists of links to journals, bibliographic databases and other sites of relevance (http://stlis.thenhs.com/hln/s_london/lsw/main/). The United Kingdom Psychiatric Pharmacy Group has an excellent collection of links (http://www.ukppg.org.uk/links/), as does Robert Hsiung's site Mental Health Links (http://www.dr-bob.org/mental.html) (see Chapter 5).

There are very few sites that focus specifically on evidence-based practice and resources in mental health. The Centre for Evidence-Based Mental Health (http://www.cebmh.com) stands out in this category. Otherwise there is the Expert Consensus Guidelines Series reproduced online at http://www.psychguides.com, and the Evidence-Based Psychiatry Center site produced by Nagoya City University Medical School, Japan, which includes a variety of clinical tools (http://www.med.nagoya-cu.ac.jp/psych.dir/ebpcenter.htm).

Bibliographic databases

While a number of the major bibliographic sources for mental health are available only as fee-based services, there are several significant freely available databases covering specific areas. The American Psychoanalytic Association maintains Jourlit and BookRev (http://www.apsa.org/lit/index.htm), which are large bibliographies of journal articles, books and book reviews related to psychoanalysis. CounselLit (http://www.cpct.co.uk/cpct/index.htm) is a UK database of counselling literature maintained by the Counselling in Primary Care Trust. The PsycheMatters site (http://www.psychematters.org.uk) offers bibliographies, full text articles, conferences and other links related to psychoanalysis and psychotherapy (including group therapy, family therapy, and child mental health). PILOTS (http://www.ncptsd.org/research/pilots/) is a database of worldwide literature on post-traumatic stress. The caredata database of social work and social care management literature (http://www.elsc.org.uk) provides substantial coverage of mental health issues. The US education database ERIC (http://ericir.syr.edu/Eric) has comprehensive coverage of child development, child psychology and special needs issues. MEDLINE (http://www.pubmed.gov) has some mental health coverage. Infotrieve (http://www4.infotrieve.com), the Zetoc article database (http://zetoc.mimas.ac.uk) and UnCover Plus (http://www.ingenta.com) are all worthwhile sources of mental health-related literature.

In searching for books and reports, library catalogues should be the first port of call. The URLs of several major libraries are given below:

- BMA Library catalogue (http://www.bma.org.uk/)

- British Library Public Catalogue (http://www.bl.uk/blpc/)

- COPAC union catalogue of major UK university libraries (http://www.copac.ac.uk)

- Royal Society of Medicine Library catalogue (http://www.rsm.ac.uk)

- LOCATORplus: National Library of Medicine (US) catalogue (http://www.nlm.nih.gov/)

- WHOLIS: World Health Organization Library catalogue (http://www.who.int/library/database/index.en.shtml).

Full text and other reference sources

FindArticles (http://www.findarticles.com) and MagPortal (http://www.magportal. com) provide free full-text access to many popular health sciences periodicals. The material covered by both is mostly of US origin. Education Online is a small full-text database run by the University of Leeds that covers UK education topics. There are several important references relating to therapeutics available: the Merck Manual (http://www.merck.com/pubs/mmanual/), WeBNF (http://www.bnf.org.uk/ Index.htm) and the drug information pages at the Glasgow Royal Infirmary Area Medicines Information Centre and DrugInfoZone sites (http://www.ngt.org.uk/ medicinesinformation/service.htm, http://www.druginfozone.org/). The US Pharma-copeia can be found at http://www.usp.org. Other useful references include PharmaLexicon: medical and pharmaceutical abbreviations (http://www.pharma-lexicon.com/) and the On-Line Medical Dictionary (CancerWEB) (http://cancerweb. ncl.ac.uk/omd/). The DSM-IV-TR diagnostic criteria for mental disorders may be found online at http://www.behavenet.com. Most of the general and specialist portals also provide links to full text resources such as practice guidelines and dictionaries.

E-journals, TOC services

An increasing number of professional journals are available online in some form. Most have full text available on a subscription-only basis, but many significant titles are free or have free content available from a certain period after publication. It is common to find tables of contents, abstracts and searchable archives. Increasingly it is possible to purchase access on a pay-per-view basis to material that would otherwise be subscription-only.

The pre-eminent site for mental health e-journals is Armin Günther's searchable and browsable directory of psychology and social science journals, now known as PsycLine (http://www.psycline.org/journals/psycline.html). Other noteworthy sites are Links to Psychological Journals (http://psych.hanover.edu/Krantz/journal.html), MedBioWorld's psychiatry list, formerly ScienceKomm (http://sciencekomm.at/ med/journals/psych.html), Highwire (highwire.stanford.edu) and the Italian site Periodici Elettronici Biomedici (=Biomedical e-journals) (http://aib.it/aib/commiss/ cnur/peb/peb.htm). PsycLine incorporates a meta-search facility for articles using other psychology databases, while Highwire offers advanced search functionality at article level, with a considerable amount of material being available in full text (via trials, free archives, sample free articles and issues). Many of the major libraries and specialized portals also incorporate lists of links to the home pages of major journals.

In addition to the table of contents (TOC) services available from publishers, there are a number of other useful free TOC and current awareness services. Highwire and Infotrieve (http://www3.infotrieve.com) provide the facility to register for TOCs of the journals it indexes. Highwire also offers a content tracking service for its journals, CiteTrack. AMEDEO (http://www.amedeo.com) provides content tracking of preselected journals for the topics depression and schizophrenia; rather than setting up individual TOC alerts for numerous individual journals, the user can set up alerts on these subjects, or regular TOC alerts, for material in any of 28 core psychiatry titles.

E-books

E-books have been a recent growth area for Internet resources. Apart from the commercial services, the most useful collections of free e-books for health sciences are available at the National Academy Press site (http://www.nap.edu/) and at MedWeb. eMedicine.com (http://www.emedicine.com) provides, among other things, a detailed reference source for most clinical specialities. The South London and Maudsley NHS Trust library website provides a further select list of individual useful e-book titles (http://stlis.thenhs.com/hln/s_london/lsw/main/). It should be noted that many organizations provide downloadable full-text versions of their publications, often in PDF format, on their websites.

Organizations

For anyone connected with the UK National Health Service the Department of Health pages are a major information source (http://www.doh.gov.uk). Particularly noteworthy are the mental health page, the National Service Frameworks pages and the publications databases. Other relevant government sites (such as those of the Home Office, Department for Education and Social Exclusion Unit) may be located via http://www.ukonline.gov.uk. Another major organizational website is that of the Royal College of Psychiatrists (http://www.rcpsych.ac.uk), which offers information about the College and its activities, extensive links to mental health information for patients and professionals, information about campaigns, lists of publications, and the texts of recent press releases and policy statements. The Sainsbury Centre for Mental Health site (http://www.scmh.org.uk) has extensive information on mental health research and policy initiatives, databases of publications and good practice, a discussion board, analysis and audit tools, overviews of major current topics, and extensive lists of links. The Institute of Psychiatry (http://www.iop.kcl.ac.uk) provides detailed information via its site about its research and teaching activities. The MIND site (http://www.mind.org.uk) is useful for its downloadable fact sheets, policy briefings and online bookshop. Among non-UK organizations, the American Psychiatric Association (APA) site holds the full text of numerous guidelines and a database of APA publications (http://www.psych.org/). The National Institute of Mental Health site (http://www.nimh.nih.gov) includes the full text of the Surgeon General's reports on mental health topics, consensus conference reports, factsheets for clinicians and research reports. The World Health Organization site (http://www.who.int) now incorporates an atlas of mental health services worldwide, as well as downloadable versions of reports.

A number of outstanding sites in specialist areas of mental health are worth listing:

▶ Addictions: DrugScope (http://www.drugscope.org.uk); Alcohol Concern (http://www.alcoholconcern.org.uk); BehaveNet – brief definitions, book lists, directories (http://www.behavenet.org); Behavioral Health World for Professionals (http://www.bhworld.com) resource library – research reports, treatment guidelines, clinical cases.

▶ Child and adolescent psychiatry: American Academy of Child and Adolescent Psychiatry (http://www.aacap.org).

▶ Depression and anxiety: Neurolink (http://www.neurolink.co.uk).

▶ Early psychosis: EPPIC (http://www.eppic.org.au).

▶ Forensic psychiatry: Forensic Nursing Resource Homepage (http://www.fnrh.freeserve.co.uk/index1.html); David Willshire's Forensic Psychology and Psychiatry Links (members.optushome.com.au/dwillsh/).

▶ Geriatric psychiatry: American Association for Geriatric Psychiatry (http://www.aagpgpa.org/); Alzheimer's Society (http://www.alzheimers.org.uk).

▶ Learning Disabilities: British Institute of Learning Disabilities (http://www.bild.org.uk); Tizard Centre (http://www.ukc.ac.uk/tizard/).

▶ Informatics: Computers in Mental Health (http://www.ex.ac.uk/cimh).

▶ Psychopharmacology: Dr Bob's Psychopharmacology Tips (http://www.dr-bob.org/tips/).

▶ Transcultural psychiatry: Australian Transcultural Mental Health Network (http://www.atmhn.unimelb.edu.au/).

Email discussion lists

Behavior Online (http://www.behavior.net/) and InterPsych (University of Sheffield) both host many ongoing discussions of topics in clinical psychology, psychiatry and psychotherapy. JISCmail, the UK academic list hosting service, is another good place to look for 'respectable' mailing lists (http://www.jiscmail.ac.uk). Topica.com (http://www.topica.com) is a large browsable and searchable source of mailing list information; it can be used to establish new mailing lists.

Conclusion

The World Wide Web provides a plethora of high-quality information resources of various kinds for mental health professionals. Basic familiarity with Web-based sources should be considered as part of everyone's 'information mastery'.

References

1   Palmer K, ed. *Signposts to Information for Community Mental Health Workers.* Bournemouth: Bournemouth University Library and Information Services, 1999.

2   Bawden D, Robinson K. Information behaviour in nursing specialities: a case study of midwifery. *Journal of Information Science* 1997;**23**:407–421.

3   Fakhoury WFH, Wright D. Communication and information needs of a random sample of community psychiatric nurses in the United Kingdom. *Journal of Advanced Nursing* 2000;**32**:871–880.

4   Obst O. Use of Internet resources by German medical professionals. *Bulletin of the Medical Library Association* 1998;**86**:528–533.

5   Westberg EE, Miller RA. The basis for using the Internet to support the information needs of primary care. *Journal of the American Medical Informatics Association* 1999;**6**:6–25.

6   Moffat MO, Moffat KJ, Cano V. General practitioners and the internet – a questionnaire survey of internet connectivity and use in Lothian. *Health Bulletin* (59), 2001. Available at http://www.scotland.gov.uk/health/cmobulletin/hb592-10.asp. [last checked 2 September 2002].

7   Health on the Net Foundation. Available at http://www.hon.ch [last checked 2 September 2002].

8   Marriott S, Palmer C, Lelliott P. Disseminating healthcare information: getting the message across. *Quality in Health Care* 2000;**9**:58–62.

9   Geddes J, Reynolds S, Streiner D, Szatmari P. Evidence-based practice in mental health. *British Medical Journal* 1997;**315**:1483–1484.

10 Brettle AJ, Long AF. Comparison of bibliographic databases for information on the rehabilitation of people with severe mental illness. *Bulletin of the Medical Library Association* 2001; **89**:353–362.

11 McDonald S, Taylor L, Adams C. Searching the right database. A comparison of four databases for psychiatry journals. *Health Libraries Review* 1999;**16**:151–156.

12 Smith R. What clinical information do doctors need? *British Medical Journal* 1996;**313**:1062–1068.

13 Gorman PN, Ash J, Wykoff L. Can primary care physicians' questions be answered using the medical journal literature? *Bulletin of the Medical Library Association* 1994;**82**:140–146.

14 Jadad A. Promoting partnerships: challenges for the internet age. *British Medical Journal* 1999;**319**:761–764.

15 Nesbitt TS, Jerant A, Balsbaugh T. Equipping primary care physicians for the digital age. The Internet, online education, handheld computers, and telemedicine. *Western Journal of Medicine* 2002;**176**:116–120.

16 The Virtual En-psych-lopedia at Dr Bob. Available at http://www.dr-bob.org/quality.html [last checked 2 September 2002].

17 Jadad AR, Haynes RB, Hunt D, Browman GP. The Internet and evidence-based decision-making: a needed synergy for efficient knowledge management in health care. *Canadian Medical Association Journal* 2000;**162**:362–365.

17

From Websites to E-communities – the Internet and mental health service users

Paul Baker

Introduction

The Internet is a powerful tool, offering a whole range of possibilities for people concerned about mental health issues, especially service users. This relatively new medium has already had an effect on the way that people can access information about their diagnoses, treatments and health care options and its importance is set to increase as the availability of the Internet expands each year and websites become more sophisticated.

It is important to define the term 'service user'. This is because the term means different things to different people. It is a potentially loaded and contentious phrase because it groups together an otherwise diverse community of individuals with very different needs. Some 'users' also have strong views about the appropriateness of the term itself, believing it to have negative connotations. This is particularly significant within the context of the Internet, where information about mental health is addressed to a broad audience, including those of us not currently using mental health services.

Furthermore, 'users' can have very different relationships to mental health services, as Box 17.1 illustrates. It is also useful to give an example of the diversity of terms employed to describe people with mental health problems – some that are regularly

---

Box 17.1. Relationships between services and people experiencing mental distress

- Primary care clients utilizing the services of GPs and/or taking prescribed medications
- Clients of community-based counselling and therapeutic services for problems such as depression, anxiety or stress-related conditions
- Clients in need of short-term and/or crisis support
- 'Ex'-patients whose relationship with services is sporadic or has ended
- Clients of complementary, holistic, alternative treatment systems concerned with the maintenance and promotion of positive mental health
- Long-term clients of psychiatric services including hospital and outpatient care, often with diagnoses for 'serious' mental illnesses

Note: Consideration should also be given to those people who may need to use services in the future and to 'secondary' users, such as family members, carers and friends of the person with the mental health problem

---

used on the Internet are listed in Box 17.2. 'Service user' is only one way of describing people with mental health problems and the nature of their relationship to the services they use. The importance of this becomes apparent when you consider that the choice of terminology used by website hosts often reveals something of their underlying philosophy and the role they play in providing information.

For instance, websites providing information about mental health often have a target audience. Some sites aim to meet the needs of the general public and provide information on issues such as stress, anxiety and depression, trauma, eating disorders and substance abuse. They are often concerned with harm reduction and health promotion, or increasing pubic awareness about mental illness and the issues of discrimination and stigma. Others focus on the needs of carers and family members who are providing support to individuals with mental health problems, sometimes with

---

Box 17.2. Terms used on the Internet to describe people experiencing mental distress

Clients: emphasizes the professional nature of the relationship most often used by psychotherapeutic services and within the private sector

Consumers: borrowed from the market place, emphasizing the concept of service users as consumers of products such as medications or care services

Ex-patients: used self-referentially by service users no longer in contact with services and by psychiatric services as a broad definition of a person's status after having been discharged from hospital

Experts of experience: a more recently coined term used by the *recovery*[18] movement to draw attention to the value of working alongside service users, a participative approach acknowledging the service user's capacity to work towards their own rehabilitation. In this model *experts of experience* are considered to be in partnership with *experts by profession* in identifying and addressing recovery strategies

Patients: widely used by psychiatric services and personnel. A term which stresses the medical focus of an ongoing relationship between the service user and services

Psychiatric survivors: a 'rights'-based term used by activist service users who assert that some forms of psychiatric treatment can be considered abusive and who campaign for reforms to end the powers of psychiatry in compulsorily detaining patients and enforcing treatment

Sufferers: a term often used by agencies and organizations that are seeking to draw attention to the consequences to the quality of life for people experiencing mental health problems. Often used by 'carer', parent and diagnosed individuals

Survivors: a term used to describe people experiencing/living through mental health problems and/or the consequences of a life event (such as sexual abuse). Regarded as more empowering than the more passive 'victim' connotation of the term 'sufferer'. Often used by self-help and mutual assistance organizations. Not to be confused with 'psychiatric survivors' (see above)

Service users: popular with service providers, particularly with the public sector, employed as a generic description of the people who use services

Users: shorthand for service users, although also employed as term for people using illicit substances

---

a focus on fundraising for research into causes and treatments, and providing support through self-help groups. Still others aim to meet the needs of people with mental health problems and address specific age groups or people with the same diagnoses (e.g. eating disorders, dementia, mood disorders, psychoses, phobias) (Fig. 17.1).

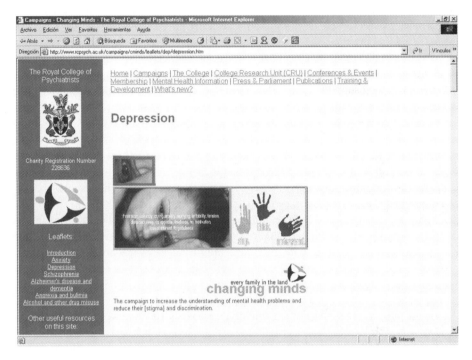

Fig. 17.1. Royal College of Psychiatry: Changing Minds Campaign on Depression.

Web-based information – an overview

In the early days of the Internet most home pages and websites of mental health organizations were little more than electronic annual reports, and communication between people concerned about mental health issues was confined to email-based news groups. The first general mental health information sites to exploit the medium were launched in North America, notably the pioneering Mental Help Net (1995)[1] and Internet Mental Health (1994),[2] alongside the more focused sites like Schizophrenia.com (1996),[3] a discussion forum providing a means for people diagnosed with schizophrenia to share information, advice and support. European site hosts followed the North American lead a few years later, as they too recognized the potential of the Internet as more people went online. From being a predominately US-based medium the Internet has now become an important means of disseminating information for many agencies (from national organizations to local user groups) in many countries, especially in the industrialized world. The availability of Internet-based information sourced from different countries of origin is important not only because the dominance of the English language on the Internet is diminishing, but also because there are inevitable cultural differences in the way mental health issues are tackled and services provided.

The importance of the Internet as a source of information for people with mental health problems appears to be increasing. As the Internet has become more sophisticated there has been a rapid increase in the number of sites aimed at service users worldwide. As the number of Internet subscribers has grown, so has the number of visits to mental health sites. Although statistics on the level of usage of the Internet as a source of information by mental health users are difficult to obtain, the indications are that it is increasing. The surge in the development of sites is a consequence of the potentially high numbers of people that organizations can reach through the Internet.

In early 2001 I conducted some research into the numbers of people with mental health problems visiting mental health sites for an article[4] on mental health information available on the Internet. The findings proved to be inconclusive, as one of the important features of using the Internet is that the person accessing information can, if they choose, remain anonymous. For many people with mental health problems, this is important, as the social stigma associated with having a mental health problem can be a disincentive to seeking information and advice. The comfort factor of being able to browse for information without the expectation of revealing your identity or status has proved to be important, but makes statistical analysis difficult.

What can be analysed are the number of visits a website is receiving through software that enables site hosts to analyse their 'traffic'. This will not confirm that the person accessing the site is a service user, but it is not unreasonable to deduce that if the site or page visited is aimed specifically at service users, that a proportion of the visitors would be likely to be service users. Using this approach, I was able to discover that the sites of UK agencies such as the Mental Health Foundation[5] and Mind[6] – both of whom provide information targeted at people who use services – receive hundreds of thousands of site visits annually. Whilst these are quite modest figures compared to those for popular sites like the BBC,[7] the agencies themselves said they were impressed at the reach this medium had given them, something that would have been quite impossible without the Internet.

Although numbers are not everything, the Internet has provided an opportunity for all kinds of mental health organizations to reach far larger numbers of people than would have been possible before. The cost of reaching a mass audience is no longer prohibitive (it does cost something, but it is affordable even for small organizations and individuals) and imaginative, well-constructed sites can have a considerable effect.

Over the last few years there has been a rapid growth in the number of new sites and in the development of existing ones, for instance in the UK organizations as diverse as the Royal College of Psychiatry,[8] the National Health Service,[9] Mind (National Association for Mental Health), SANE[10] and the Mental Health Foundation have all recently launched or redeveloped their websites to provide information for service users and the general public (Fig. 17.2). In addition the voluntary, statutory and

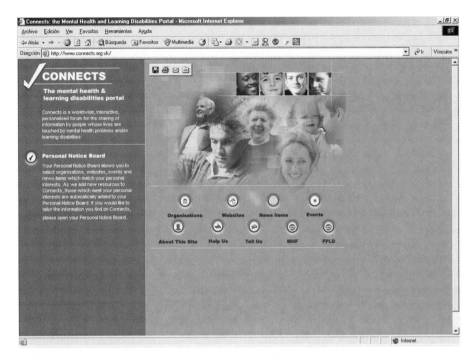

Fig. 17.2. Connects Mental Health and Learning Disabilities Portal, a comprehensive directory of mental health on the Web.

commercial sectors have also been developing new sites, as have smaller organizations and individuals.

Information and power – the 'democratization' of information provision

It is no longer the case that service users have to rely solely on information provided by their clinicians or other health care professionals. This process of information 'democratization' has been an increasingly important feature in the relationship between service users and professionals over the last 40 years and this process is being speeded up by the Internet. The Internet has become a place to get a second opinion; to share experiences with other people who have the same problems; to carry out research into diagnoses and treatments; and to find out about patients' rights. Before the invention of the Internet it was always possible to obtain this information from books, leaflets and magazines, or by seeking advice by telephone or in person. However, there is something about the accessibility, immediacy and diversity of the information on the Internet that has opened up a whole range of new possibilities.

People experiencing mental distress and their family and friends have often sought information about the nature of the help available to them before approaching services directly. This is prompted both by the anxiety most people feel about the issue of mental illness generally and the uncertainty and fear about what might happen to them if they seek assistance from a service, especially a statutory service. Because psychiatric services have the legal responsibility and power to detain, monitor and treat patients, sometimes against their will, it is not surprising that where possible, people seek reassurance about the consequences of requesting help. The Internet has become one of the places that people use to seek this information.

The Internet then, can be considered a great equalizer, a tool for the empowerment of service users and a potential means of breaking down the stigma of mental illness in the wider community. Having said that, it would be wrong to conclude that it represents problem-free innovation. Although, as the saying goes, 'information equals power', it does depend on the quality of the information being provided. Is it authoritative? Is it accessible to the lay person? Is it helpful? Is it accurate?

The answer depends as much on your beliefs and values as it does on the scientific credibility of the information. Mental health on the Internet is a broad church. You can find information promoting all the different types of psychotherapy and counselling, whilst others promote medical solutions (especially pharmaceutical ones) and still others are critical of the whole psychiatric system, from Pharmacy Companies (pro) to sites sponsored by the Scientologists (anti).

Take for example electroconvulsive therapy (ECT), a controversial treatment, which has both supporters and detractors. There are at least 18 websites (as of June 2002) specifically dealing with ECT. These range from the Association for Convulsive Therapy,[11] an international organization dedicated to promoting the safe, ethical and effective use of ECT through to Ban Shock,[12] which unsurprisingly in view of its name is in favour of banning any form of 'shock' treatment. Taking the middle ground are ECT.ORG[13] and Electroboy,[14] a personal site on manic depression and ECT, and ECT On-line,[15] which provides information both for and against the treatment (Fig. 17.3). Having obtained information from these sites (which can be downloaded and printed), it is then possible to discuss any anxieties with the psychiatrists and nursing staff. That is not to say that the staff will always welcome an informed user requesting answers that they may not have themselves, but it might help to ensure that mental health care staff will take care to explain the benefits and potential risks of treatments in an open way.

This can work to the advantage of patient and doctor alike. Recently, I was working with a day service for people with long-term mental health problems. After a staff and member discussion we agreed to set up a computer connected to the Internet and encouraged the clients of the service to make use of it. One of the most popular uses was for people to check the medication they had been prescribed. Concerns such as unwanted side-effects of medication (anything from feeling thirsty to putting on weight), the dosage level prescribed by their doctor, the way the medication worked and the condition it was prescribed for could be addressed and answered quickly by accessing sites designed specifically for this purpose.[16]

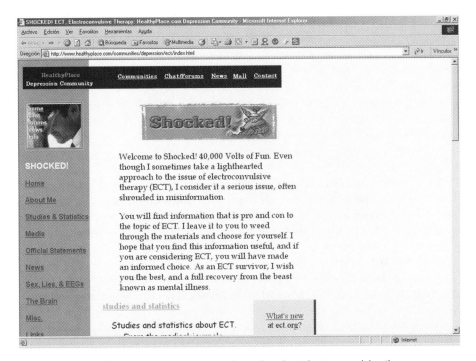

Fig. 17.3. ECT.ORG: information on the case for and against electroconvulsive therapy.

Using the Internet in this way proved to be an enlightening process for many of the members, who were not only better informed about treatments that had a significant effect on their quality of life, but were also more confident in sharing this information with other members, their families and friends, and their doctor. This led to more commitment in complying with the treatment plan on the part of the service user and a willingness on the part of the clinician to listen to the views of the patient and if necessary alter dosage or change the type of medication.

It had one other significant, if unintended, consequence. The day service itself responded to the information gained from the Internet when we realized that many of our members were on forms of medication that caused dehydration. Surprisingly perhaps (but in common with many other mental health services) the staple drinks provided by the centre were tea, coffee and soft drinks (some of them diuretic) – but not filtered, chilled water. So, we bought a water cooler and made sure that water was available at all meals and as an alternative to the other drinks. We also promoted the drinking of water amongst the members. This became part of an overall 'healthy living' strategy, including the kinds of meals prepared, the scheduling of relaxation and exercise classes. Our ambition was to improve the quality of people's lives through the promotion of healthy lifestyles and resulted in the service users reporting that they felt mentally and physically healthier.

Developing web-based information on mental health

I believe that there is an increasingly important role for services in supporting the constructive use of the medium. This is not only by making the Internet available to service users (and providing training and support in using the web) within psychiatric care establishments, although this is an important step, but also by hosting sites themselves. Sites hosted by services can describe the nature of the service they provide, the criteria for admission, and can provide feedback from service users and other more creative content, perhaps arising from the interests of service users and staff. There are already significant numbers of services, particularly community-based projects that have involved their service users in the creation of websites. These sites include those which are hosted by the users themselves. In doing so these agencies have recognized the value assisting service users to develop new skills and interests and promoting working partnerships for the benefit of the individuals involved and the wider community.

The effect of the Internet on service users is not only limited to the availability of information about mental health issues or the ability to join online communities to discuss issues with people who have similar needs. Most service users have periods when they are not experiencing a mental health crisis and their relationship to services is low. However for many service users, the social stigma attached to mental illness and the consequences of periodic incapacitation leads to unemployment, low income and social exclusion. It is possible that having the status of a mentally ill person can in some circumstances lead to loneliness, isolation and withdrawal from society. The consequences of social exclusion are in themselves damaging to self-esteem and bad for mental health. In some cases the Internet, because of the wide range of information available, can provide solutions to these problems. For instance it can enable service users to develop friendships online, investigate new interests and hobbies. It can be part of a process of opening up one's life again.

Websites providing information about mental health are becoming more focused (Box 17.3). Some sites are aiming to meet the needs of the general public and provide information on issues such as stress, anxiety and depression, trauma, eating disorders and substance abuse. They are often concerned with harm reduction and health promotion or increasing public awareness about mental illness and the issues of discrimination and stigma. Others focus on the needs of carers and family members who are providing support to individuals with mental health problems, sometimes with a focus on fundraising for research into causes and treatments, and providing support through self-help groups. Still others aim to meet the needs of people with mental health problems and address specific age groups or people with the same diagnoses (e.g. eating disorders, dementia, mood disorders, psychoses, phobias). By book-marking the most useful sites on the browser for easy access, service users can be assisted in finding the sites that will be useful to them. Developing a sense of community among visitors is now considered essential for success. The sense of belonging to a particular interest group fosters the credibility of a site which encourages visitors to return.

Some of the ways in which services can evaluate the quality of websites (including their own) and determine their usefulness to service users are listed in Box 17.4.

Box 17.3. Information for service users available on the net[19,20]

Advice and information: medication and treatments; mental health law and rights; health and social care services

Issues: addiction and recovery; child and adolescent; grief, loss and bereavement; diagnoses and disorders; symptoms

Campaigns and public awareness: reducing stigma; promoting positive mental health; critical and anti-psychiatry; issues and controversies; psychological abuse; policy and advocacy

Support: chat rooms; discussion forums; talking therapies; counselling services; mutual support and self-help groups; alternatives and complementary approaches; help-lines

Others: humour; history; organizational information; products; research

---

Box 17.4. A website evaluation guide to meeting the needs of service users

Accessibility: text-only versions of graphic image-based sites are important for those people using slower computers and/or with visual impairments. Sites using Macromedia Flash Shock Wave[21] technology should be aware that these features can take a long time to download via slow modem connections

Authority of information: whatever the position adopted by the site, it is important that the information is authoritative, consistent and where possible sourced. This is particularly the case for advice services. A useful resource is the 'Hon Code', the Health on the Net Foundation Code of Conduct (HONcode) for medical and health websites. This organization addresses one of Internet's main healthcare issues: the reliability and credibility of information[22]

Features: the application of technology should be directed to the needs of the people using the site. Increasing numbers of sites have invested in features to make themselves more distinctive and interesting to their visitors by including internal search engines, chat rooms, message boards, email newsletters, auto-responders, online shopping, etc. It is important that these features enhance the visitor's experience rather than detract from it

Language: this should be appropriate for the target audience and wherever possible be understandable to lay people. Some sites have made great efforts to ensure that medical-based information is written in plain language

Transparency: the street address, telephone number and email address of the site host should be displayed prominently

---

What does the future hold?

What does the future hold for the Internet as a means of delivering information about mental health to service users? Whilst it should be acknowledged that the medium is still in its infancy and the potential it holds remains to be fully realized, it is clear that the way the Internet is being used has changed. For instance, the gradual move from modem access to the higher speed, permanent broadband access is encouraging greater use and enabling more sophisticated use of audio, video and animation. This makes the sites less reliant on text and should result in more interesting ways of delivering information. A good example of this is the @ease[17] site, a mental health resource for young people under stress or worried about their thoughts and feelings (Fig. 17.4). It is hosted by the UK National Schizophrenia Fellowship, and uses a cartoon format with animation. The site involves the visitor in undertaking an interactive journey. By using new technology with a narrative style and backed up with facts about mental health, the issue of mental health is made much more interesting and relevant to the young people that it is attempting to reach.

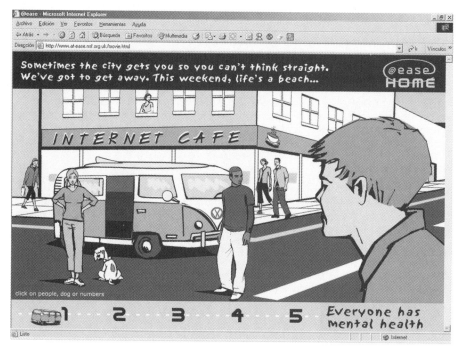

Fig. 17.4. The @ease site for young people, which uses a cartoon format with animation.

There are signs that the way the Internet is being used to provide information is undergoing further change. More emphasis is being placed on the interactive capacities of the Internet. The website itself is now only part of a package of information provision services that hosts can provide (Box 17.5).

In conclusion the Internet and other digital forms of delivering information about mental health issues is, on the whole, a positive development for service users. The Internet could become an important force for bridge-building between otherwise socially excluded service users and the rest of society. By providing service users a presence in this new 'mass' medium (previously only possible through the editorial control exercised by newspapers and television) there is scope for challenging inaccurate stereotyping and showing that people with mental health problems are

---

Box 17.5.   Creating e-communities: enhancing interactivity with website visitors

- Email newsletters to inform interested visitors about new developments on their sites, news items and events

- e-broadcasting (for Internet-based radio/video) either streamed for live programming or archived to enable ongoing access to documentaries

- Live 'online' discussions hosted by experts on a wide range of topics are an increasing feature of many of the larger sites

- Online conferencing facilities enabling conferences to be 'attended' virtually, with considerable savings in travel and accommodation costs. These online conferences are often held in parallel with a venue-based conference

- Online consultancy: scheduled telephone and email consultation with experts from different fields

- Viral marketing: which can be as simple as a 'Tell a friend about the site' option on the home page to more sophisticated campaigns, such as the recent Cuppa Campaign[23] on Stress Awareness sponsored by the Mental Health Foundation. This took the form of an animated postcard which was sent out to subscribers, who were encouraged to post it on to friends and colleagues (Fig. 17.5.)

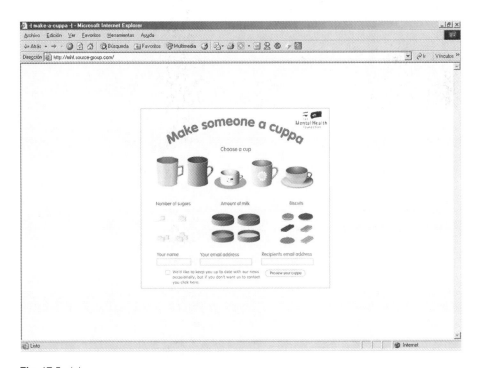

Fig. 17.5. (a)

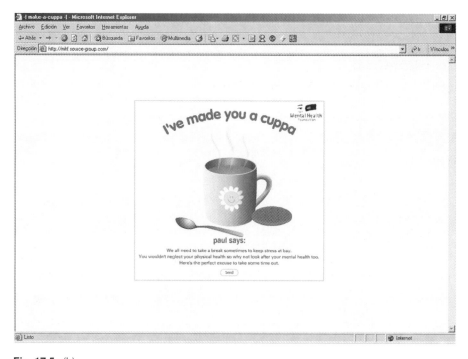

Fig. 17.5. (b)

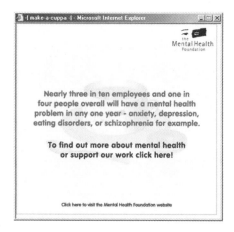

Fig. 17.5. (a–c) The Cuppa Campaign – an example of using the 'viral marketing' method to promote awareness of stress.

'people' first. The raised profile that mental health issues have gained through the Internet could also lead to a lessening of stigma faced by people experiencing mental health problems and more openness in society about the causes and consequences of mental distress.

Services in alliance with the people who use services have an exciting opportunity to play a part in the development of these new e-communities and to ensure they are inclusive and help promote positive mental health – so let's embrace it!

References

1   Mental Help Net. Available at http://mentalhelp.net/ [last checked 2 September 2002].
2   Internet Mental Health. Available at http://www.mentalhealth.com/ [last checked 2 September 2002].
3   Schizophrenia.com. Available at http://www.schizophrenia.com/ [last checked 2 September 2002].
4   Baker P. Net gains: mental health on the internet. *Open Mind: The Mental Health Magazine* 2001;**109**(May/June):10–11.
5   Mental Health Foundation. Available at http://www.mentalhealth.org.uk/ [last checked 2 September 2002].
6   Mind: The Mental Health Charity. Available at http://www.mind.org.uk/ [last checked 2 September 2002].
7   BBC (British Broadcasting Corporation). Available at http://news.bbc.co.uk/ [last checked 2 September 2002].
8   Royal College of Psychiatry: mental health information. Available at http://www.rcpsych.ac.uk/info/index.htm [last checked 2 September 2002].
9   National Health Service (NHS Direct). Available at http://www.nhsdirect.nhs.uk/index.asp [last checked 2 September 2002].
10 SANE. Available at http://www.sane.org.uk/default.htm [last checked 2 September 2002].
11 Association for Convulsive Therapy. Available at http://www.act-ect.org/act/index.php [last checked 2 September 2002].
12 Ban Shock. Available at http://www.banshock.org/ [last checked 2 September 2002].
13 ECT.ORG. Available at http://www.ect.org [last checked 2 September 2002].
14 Electroboy. Available at http://www.electroboy.com/ [last checked 2 September 2002].
15 ECT On-line. Available at http://www.priory.com/psych/ectol2.htm [last checked 2 September 2002].
16 Norfolk Mental Health Care NHS Trust: pharmacy medicine information website. Available at http://www.nmhct.nhs.uk/pharmacy/drug_idx.htm [last checked 2 September 2002].
17 @ease. Available at http://www.at-ease.nsf.org.uk/siteindex.htm [last checked 2 September 2002].
18 Mental Health Recovery Self-Help Strategies. Available at http://www.mentalhealthrecovery.com/ [last checked 2 September 2002].
19 Connects: the mental health portal. Available at http://www.connects.org.uk/ [last checked 2 September 2002].
20 (DMOZ): The Open Directory Project. Available at http://dmoz.org/Health/Mental_Health/ [last checked 2 September 2002].
21 Macromedia: flash shock wave. Available at http://www.macromedia.com/software/ [last checked 2 September 2002].
22 Health On the Net Foundation (HON) Hon Code. Available at http://www.hon.ch/HONcode/Conduct.html?HONConduct227226 [last checked 2 September 2002].
23 Cuppa 23. Cuppa Campaign. A stress awareness campaign run by the Mental Health Foundation, London, UK. Available at http://mhf.source-group.com/ [last checked 9 September 2002].

18

Online Counselling and Psychotherapy

Robert King, Darren Spooner and Wendy Reid

Introduction

Online counselling psychotherapy refers broadly to any form of psychological treatment that uses the Internet as a primary or substantial means by which therapist and client communicate with each other. The term therapist and client are used a little loosely in this context because we include self-help therapies where there is no active professional therapist, including peer-conducted self-help groups. As with standard psychotherapy, treatment may be directed towards the individual or it may involve a group of people.

One important difference between online and standard psychotherapy relates to synchronicity. Aside from self-help books, standard therapy is provided in 'real time' with the therapist and client being present in person or by telephone at the point of communication. Online therapies may be in real time (synchronous) or the transmission and receipt of communications may occur at different times (asynchronous).

Taking into account the variables of synchronicity/asynchronicity and individual/group there are four permutations of online therapy:

- real-time individual therapy
- real-time group therapy
- asynchronous individual therapy (using email)
- asynchronous group therapy (using a bulletin board or listserve).

Self-help sites, based on use of the Internet, represent a fifth distinctive form. In practice it is not unusual to find hybrid online therapies that combine two or more of these forms.

Real-time individual therapy

Real-time counselling is currently based on text message exchange. The user sends text messages identifying their problems and the counsellor responds. Unlike self-help or email therapy, real-time professional counselling simulates standard face-to-face counselling in that it is fully interactive and provided by a professional counsellor using standard counselling techniques, adapted to a text exchange format.

Real-time counselling can be contracted through an individually scheduled contact time, which simulates an individual appointment. Private practitioners can and do advertise services through the Internet and arrange 'appointments' for real-time counselling. Therapist and client use a chat protocol to exchange messages. Little is known about the take up or effectiveness of such services. Qualifications and experience of therapists may be difficult to verify and there is certainly potential for exploitation and unethical practice.

The capacity of government or not for profit organizations to provide real-time service depends on availability of counsellors as well as a suitable text exchange protocol. The organizational requirements for such a service make it difficult to provide except in the context of a substantial infrastructure. The Kids Help Line organization in Australia has developed a real-time counselling service as a supplement to its national telephone hot-line service for young people (see the case study in Appendix 18.1).

Real-time group therapy

Real-time group therapy makes use of a chatroom environment for message exchange between people who enter the chatroom. This form of therapy can be quite formal and structured or can be quite informal.

In its more formal mode, groups are scheduled for particular times and have memberships that are controlled through some form of screening or entry process. A professional counsellor or therapist who facilitates the exchange of messages both by commenting on messages and by ensuring that the group functions cohesively usually moderates this kind of group. This may involve establishing standards for the way group members communicate with each other and ensuring that all participants have the opportunity to contribute.

Real-time therapy groups can however be quite informal and entirely composed of peers. These are chatrooms that anyone can enter or leave at any time and are often linked to self-help sites (see above).

Chatrooms cannot accommodate large numbers of people at a time unless many are prepared simply to be observers.

Asynchronous individual therapy – email

Email therapy involves exchange of messages. It is asynchronous and requires the client to be able to articulate their problems or issues in reasonable detail so that the therapist can respond with suggestions, interpretations or requests for clarification or further information. It is analogous to traditional correspondence by letter but with considerably improved efficiency in transmission.

In the early development of psychoanalysis, therapeutic exchanges often occurred by letter because of the geographical isolation of early practitioners. Some consider Freud's correspondence with his friend Fliess to have been his personal therapy. Email therapy enables both client and therapist to provide thoughtful and carefully considered communications. It has the limitation of being unable to deal with emergent thoughts as is possible in a real-time dialogue.

Asynchronous group therapy – bulletin board or listserve

Bulletin boards and listserves provide mechanisms by which a group of people can exchange messages. The messages are posted either on a website (bulletin board) or by direct delivery to each member's email account (listserve). Group members are required to register on a listserve whereas bulletin boards may be either open or accessible only to registered members.

Asynchronous group therapy has the advantage of not requiring scheduling. Participants can access and send messages when it suits them by either logging onto the relevant website or opening their email account. Asychronous group therapy is also able to accommodate quite large groups, although at any particular moment message exchange is likely to be restricted to a subset.

Several research sites have introduced bulletin boards or listserves as adjuncts to self-help sites. The effectiveness of asynchronous group therapy is not known but anecdotal accounts and as yet unreported surveys suggest that these processes engender a sense of participation and belonging, and therefore commitment to treatment and recovery. They therefore contain at least some of the dynamics that are thought to contribute to the therapeutic value of groups.

Self-help – Internet

Self-help is a well-established form of psychological treatment. It is best known in the form of bibliotherapy, whereby help is provided through a self-help book or manual. These books typically provide information, advice and structured exercises designed to assist the reader to overcome general or specific difficulties. Bibliotherapy has not been as extensively researched as standard therapist-provided treatment, but such research as exists suggests that bibliotherapy based on standard psychological treatment manuals may be as effective as equivalent face-to-face treatment.

Some Internet-based self-help uses similar principles and is little more than an alternative form of publication and distribution to bibliotherapy. However most Internet self-help is unlike bibliotherapy in important respects and offers a rather different kind of therapy experience, the value of which is more difficult to judge.

The Internet is a more accessible medium than book publishing, which means that individuals and groups who lack resources to publish a self-help book can and do mount Internet self-help sites. Whereas self-help books are mostly written by professional therapists, Internet self-help sites are often developed by people who have experienced emotional problems or have had a history of treatment for mental illness. The creation and operation of self-help sites may in fact be a form of therapy in itself. Self-help sites may be the product of self-help groups or may be the creation of an individual.

As well as being less dominated by professional providers, Internet self-help is likely to be more interactive than bibliotherapy. Internet self-help sites often include links to other sites as well as invitations to post messages or comments. The site user may be invited into the personal world of the site creator, having access to favourite poetry or other personal mementos. Self-help sites may also include casual chatroom options that enable site users to communicate with each other in real time using standard chatroom protocols.

These distinctive features of Internet self-help make for weak quality control in respect of content and variable site maintenance standards. Sites may be ephemeral or idiosyncratic. However this does not imply that they are useless or even that they are less effective than professional bibliotherapy or its Internet equivalent. It may be that engagement through the Internet with people who have experienced mental illness is a source of hope or even inspiration. However, there is no empirical basis for assuming that they promote recovery.

Why should online therapy be therapeutic?

While there is substantial evidence to show that psychotherapy in general is both objectively helpful and highly valued by people experiencing a broad variety of emotional problems, including episodes of mental illness such as depression, the precise mechanism of its operation is not well understood. It would appear that only about 15% of the effect of psychotherapy can be attributed to the specifics of technique and that specific technique has almost no relevance in the case of some common disorders. About 30% of psychotherapy affect appears to result from what are termed 'common' or non-specific factors. These relate to the capacity of therapy to engender hope for recovery and expectation of change as well as qualities usually attributed to the therapeutic relationship such as trust and empathy. About 55% is associated with client factors and external events.

Those who doubt the capacity of online therapies to be effective usually do so because they over-rate the importance of the physical presence of the therapist to recovery and under-rate the importance of what are sometimes termed 'virtual' relationships. They take the view that an effective therapeutic relationship must be a 'real' relationship – meaning that it must involve both non-verbal and verbal components. They are particularly concerned that relationships that rely entirely on exchange of verbal messages will be overly intellectualized and ultimately sterile.

However this overlooks the fact that most therapies in their procedure and framework seek to maximize the verbal component of the relationship and minimize non-verbal and conventional social components by setting clear limitations to intimacy beyond the therapy hour and by minimizing the use of touch or any form of communication that might be incongruent with verbal message exchange. Freud invented a form of communication (the patient on the couch) that ensured that therapist and client did not even have eye contact.

It also overlooks the clear evidence that powerful and highly emotional relationships can and do develop through Internet-based communication by email or listserve and that such relationships can develop into lasting friendships and sometimes marriage (or, equally, can develop into bitter enmity). The interpersonal and emotional quality of online communication is in reality more prominent than people unfamiliar with the medium imagine.

In summary, online therapy is able to capitalize on the common therapeutic factors such as the development of hope and expectation of recovery and may make more use of interpersonal alliance than is commonly thought. As we will see below, online therapy also has specific advantages with respect to the less important technique factors that contribute to therapeutic outcomes.

Specific advantages of the Internet in the delivery of psychotherapy

Access

Most conventional psychotherapies require the client to attend the consulting rooms of the psychotherapist. Access to therapy is contingent upon local availability and capacity of the client to attend at times determined by the practitioner. People are usually more comfortable working in psychotherapy with a professional from a broadly similar background with respect to culture and values, with the result that cultural minorities and minority language groups have particular problems with access to conventional psychotherapy.

Online therapy is substantially free of restrictions imposed by geographical location or time zone. Online therapy is also potentially accessible to people who are housebound as a result of physical or psychological impairment and to people with impaired hearing. People living in more remote or rural areas and members of minority language or cultural groups are likely to particularly benefit from the ability to access therapists online.

People who wish to retain anonymity when accessing therapy may find online therapy especially advantageous. Groups that feel particularly vulnerable, such as children and persecuted minorities as well as people that suffer from especially strong feelings of shame about seeking help, are more likely to access a service where they are not required to disclose their identity.

Cost

Start-up costs for delivery of online therapy are highly variable. Sophisticated self-help sites require substantial development costs and involve some maintenance costs. By contrast, the capital costs associated with provision of therapy by email can be relatively small. Even where start-up costs are relatively high, the potential to deliver treatment to large numbers of people means that the unit cost of the therapy may be very low. It is likely that the cost of provision of an Internet therapy will be lower than its equivalent when not delivered online.

A moderately sophisticated self-help site will be less expensive than publication and distribution of a self-help book. Site maintenance is likely to be less costly than publication of a revised edition. Individual therapy by email or group therapy by chatroom does not require the overheads necessary to maintain a standard consulting room environment.

Standardization and updating of technical components of therapy

Although, as indicated above, therapy technique is usually less important than is commonly believed to be the case, provision through an Internet site increases the likelihood that the technical aspects of therapy will be both standard and reflect recent research developments. This applies especially to the professionally developed self-help sites. Insofar as online delivery increases fidelity to standard procedures it increases the extent to which a therapy will be 'evidence based', a factor that is of developing importance in the decisions of third parties such as insurance companies in relation to funding of treatment.

Record-keeping

Conventional psychotherapies usually rely on brief notes recorded some time after a session as a record of what has taken place. Such notes are inevitably inadequate records. They provide a poor reference point for the therapist who wants to keep track of the progress of a therapy or who is required to produce a record of a therapy for a court or other third party. They provide no record for the client.

By contrast, online therapies usually enable both therapist and client to retain a complete record of all interactions. Clients can and, in our experience, do review detailed therapy records to refresh the experience and clarify whatever learning occurred. While some therapists may be a little uneasy about the prospect of such a complete record being available, it introduces a transparency into psychotherapeutic work that will for the most part serve the interests of both therapists and clients. One particular advantage for therapists is the capacity to utilize records to improve practice through either personal reflection or external supervision.

Risks and disadvantages of online therapy

Engagement and attachment

Psychotherapy is an inherently difficult process as it usually involves some challenge to the client's usual approach to thinking or responding. Resistance to change is a common phenomenon and the simplest form of resistance is disengagement from the therapy. In conventional psychotherapy, the therapist works on the development of a human bond with the client that is sufficiently robust to overcome tendencies towards disengagement. As social animals, we are prone to develop attachments and alliances. However these may be mediated by a variety of non-verbal processes. It is possible that the purely verbal communication that occurs online is less robust than non-verbal communication with respect to the development of engagement and attachment. However, as discussed above, the capacity of people to the development of alliances and attachments online may be greater than is often supposed.

Crisis intervention

Psychotherapists not infrequently encounter clients who need crisis intervention in the context of suicidality or exacerbation of symptoms. Crisis intervention may involve the activation of local resources including police, mental health teams and hospitals. Online therapists are at a significant disadvantage in such situations; especially if local resources are unknown to the therapist and even more so if the full identity of the client is unknown. Online therapists may need to develop a crisis intervention contingency plan as part of the initial contracting with an online client. Similar limitations exist with telephone counselling.

Lack of non-verbal cues

While psychotherapies are primarily verbal, therapists do make use of non-verbal information including tone of voice when interpreting verbal information. This is particularly important when there is some inconsistency between the content of the message and the way it is delivered. In the absence of non-verbal cues, the therapist must rely on the broader context of the communication or subtle variations in use of language to detect incongruence. As therapies develop this becomes easier, but in the early stages of a therapy in particular, online therapists are likely to be at a disadvantage in assessing and interpreting the content of purely verbal messages.

Technical limitations and failures

Online therapy presupposes that both therapist and client have access to Internet communication and the basic knowledge to use email, chatrooms, etc. Older, poorer and less well-educated people are disadvantaged in many cases by lack of access to facilities or lack of confidence to develop skills in use of facilities. Online communication also remains susceptible to a variety of technical failures including line drop out, local computer failures and server failures. Real-time therapies are especially vulnerable and even more so when one of the connected parties is dependent on telephone lines.

The evidence base for online therapy

Despite widespread enthusiasm for the use of information technology in the delivery of psychological therapies, the evidence in support of its efficacy and feasibility is limited compared to IT applications for medical health problems. Nevertheless, research suggests that computers and the Internet may well provide an effective platform for the delivery of psychological therapies.

The Internet can be used psychotherapeutically by either facilitating access to information such as self-help and self-management sites (see Chapters 15 and 16), or by facilitating communication between people such as a patient and therapist or between supportive peers (see Chapters 17 and 19). Person-to-person communication on the Internet can be live, in 'real time', or asynchronously using email or discussion forums. Some outcomes data exist for each mode of delivery, for combinations of the two, of for the use of these interventions as adjuncts to other therapies. These data are limited, and the quality of the research is variable.

Psychological self-help and self-management information for mental health problems is voluminous on the Internet. The quality and accessibility of self-help information is inconsistent, and there has been little evaluation of its effect. Given that such information is generally used to inform treatment decisions and self-management of illness, quality and consistency is vital. Griffiths and Christensen[1] reviewed 21 frequently accessed depression websites and found a generally poor quality of information. Clinical evidence was not often cited for conclusions and recommendations, information was sometimes inaccurate, most of the sites provided information that was inconsistent with National Health and Medical Research Council clinical practice guidelines for the management of depression, and these inconsistencies were not related to the prestige of the publishing institution or credentials of the author (see Chapter 15).

Some studies have attempted to formally evaluate the effect of Internet self-help. For example, Carlbring et al[2] delivered a treatment for panic disorder via the Internet. Cognitive behavioural self-management information was provided via a website and augmented by therapeutic email contact, and subjects were randomized to treatment or waitlist conditions (where patients are told they will receive treatment at a defined future time, but are compared with the intervention group prior to this). Significant effects were reported for the treatment condition on all outcome measures, but there were no follow-up data. Despite some methodological weaknesses such as small sample size and stringent inclusion/exclusion criteria, these data are promising. The authors also reported that lack of face-to-face contact was expressed as a positive feature of treatment for some of the sample of panic-ers.

Klein and Richards[3] found similar outcomes for their sample of panic disorder sufferers compared to waitlist, but this study did not involve email contact. It did, however, include an element of face-to-face computer training, and this could confound treatment effects of the Internet programme.

J. Kenardy, K. McCafferty and V. Rosa (unpublished results) used a simple text-based interactive Internet site to offer early intervention cognitive behavioural information to people at risk of developing anxiety disorders. They found significant effects of the intervention on measures of anxiety sensitivity, agoraphobic cognitions, catastrophic cognitions and symptoms of depression. The authors reported good effect sizes, high user satisfaction and maintenance of change at follow-up.

Kovalski and Horan[4] found that their Internet-based cognitive restructuring programme was effective in changing the irrational career beliefs of a small sample of adolescent girls. The effect was only seen in Caucasian girls and not in those from ethnic minorities. Although some changes in beliefs were observed, it is unclear whether the programme was based on cognitive therapy principles or on basic education.

Similar to Carlbring et al,[2] Strom et al[5] claimed that their Internet-based self-help treatment was successful in the management of recurrent headaches. The treatment consisted of an interactive educative website based on behavioural self-management principles, and email support during treatment. Although there were significant improvements in headache in the treatment group, the study had no follow-up and a large attrition rate (56%). There were also some anomalies in the data such as a large, but non-significant, pretreatment difference between treatment and waitlist groups on headache index scores. At post-treatment the active treatment groups' headache index scores had dropped significantly compared to the waitlist, but the post-treatment means for both groups were comparable, confusing the issue of clinical meaningfulness of the outcomes.

Good outcomes were found for a multi-component Internet-based programme for the reduction of risk factors for eating disorders in female university students.[6] At 3-month follow-up active treatment participants ($n = 24$) showed a significant reduction in a drive for thinness and a significant improvement in body image compared to waitlist controls. Treatment consisted of an interactive cognitive behavioural therapy website, online discussion forum, supportive email contact and face-to-face contact. In addition to waitlist control, the Internet programme was compared to a classroom-delivered programme and was found to be superior.[7] Despite a favourable outcome for the Internet-based intervention, it is unclear to what extent the Internet component was therapeutic given that each participant was also given three face-to-face sessions during the active treatment phase. However, participants in the Internet condition rated the online discussion forum as favourably as participants in the classroom condition.

Although email has obvious applications in facilitating psychotherapeutic contact between a client and therapist, there is little information available in support of its effectiveness owing to a paucity of empirical research in this area. King et al[8] discuss the use of email for conducting family therapy, suggesting its usefulness in facilitating communication between geographically dispersed family members, or estranged family members who are unwilling to engage in face-to-face therapy in the same consulting room. However, the authors' report is anecdotal and impressionistic rather than empirical.

Robinson and Serfaty[9] used an uncontrolled email therapy intervention with 23 sufferers of bulimia who were recruited through the Internet. From an online screen all subjects appeared to meet DSM-IV[10] diagnostic criteria for bulimia nervosa. At 3-month follow-up significant reductions in outcome measures were observed.

Murdoch and Connor-Greene[11] used email as an adjunct to face-to-face therapy and reported on outcomes for two cases, one with depression and the other an eating disorder. Although formal outcomes were not reported, there were transcripts of the clients' reports of satisfaction and the benefits of email. These testimonies suggest that email contact bolstered the therapeutic alliance, increased compliance and gave greater flexibility and opportunity to reflect on the content of therapy.

Lange and colleagues[12,13] supported Internet-based self-help with email feedback immediately following the completion of each therapy task. The sample consisted primarily of people with a diagnosis of post-traumatic stress disorder or pathological grief, but there it was not homogeneous with regards to the nature of the trauma or trigger event. Although the intervention was piloted prior to the trial, and although outcomes generally appeared favourable, there were a number of weaknesses in methodology that limit the generalizability of the study. The sample was small and consisted of students who were being given course credit for participation in the study. The follow-up period was only 6 weeks, at which only eight participants completed follow-up measures, and inclusion/exclusion criteria were particularly stringent.

Hsiung[14] reported on the use of an online support group that was supported by therapist input. Again, no clinical outcome data were reported, although utilization indicated perceived usefulness of the group for members. In an 8-month period in 2000, 1516 members posted 21 230 messages in 3028 separate discussion threads. Thus on average, every message posted received 6.7 replies. Support from peers and therapists can clearly be therapeutic during psychological difficulties, and the fact that such an online forum was so frequently used suggests that it was therapeutic, at least for some.

In addition to the above studies of Internet-based psychological intervention, there are also some limited data on psychological therapies delivered directly using a personal computer as opposed to online. Computer-based multimedia programmes usually use a video and audio-based platform over which text-based information and exercises are overlaid. Currently, Internet bandwidth usually prohibits the use of such programmes because downloading video and audio is so slow. Broadband Internet is becoming more widely available, and so the delivery of full multimedia programmes over the Internet will become much more likely in the future (see Chapter 1). An overview of these programmes is therefore relevant.

Although Stuart and LaRue[15] claimed that face-to-face support was important in any computer-based treatment, other research has shown that this is not necessarily the case. Selmi et al[16] developed computer-administered interactive cognitive behavioural treatment for depression and tested it with a sample of 12 depressed adults. The computer treatment was compared to traditional face-to-face cognitive therapy and waitlist conditions of equal size. The computer-based treatment was shown to be as effective as the face-to-face therapy, and significantly more effective than the waitlist control. There were also few differences in participant evaluations of the two active treatments. Similarly, White et al[17] found that a cognitive behavioural CD-ROM treatment was both effective and rated favourably by a sample of chronically anxious adults. Additionally, at least two multimedia CD-ROM packages for the cognitive behavioural self-treatment of depression and anxiety have recently become commercially available. The promotional literature for these two packages (Good Days Ahead and Beating the Blues) suggests that they are as effective as face-to-face cognitive behavioural therapy for some people, but clinical outcomes are currently awaiting publication.

The above research warrants cautious optimism for the use of Internet and computer-based psychological therapies. These techniques are still in their infancy and therefore the evidence base is limited. Further research should focus on the comparative efficacy, cost effectiveness and consumer acceptability of IT-based psychotherapy compared to face-to-face therapy, and justification for its use either as a stand-alone intervention or a supplement to other treatment should be based on robust evidence rather than unbridled enthusiasm and thirst for the state-of-the-art.

References

1   Griffiths KM, Christensen H. Quality of web-based information on treatment of depression: cross sectional survey. *British Medical Journal* 2000;**321**:1511–1515.
2   Carlbring P, Westling BE, Ljungstrand P, Ekselius L, Andersson G. Treatment of panic disorder via the internet: a randomized trial of a self-help program. *Behavior Therapy* 2001;**32**:751–764.
3   Klein B, Richards JC. A brief Internet-based treatment for panic disorder. *Behavioural and Cognitive Psychotherapy* 2001;**29**:113–117.
4   Kovalski TM, Horan JJ. The effects of Internet-based cognitive restructuring on the irrational career beliefs of adolescent girls. *Journal of Cognitive Psychotherapy* 1999;**13**:145–152.
5   Strom L, Pettersson R, Andersson G. A controlled trial of self-help treatment of recurrent headache conducted via the Internet. *Journal of Consulting and Clinical Psychology* 2000;**68**:722–727.
6   Winzelberg AJ, Eppstein D, Edlredge KL, et al. Effectiveness of an Internet-based program for reducing risk factors for eating disorders. *Journal of Consulting and Clinical Psychology* 2000;**68**:346–350.
7   Celio AA, Winzelberg AJ, Wilfley DE, et al. Reducing risk factors for eating disorders: comparison of an

Internet- and a classroom-delivered psychoeducational program. *Journal of Consulting and Clinical Psychology* 2000;**68**:650–657.

8   King SA, Engi S, Poulos ST. Using the Internet to assist family therapy. *British Journal of Guidance and Counselling* 1998;**26**:43–52.

9   Robinson PH, Serfaty MA. The use of e-mail in the identification of bulimia nervosa and its treatment. *European Eating Disorders Review* 2001;**9**:182–193.

10 American Psychiatric Association. *Diagnostic and Statistical Manual of Mental Disorders*, 4th edn. Washington, DC: American Psychiatric Association, 1994.

11 Murdoch JW, Connor-Greene PA. Enhancing therapeutic impact and therapeutic alliance through electronic mail homework assignments. *Journal of Psychotherapy Practice and Research* 2000;**9**:232–237.

12 Lange A, van de Ven JP, Schrieken B, Bredeweg B, Emmelkamp PMG. Internet-mediated, protocol-driven treatment of psychological dysfunction. *Journal of Telemedicine and Telecare* 2000;**6**:15–21.

13 Lange A, van de Ven JP, Schrieken B, Emmelkamp PMG. Interapy. Treatment of posttraumatic stress through the Internet: a controlled trial. *Journal of Behaviour Therapy and Experimental Psychiatry* 2001;**32**:73–90.

14 Hsiung RC. The best of both worlds: an online self-help group hosted by a mental health professional. *CyberPsychology and Behaviour* 2000;**3**:935–950.

15 Stuart S, LaRue S. Computerized cognitive therapy: the interface between man and machine. *Journal of Cognitive Psychotherapy* 1996;**10**:181–191.

16 Selmi PM, Klein MH, Greist JH, Sorrell SP, Erdman HP. Computer-administered cognitive-behavioral therapy for depression. *American Journal of Psychiatry* 1990;**147**:51–56.

17 White J, Jones R, McGarry E. Cognitive behavioural computer therapy for the anxiety disorders: a pilot study. *Journal of Mental Health UK* 2000;**9**:505–516.

18 National Board of Certified Counsellors, Inc. and Center for Credentialing and Education, Inc. *The Practice of Internet Counselling*. Available at http://www.nbcc.org/ethics/webethics.htm [last checked 17 September 2002].

Appendix 18.1 Case study. Online therapy – The Kids Help Line Web Counselling Service

Overview

The Kids Help Line is Australia's only free, national telephone and web counselling service for children and young people aged between 5 and 18 years. The telephone counselling service has been operating since 1991 and is available 24 hours a day from anywhere in Australia. Approximately 90 paid, highly trained counsellors work from the call centre in Brisbane, Queensland on a part-time, casual basis. The service maintains a significant data collection and research unit. The Kids Help Line is funded by a mixture of lottery sales, government and corporate support.

Independent evaluation has found that over 90% of Australian secondary students know of the service, how to contact it and what the service can provide. Each year approximately 1.3 million attempts are made by young people to reach a counsellor, of which about half are successful. The principles that underpin the management of the help line and service delivery are:

▶   no gate keeping – counsellors will respond to any problem, the service is not specifically for 'crisis' or particular types of problems and young people get straight through to a counsellor when they call

▶   clients have a choice of gender of counsellor

▷ clients can call back and speak to the same counsellor as often and as long as they need

▷ feedback from young people about the service is encouraged.

History of web-based interactions with young people

In 1995 the Kids Help Line developed its website and provided an email address encouraging young people to contact the service. Email messages came from around the world, many seeking help for problems. The policy at the time was to acknowledge the issue, and refer these clients back to services and resources in their own communities.

However, in line with the fourth operational principal of feedback, and repeat email messages from young people, it became clear that they were seeking a more comprehensive response from the service. By 1997 chatrooms were becoming more common on the World Wide Web, and young people began to request that the Kids Help Line provide counselling in this form. At the same time, feedback from counsellors revealed increasing use of the Internet to share visual, web-based materials with clients while counselling them by telephone (i.e. counsellors and clients would be looking at the same web-page while counselling took place – perhaps to seek further, more specific information on particular issues).

By 1998 it was clear that young people were seeking a choice of modality across voice and text-based applications for seeking help. At this time a formal commitment was made to provide counselling by email, and to develop a real-time web-based counselling service.

The development of online counselling

Several areas of concern were identified as being crucial in the development of the service: development and access, legal and insurance, ethical and counselling practice.

Development and access

The briefing provided to the software programmer for Kids Help Line's web counselling service included:

▷ users should not need to download any software to access the service

▷ the program should work with any computer and any browser

▷ the interaction with the counsellor should not leave any 'footprint' on the client's computer (i.e. no record of the transcript would remain on the hard drive)

▷ the program should behave as if the client was in a queue in the same way as the telephone service does

▷ the program should provide management information.

These were seen to be the key aspects to ensure the service was accessible, protected young people's privacy and treated them with respect in all phases of their contact. The resulting screens are shown in Figures 18.1 and 18.2.

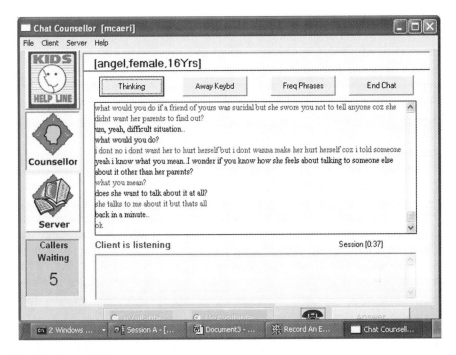

Fig. 18.1. Counsellor's screen.

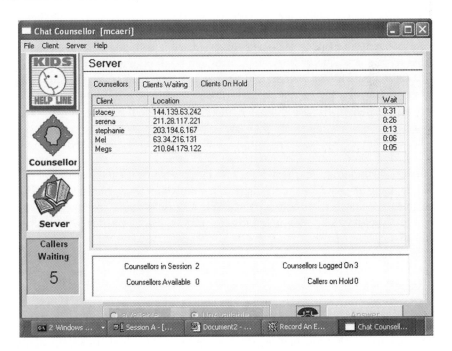

Fig. 18.2. Counsellor's management information screen.

Legal and insurance

An interview with lawyers confirmed that many of the same procedures and policies that protected the telephone service would also apply to web counselling. High standards of counsellor training and supervision, clear policy and procedures for compliant management and duty of care situations, security of data, and a commitment to data collection and dissemination, as well as knowledge development were the most important considerations.

Ethical issues

Ethical issues included having predisclaimer information and clear disclaimers, both written in language that could be easily understood by young users. Predisclaimers state what the service is and can do, while the disclaimers outline confidentiality, anonymity and security. Feedback from young people about the disclaimers indicates that they understand them clearly, and they give a sense of safety and confidence in the service. Other ethical issues include clear policy and procedures outlining counsellor obligations and client rights. The Kids Help Line also used the NBCC Ethical Standards.[18]

Counselling practice

The key areas identified by counsellors as important for text-based counselling included the transferability of skills, the practical differences of using telephone, web and email modalities, how to manage duty of care situations and risk assessment for child abuse, mental health and suicidality, moving clients from one modality to another, and research and evaluation (both client and counsellor) processes.

The process for resolving the issues identified above included extensive counsellor discussion and consultation, the engagement and briefing of a software programmer, and consultation with lawyers. Extensive searches were undertaken to identify other web-based counselling services and any literature that would inform both development and practice, resulting in a comprehensive set of readings for counselling staff.

The selection process requires interested staff to have completed the Kids Help Line training and probationary process, ensuring consolidated skills and extensive experience. This is complemented by a short induction process to the web-counselling software, an extensive range of readings, and a probationary period lasting 100 hours with intensive supervision and support. Web counsellors also meet regularly as a group to share practice wisdom and discuss various practice and case management issues.

The service began in May 2000 and currently operates between the hours of 15:00 and 21:00, from Monday to Friday. These limited hours are due to resource constraints.

Service demand

Since opening 14 000 attempts have been made by young people to get through to a web counsellor (to August 30, 2002), of which 7216 interactions have been completed.

This response is due to a constraint on staff resourcing due to funding limitations, limited hours of operation and the length of each interaction, which is an average of 43 minutes. Despite no marketing (young people find the service either on the Kids Help Line website, or by word of mouth), between the years 2000 and 2001, there was a 35% increase in completed interactions, and this trend seems likely to continue. Kids Help Line is currently looking at ways of increasing its capacity to respond to young people via its web service.

Client profile

Contrary to the expectation that a web-based service would attract more boys and young men to seek help, the gender breakdown of web-counselling clients in 2001 was 84% females and 16% males. While this reflects help-seeking trends across most human services, it differs from the pattern of use on the Kids Help Line telephone service for which 28% of clients are males. Those using the web service are more likely to be older than is the case by telephone, with 72% of callers aged between 15 and 18 (44% by telephone). This probably reflects level of access to a computer, as well as confidence in using text to communicate.

Client issues

The 10 main problems (of a possible 35) about which young people seek help via the web are shown in Figure 18.3, which compares them with the corresponding rates via telephone. While the problem types reflect the older age of clients, they also indicate

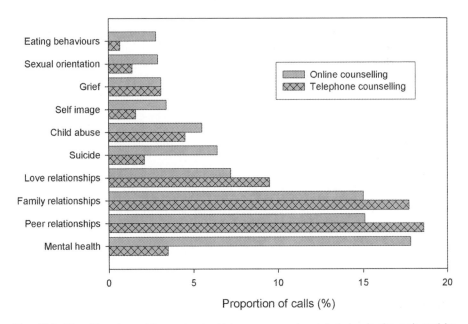

Fig. 18.3. The 10 main problems about which young people seek help via the web and by telephone.

that young people find it easier to disclose some types of issues by writing, an observation backed up by anecdotal feedback to counsellors. The nature of contacts shows that:

▶ *Mental health* – 23% are clinically diagnosed.

▶ *Family relationships* – a greater proportion experience frequent or major conflict than is the case by telephone.

▶ *Peer relationships* – a higher proportion are concerned for a friend's well-being.

▶ *Sexual abuse* – a higher proportion where the abuse is no longer current but the client is seeking counselling for unresolved issues arising from the abuse (as opposed to first-time disclosures of current abuse).

▶ *Suicide* – 71% contact about suicidal thoughts or fears, a higher proportion than is the case by telephone where young people are more likely to call about previous attempts, a current intention or a suicide in progress.

▶ *Eating behaviours* – 64% are experiencing continued disordered eating behaviours or a severe health problem.

▶ *Sexual orientation* – the only problem type about which males make the majority of contacts. Of these, one third are experiencing problems as a consequence of their sexuality.

Of the contacts made via the web, 13% of young people undertake to contact the counsellor again, either by web or telephone. Twenty-one per cent accept a referral to another service or agency, and in 15% of cases a crisis intervention is enacted, whereby emergency services or statutory agencies are contacted for assistance.

Counselling young people online

The following observations have been drawn from focus groups and clinical supervision with counsellors. Web counselling is yet to be evaluated by independent researchers.

Young people appear to experience a greater sense of safety, anonymity and control using web counselling than is the case by telephone or face to face. Disclosing severe or traumatic events in writing gives young people greater control over their emotions, and they feel less likely to 'crack up' or 'break down'. Using text gives permission to share their experience without having to say it out loud. Furthermore, seeing the words on the screen helps young people to confront their problems and may allow greater cognitive processing of the issues. At times counsellors offer their young clients a choice to change modalities – mainly moving from email (asynchronous) to web (synchronous) or to telephone. Counsellors may suggest changing modalities when a duty of care situation arises (the telephone service is available 24 hours every day); when counselling is not progressing using text; as an interim step with a view to face-to-face referral; or in the case of multiple long emails containing multiple and complex issues.

The choice to move to telephone counselling – to 'say it' rather than 'see it' – adds a new dimension to the counselling relationship, with both parties required to renegotiate the relationship, and rebuild rapport and trust. As one young client said – 'it's like finally meeting someone you've been talking to on the phone for a while and they are nothing like what you imagined them to be'. It also appears to facilitate emotional processing of issues.

The adult–child power dynamic often evident in counselling interactions involving voice (either by telephone or face to face) is lessened in web counselling, with the young client seemingly more empowered to challenge adult interpretations of their experience and issues. Young people are more likely to correct or seek clarification of the counsellor's meanings and responses.

Compared to telephone counselling, web-based interactions are longer and more intense. As shown in Figure 18.3, and reflecting the age group of clients, the types of issues discussed are generally very serious and often involve a mental health assessment or an assessment of suicide risk. Frequently the client enters the web-counselling interaction with a sense of engagement, safety and rapport, and discloses serious issues immediately. This is a reversal of telephone or face-to-face counselling in which counsellors spend the opening part of the interaction developing rapport and trust, and assisting their clients to express their concerns.

With text-based modalities counsellors find themselves needing to slow the interaction and rate at which information is being given to them to give *themselves* time to respond effectively. Their task in the opening sequences is to validate the seriousness of the information while deciding which pieces of it to work with first, slowing the pace and preparing for risk assessment if needed.

Risk assessment is also quite different in a text-based modality. Without voice tone and pace to soften the impact of a series of questions, counsellors have found that they ask fewer questions, earlier in the interaction, and inform their client of what they are doing, effectively making the process visible. Without this preparation, a set of questions can appear to the client to be interrogative and cold, effectively breaking rapport.

With no physical or auditory cues, punctuation and layout considerations are crucial. The information gained from pitch, tone and pace during telephone and face-to-face counselling are absent – however the speed and punctuation of the client does provide considerable information about the affect of the client. For example, distressed clients type rapidly with no punctuation, many spelling mistakes and grammatical shortcuts. As the level of distress wanes in the course of the interaction, pace slows and grammar and punctuation improve. Conversely, depressed clients may be very slow in their exchange, with lots of pauses. In order to facilitate an effective exchange or maintain rapport, counsellors at times match their punctuation, pace and layout to those of the client. Interestingly, encouragers such as 'mmm' and 'uhuh' commonly used in telephone or face-to-face counselling are equally as effective when typed into the interaction.

Reflecting feelings is one of the more difficult counselling skills to adapt to a text-based modality. Fewer cues make it more difficult to get a sense of the client's emotional state, leaving counsellors reliant on questions to gather this information.

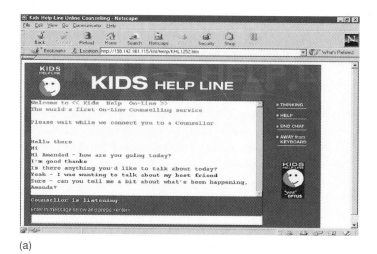

Fig. 18.4. (a) Current screen. (b) Example of new screen.

They have found original ways to give the client a sense of empathy and sensitivity when asking delicate questions about feelings by using punctuation such as brackets to 'hold' the question, dots to soften the entry into the question, and tentative expressions such as 'I guess ...'. For example: '... it sounds like ... (you are so sad) ...'

Counsellors also report that they miss not being able to laugh together during the counselling interaction, as is the case with telephone or face-to-face counselling. Laughing can be hugely beneficial in changing or releasing energy or tension during counselling, and typing 'lol' is not the same. Notwithstanding this, there are times when exchanges of humour do take place during web counselling.

Finally, the ability to scroll back and review the interaction while it is still occurring is seen as extremely useful to both counsellors and clients. Counsellors can see pieces of information that they may need to recheck or follow through with, or make visual connections between various items. The opportunity to take their young clients back to look at what has been 'said' can reinforce insights or understandings, or create a new opportunity to process information and develop insights and understanding.

Counsellors regularly review their experience and practice of text-based counselling in clinical supervision or peer support groups, often reinterpreting counselling theories and frameworks, which have largely been developed with the unspoken assumption that voice is the modality of exchange. Furthermore, counsellors are unanimous that the therapeutic alliance is alive and well in text modality.

The future

The Kids Help Line aims to support multimodal applications and integrate telephone, text and image. In the short term, interactive web-based counselling 'tools' are being developed. Part of this project involves developing new ways for young people to represent their feelings visually using barometers and slides that indicate the feeling, its intensity and frequency. The web-counselling screen is being redeveloped (Fig. 18.4.) so that young people can design their own counselling 'space' by choosing natural images and surrounds (e.g. sky, sea, fire).

Further developments will include a shared whiteboard for counsellors and clients to use for genograms, timelines and life charting, and short (1 minute) web-based films that show young people talking about various problems such as bullying, family relationships and mental health. These films are intended to show young people that they are not alone with their problems, and also model help-seeking. Young people have the fastest take-up rate of new technologies so service providers need to ensure that they are able to respond to young people no matter how they choose to seek help.

19

Developing a Programme in E-mental Health Care

Barbara Johnston

Introduction

By the year 2020, depression will represent the second largest burden of disease globally.[1] Current resources required to provide high-quality mental health care are insufficient and demand continues to increase. Part of the problem is that there is a maldistribution of psychiatrists in many countries, with most practitioners working and living in large cities. This leaves patients in many rural and remote areas with limited access to mental health services.

E-health can change the way that mental health is practised. In association with the move towards evidence-based medicine and quality-based practice, e-health can make mental health care accessible, affordable and efficient. This shift to a new model of care requires new thinking. This chapter describes an innovative, Internet-based mental health programme that is being developed in California by Kaiser Permanente.

Kaiser Permanente and mental health care

Kaiser Permanente (KP) is the largest non-profit health maintenance organization in the USA and provides health care to over eight million members, mainly in California. The organization has received international recognition for its excellence in health care outcomes. It has been shown to be more clinically and cost effective than the British National Health Service.[2] KP's investment in information technology has been cited as one reason for its efficient provision of high-quality health care.

Telemedicine, using some form of videoconferencing technology, has been used for at least 30 years.[3] A wide range of telemedicine applications has been trialled; for example, KP began using telemedicine in home health care in 1996.[4] Telepsychiatry is one of the more successful forms of telemedicine. It has been found to be clinically effective,[5–8] acceptable to patients and clinicians,[9–13] and cost effective.[14–17] Telepsychiatry is now generally accepted as a valuable technique for the provision of mental health care, in a variety of settings,[6,18–21] especially at a distance.[22–25]

One problem in treating patients with mental illnesss is their poor adherence to the medication and treatment plans prescribed by their psychiatrists. Because of the nature of the symptoms of depression it can be difficult to get patients to return to their clinic appointments, and it is common for these patients to stop taking their medications because of side effects or lack of support. In the year 2000, KP completed and published the 'Nurse Telecare' study in California.[26] Telephone outreach calls by psychiatric nurses to mental health patients were found to: (i) decrease symptoms of depression; (ii) improve satisfaction with care; and (iii) improve medication adherence. A significant number of KP members were already using the Internet. Since the use of email had been shown to be well accepted by patients and providers in other studies,[27] KP decided to implement an online mental health care programme. This was a logical way to integrate clinical face-to-face and online services.

KP Online website

The 'KP Online' website (http://www.kponline.org [last checked 7 July 2002]) allows Kaiser members to:

▶ obtain information on medications, symptoms, diseases and medical tests from a drug pharmacopoeia and health encyclopaedia

▶ find basic information about common health concerns and current health issues

▶ use the personal health assessment tool to find ways to improve their own health and prevent illness

▶ browse through links to other useful health sites on the Internet

▶ send a question to a KP advice nurse or pharmacist, or request an appointment at their local medical centre

▶ communicate with KP staff or other members using the 'discussions' section to exchange messages about subjects such as cancer, fitness and parenting

▶ obtain answers to health questions and request appointments.

The KP Online site has been heavily used. More than 100 000 of Kaiser's members have used the patient services site. Its success is proof that many patients like to use the Internet to access health care information. The next stage for KP was an e-mental health programme to provide a full range of health services online.

E-mental health programme

Like many other health care organizations, KP has problems in getting mental health patients to adhere to their prescribed treatment plans. Despite having access to mental health care services these patients frequently stop taking their prescribed medications, do not return to the mental health clinic appointments, and rarely have their families involved in their care planning. Conventional methods make it difficult to provide the ongoing education and family support that is required to support these patients and their carers.

The e-mental health programme is a voluntary option offered as an additional part of the member's usual psychiatric clinic and inpatient care. These patients are seen in

KP mental health care clinics but can also receive outreach e-mental health care with the hope of providing more support, education and follow-up. These e-mental health patients are encouraged to involve their families in the treatment plans and the education components of this online health programme. The decision to involve a family member or confidante in the programme rests entirely with the patient. Unfortunately, mental health care continues to carry a stigma for many people and this can lead to patients feeling a need to keep the illness secret or at least separate from others. Not everyone has someone available to participate and others may prefer to manage this part of their health care independently/privately.

The programme is meant to bring health care into the information age. Many patients are more familiar with using Internet functions like discussion threads and chatrooms than their health care providers. The e-mental health concept is novel and is therefore being developed under careful scrutiny. The programme is part of a research study to evaluate the implementation of an e-mental health programme to improve outcomes for KP mental health care patients and their families.

Objectives of the programme

The e-mental health programme uses the Internet to deliver personalized, comprehensive, evidence-based, convenient, accessible and confidential care to patients with mental illnesses who are under the care of a KP psychiatrist. The programme promotes involvement of a confidante (family member or friend) as a care partner and focuses on improving patients' self-management skills. Patients can go online to learn about their illness and how to recognize and better manage their symptoms. They can learn more about their medications and have access to a nurse care manager who can help them with issues related to their disease. A major goal is to reach out to members when they need the care, which for some may be after normal clinic hours. The hope is that by providing access to care, information and support via the Internet the patients will be more likely to adhere to medication and treatment plans. Another major objective is to educate and support the patient's confidante. Involvement of a confidante is recommended to the patients but not required.

The intention of the e-mental health programme is to improve treatment adherence rates, clinical outcomes and patient satisfaction. Comments are also being solicited from clinicians (psychiatrists and psychiatric nurses) on the convenience and effectiveness (or lack thereof) of the programme to explore its effects on the utilization and cost of health services.

New partners

The e-mental health programme offers members access to health education, psychiatric nursing case management and support – when and where they need it. The development of this programme required substantial resources. Key stakeholders included members from diverse departments internally, and several outside consultants and mental health organizations. To ensure a patient-focused and user-friendly outcome, representatives were included from national patient advocacy groups, patients with specific mental health conditions, psychiatrists (both Kaiser and non-Kaiser), psychiatric nurses, psychologists, physician IT experts, researchers, bioethicists, finance administrators and IT professionals. From the start, the plan was to obtain expert opinions from a wide variety of people. We needed patients and nurse care managers who could advise on functionality and systems, i.e. what made sense and what did not. The users were critical to ensure that the end product was going to be adopted by them.

The problems faced by the psychiatry department providers in particular were a frustration that 'standard care' was not producing acceptable outcomes. Patients with mental illness could come in for care in the KP clinics and could obtain the medications they needed. The problem was that these patients did not comply with return follow-up visits and frequently did not adhere to treatment plans. The psychiatrists and the psychiatric nurse care managers would make follow-up appointments for the patients to come back into the KP clinics but the patients would not keep their appointments. One of the main objectives of the e-mental health programme was to use the power of the Internet to provide more convenient and accessible care. This programme is not intended to eliminate conventional care but rather to extend that care online, where members may be more likely to use it. Building a system that works for the patients and the staff requires their involvement from the beginning.

Programme development meetings

Development of the new model of care required the cooperation of new health care and IT partners. Incorporating the Internet into health care required a team which included expertise in web-page design, IT security, government regulations, Internet-savvy patient perspectives, physician care practices, IT legal and ethical issues, nursing and case management practices, and research methods.

The meetings were structured to encourage everyone involved to speak openly. There were new characters involved and health care and IT staff were equally reliant on each other for a successful product. Communication was a key element in creating the programme. We were all committed to developing a user-friendly, effective and high-quality e-mental health care programme. This meant that the disparate groups involved in planning the research study had to learn each other's language.

There was a sense of excitement as the team embarked on creating a new way of caring for people with mental illness. People with mental illnesses often have a feeling of being stigmatized, which can add to their resistance to attending psychiatry clinics for care. Many of the team members could relate to this problem from either their own experience or that of a close friend or relative. This added to a sense of purpose within the group. The potential health benefits gave even more momentum as the group progressed forward.

Discussions about each phase of the programme brought both new challenges and new solutions. A chatroom site, which seemed an obvious forum to provide peer and provider support, led to much discussion. This was not obvious to all at the table.

Some team members had never engaged in a chatroom. This led to a dialogue on how chatrooms have worked thus far, how this could be useful to our patients, and also how to manage and supervise the site. The medical staff dealt with issues regarding the benefits to the patients' care. The web-page designers came up with a page that was suited for health care and was easy for patients and providers to navigate. The IT experts assured a secure site to meet the patient privacy laws. Each phase of the programme required this kind of collaboration, exchange of ideas and knowledge, and ultimately produced an excellent product.

The enthusiasm of the chief investigator, Enid Hunkeler, for the project kept the momentum going through many difficult days.

Planning for e-health

The goals of e-health in general include embracing the power of technology to improve health care outcomes. Planning for e-health requires being prepared to develop new partners, new technologies and most important integrating change management into the processes. This process can be threatening for all concerned. Examples of issues that were brought up during the development of the e-mental health programme are shown in Table 19.1.

Table 19.1. The strengths contributed by each team and how these affected the outcome

Core components	Strengths of health team	Strengths of IT team	Outcome
Knowledge	Health and care management	Technology	*Health team* acquired deeper knowledge of the technology and learned that e-health systems should be kept simple for the user *IT team* learned about the health area
Skills	Clinical skills User skills for basic computing and Internet email Privacy requirements	Coding and software development skills Web-page design IT Security requirements	*Health team* learned IT skills and more about IT, designing effective web pages for consumers and IT security *IT team* learned health skills, health-related graphics and more about patient privacy requirements
Attitudes	Focused on provider attitudes Experience with providing face-to-face health care Wanted a more consumer-centred focus	Focused on IT issues Experience as health care consumer Wanted a carefully designed online interface that met the users' needs	*The united team* designed an e-health system that was consumer friendly and focused

Working in the e-health environment requires flexibility, teamwork, innovation, willingness to take risks, a commitment to continuous learning and a belief in patient-centredness. It also requires something that most of us resist – change. The health care profession is conservative and can be resistant to change. That is not to say that health care cannot or will not change but that those brave enough to propose change to health care must be prepared for a challenge. In defence of the health profession it is only fair to say that we are patient advocates and frequently their guardians. We are held responsible for practices that improve the quality of life for the people who we care for. Planning will require change in management strategies to ensure participation, development, adoption and success.

Conclusion

The provision of health care is undergoing a change that has already occurred in business, government and education. All these entities have incorporated the use of technologies into their business processes so that they can remain competitive. The health industry is being forced to integrate technology for its survival also. There will be major changes in health work practice during the next 10–20 years, enabled by the Internet-driven information and communications revolution. The data capture that technology enables will drive access to improved health care when and where it is needed, and regardless of time or distance. The enormity of these changes should not be underestimated. Health care providers and organizations are a conservative group and the changes to come will be a great challenge to all. Health care professionals are known for resisting change in general which forces the 'change-agents' to prove that the effects of new health practices are in the best interests of the patients. The e-health revolution will require research to ensure that patient care is not only safe but also improved.

Research in e-health has so far been primarily done on pilot studies and '… challenges remain in providing credible assessments of telemedicine applications and in finding the resources necessary to undertake them'.[28] The KP e-mental health programme is based on scientific research. The KP e-mental health research study has brought together diverse groups who have become a team working together in a new environment. One of the most important factors in this successful team has been the passion and commitment of the principal investigator.

The introduction and acceptance of e-health requires new partnerships that bring health care providers, web designers, information technology specialists and consumers together for a common goal – better health care and improved access. Future health care clinics and boardrooms will be more likely to include colleagues from medicine, nursing, administration, information technology, ethics, design, consumers and finance. All these disparate entities must work together to embrace the power of the Internet and to promote information-age health care. It is crucial that this process occurs in a carefully evaluated manner so that the lessons learned can be properly measured and then applied to other areas of health care.

References

1 Yellowlees P. *Your Guide to E-Health – third millennium medicine on the Internet.* Brisbane: University of Queensland Press, 2001.
2 Feachem RGA, Sekhri NK, White KL, Dixon J, Berwick DM, Enthoven AC. Getting more for their dollar: a comparison of the NHS with California's Kaiser Permanente. *British Medical Journal* 2002;**324**:135–143.

3   Baer L, Elford DR, Cukor P. Telepsychiatry at forty: what have we learned? *Harvard Review of Psychiatry* 1997;**5**:7–17.

4   Johnston B, Wheeler L, Deuser J, Sousa KH. Outcomes of the Kaiser Permanente Tele-Home Health Research Project. *Archives of Family Medicine* 2000;**9**:40–45.

5   Kennedy C, Blignault I, Hornsby D, Yellowlees P. Videoconferencing in the Queensland health service. *Journal of Telemedicine and Telecare* 2001;**7**:266–271.

6   Zaylor C, Nelson E-L, Cook DJ. Clinical outcomes in a prison telepsychiatry clinic. *Journal of Telemedicine and Telecare* 2001;**7**(suppl 1):47–49.

7   Preston J, Brown FW, Hartley B. Using telemedicine to improve health care in distant areas. *Hospital and Community Psychiatry* 1992;**43**:25–32.

8   Hilty DM, Servis ME, Nesbitt TS, et al. The use of TeleMedicine to provide consultation-liaison service to primary care setting. *Psychiatric Annuals* 1999;**29**:412–417.

9   Frueh BC, Deitsch SE, Santos AB, et al. Procedural and methological issues in telepsychiatry research and program development. *Psychiatry Services (Washington DC)* 2000;**51**:1522–1527.

10   Simpson J, Doze S, Urness D, Hailey D, Jacobs P. Evaluation of a routine telepsychiatry service. *Journal of Telemedicine and Telecare* 2001;**7**:90–98.

11   Mielonen M-L, Ohinmaa A, Moring J, Isohanni M. The use of videoconferencing for telepsychiatry in Finland. *Journal of Telemedicine and Telecare* 1999;**4**:125–131.

12   Blackmon LA, Kaak HO, Ranseen J. Consumer satisfaction with telemedicine child psychiatry consultation in rural Kentucky. *Psychiatric Services* 1997;**4**:1464–1466.

13   Callahan EJ, Hilty DM, Nesbitt TS. Patient satisfaction with telemedicine consultation in primary care: comparison of ratings of medical and mental health applications. *Telemedicine Journal* 1998;**4**:363–369.

14   Trott P, Blignault I. Cost evaluation of a telepsychiatry service in northern Queensland. *Journal of Telemedicine and Telecare* 1998;**4**(suppl 1):66–68.

15   Elford DR, White H, St John K, Maddigan B, Ghandi M, Bowering R. A prospective satisfaction study and cost analysis of a pilot child telepsychiatry service in Newfoundland. *Journal of Telemedicine and Telecare* 2001;**7**:73–81.

16   Lyketsos CG, Roques C, Hovanec L, Jones BN 3rd. Telemedicine use and the reduction of psychiatric admissions from a long-term care facility. *Journal of Geriatric Psychiatry and Neurology* 2001;**14**:76–79.

17   Kennedy C, Yellowlees P. A community-based approach to evaluation of health outcomes and costs for telepsychiatry in a rural population: preliminary results. *Journal of Telemedicine and Telecare* 2000;**6**(suppl 1):155–157.

18   Johnston D, Jones BN 3rd. Telepsychiatry consultations to a rural nursing facility: a 2 year experience. *Journal of Geriatric Psychiatry and Neurology* 2001;**14**:72–75.

19   Frueh BC, Deitsch SE, Santos AB, et al. Procedural and methodological issues in telepsychiatry research and program development. *Psychiatric Services* 2000;**51**:1522–1527.

20   Zimnik PR. A brief survey of Department of Defense telemedicine. *Telemedicine Journal* 1996:**2**:241–246.

21   Zaylor C, Whitten P, Kingsley C. Telemedicine services to a county jail. *Journal of Telemedicine and Telecare* 2000;**6**(suppl 1):93–95.

22   Rohland BM. Telepsychiatry in the heartland: if we build it will they come? *Community Mental Health Journal* 2001;**37**:449–459.

23   Vought RG, Grigsby RK, Adams LN, Shevitz SA. Telepsychiatry: addressing mental health needs in Georgia. *Community Mental Health Journal* 2000;**36**:525–536.

24   Brown FW. Rural telepsychiatry. *Psychiatric Services* 1998;**49**:963–964.

25   Watts LA, Monk AF. Telemedicine. What happens in remote consultation. *International Journal of Technology Assessment in Health Care* 1999;**15**:220–235.

26   Hunkeler EM, Meresman JF, Hargreaves WA, et al. Efficacy of nurse telehealth care and peer support in augmenting treatment of depression in primary care. *Archives of Family Medicine* 2000;**9**:700–708.

27   Roine R, Ohinmaa A, Hailey D. Assessing telemedicine: a systematic review of the literature. *Canadian Medical Association Journal* 2001;**165**:765–771.

28   Haily D, Roine R, Ohinmaa A. Systematic review of evidence for the benefits of telemedicine. *Journal of Telemedicine and Telecare* 2002;**8**(suppl 1):1–30.

20

Empirically Supported Computerized Psychotherapy

Kate Cavanagh, Jason Zack and David Shapiro

Introduction

Computer systems are now widely used and accepted in psychotherapeutic practice to assist in assessment, diagnostic interviewing, history taking, consumer health education, mental health consultation, clinical training and specific forms of behavioural modification.[1] However, their most complex and controversial role is as psychotherapist — where the computer delivers the core treatment without input or direction from a human clinician.

For four decades, clinicians and researchers have attempted to identify and isolate the replicable ingredients of the psychotherapeutic encounter and to translate these features into computer-delivered behavioural health interventions. Attempts to mimic the ingredients of the psychotherapeutic encounter using computers have been characterized by four waves, largely mirroring the zeitgeist in non-dynamic schools of psychotherapeutic thought: client-centred (dialogue), behavioural (training and instruction), cognitive (restructuring and problem solving) and cognitive behavioural (combining the latter two techniques). These therapeutic approaches are particularly suitable for computer adaptations because they tend to be structured and non-interpretive (not requiring clinical insight).

In this chapter we review packages which are designed for the management of mental health problems, especially anxiety and depression (Table 20.1). We have excluded any discussion of computerized behavioural health programmes targeting physical health problems, even where there may be a strong psychosomatic component (e.g. asthma, psoriasis) or general health behaviours such as smoking or dieting, although some of the techniques and delivery mechanisms overlap between these and computerized mental health packages. We have also excluded from consideration any programmes that have personal growth or enlightenment as their primary goals. A discussion of the legal and ethical considerations of the implementation of computerized psychotherapies is also beyond the scope of this review.[2] Lastly, we do not discuss interactive voice response (IVR) systems developed for self-treatment of mental health problems.[3]

Table 20.1. Computer tools for psychotherapy included in this chapter

Application	Authors	Features
ELIZA: general therapeutic interview	Weizenbaum[5]	Uses natural language to simulate therapeutic dialogue
SUBABGOL: general therapeutic interview	Colby et al[4]	Uses natural language to simulate therapeutic dialogue
DILEMMA COUNSELLING SYSTEM (DCS)	Wagman[7]	Teaches problem-solving skills
DAD: desensitization for snake phobia	Lang et al[12]	Self-directed graded exposure with relaxation
Graded exposure for test anxiety	Biglan et al[13]	Graded exposure with relaxation to a standard test-anxiety hierarchy
Cognitive therapy for depression	Selmi et al[48]	Structured information and education, cognitive strategies
Systematic desensitization for phobias	Ghosh and Marks[15]	Multiple choice questions, relaxation training, self-directed exposure, homework
Systematic desensitization for phobias	Chandler et al[14]	Relaxation training, systematic desensitization, self-directed exposure, homework
THERAPEUTIC LEARNING PROGRAMME (TLP)	Colby et al[40]	Computer plus group therapy programme, multiple choice questions, identification of problems, target setting, homework
OVERCOMING DEPRESSION	Colby[49]	Psychoeducation and dialogue using natural language
MINDSTREET	Wright et al[50]	Interactive video, multiple choice questions, homework manual, feedback to clinician
Virtual reality graded exposure	Rothbaum et al[26]	Therapist-guided virtual reality exposure for acrophobia
Cognitive behavioural therapy for panic	Newman et al[44]	Palmtop computers used as an adjunct to cognitive behavioural therapy, psychoeducation, self-monitoring, positive reinforcement
FEARFIGHTER	Kenright et al[22]	Multiple choice questions, self-directed exposure, relaxation training, homework
BEATING THE BLUES	Proudfoot et al[51]	Multiple choice questions, interactive multimedia cognitive and behavioural therapy modules, case vignettes, progress reports to clinician, homework.

The first wave: tickertape therapists

The first generation of computerized psychotherapies were characterized by attempts to simulate the 'talk' of 'talking therapists'. Colby and colleagues[4] designed a program to 'communicate an intent to help, as the psychotherapist does, and to respond as he does by questioning, clarifying, rephrasing and occasionally interpreting' and conveyed a hope that this application might offer a widely available psychotherapeutic tool. The same year at the Massachusetts Institute of Technology, Weizenbaum[5] described his software ELIZA, a similar system, which allowed people to discuss their problems using natural language: ordinary words, phrases and sentence structure with their tickertape therapist.

Weizenbaum considered his system a straw-man, a tool for exploration of the possibilities and limitations of computer-simulated natural language using conversational rules based on non-directive, client-centred, Rogerian techniques featuring restatement, empathic reflection. He never intended ELIZA to function as a true psychotherapist.[6] He was primarily concerned with the ethical issues associated with computerized psychotherapy, and concluded that it would be immoral to substitute a computer for a psychotherapist, whose role 'involves interpersonal respect, understanding, and love'.

Although a precipitator of great discussion, the use of natural language simulation in computerized psychotherapy has not been widely adopted in health care to date. Rather than offering empirical support for the use of such systems, over the next decade, computer scientists and psychotherapists alike exploited the limitations of these programs, emphasizing their shortfalls in generating meaningful therapeutic dialogue[7] and more generally arguing the folly of using computers in psychotherapy.[8]

After computerized psychotherapy's early foray into the simulation of natural language and the psychotherapeutic dialogue, researchers argued that computerized psychotherapies were 'more attuned to brief, focused interventions of a cognitive or behavioural inclination, those that claim to be independent of non-specific aspects of therapy and that expect new relationships or behaviours to be experienced mainly outside the therapeutic setting'.[9] Acknowledging their limitations, researchers focused on the translation of specific cognitive and behavioural techniques to be delivered by computer systems.

The second wave: simple behavioural techniques

Behavioural psychotherapies have enjoyed considerable success in the treatment of anxiety and are recognized as a treatment of choice for specific fears by health professionals.[10,11] In combating specific fears, graded exposure with relaxation training is a highly effective and rapid intervention. The technique, ubiquitous in behavioural treatment of anxiety disorders, involves identifying and encountering a hierarchy of feared stimuli until no further anxiety is experienced in their presence. The structured and systematic nature of this psychotherapeutic technique lends itself particularly well to computerization, a key principle that has been seized upon by the authors of therapeutic computer packages. This section describes a number of programmes delivering this technique and evaluates their effectiveness in the management of agoraphobia and other anxiety disorders.

Automated graded exposure

The earliest computerized desensitization programmes were automated prototypes. The first automated desensitization procedure to be evaluated in a controlled trial was a system called DAD.[12] Following four sessions of therapist-guided relaxation training, the DAD system presented a 20-item snake-fear hierarchy, where exposure and relaxation episodes were controlled by the snake-phobic participants using switches attached to the arms of their chair. Outcome measures indicated marked improvement in participants using the DAD system comparable to those experiencing therapist-guided desensitization. Indeed on some measures DAD outcomes excelled live therapy, leading the authors to conclude that live therapist involvement in desensitization may not only be an unnecessary luxury, but a hindrance!

Computerized graded exposure: standardized hierarchies

The first truly computerized graded exposure programme was developed by Biglan et al for the management of test anxiety.[13] Their programme included audiotaped relaxation training and a computer-controlled desensitization system. Prior to using the programme, students were trained to relax. In the computer-controlled programme, a standard hierarchy of 20 textual descriptions of items related to test anxiety was presented one at a time on a video display terminal. Anxious students were instructed to imagine the item while relaxing for a 30-second period. If during that period the students felt discomfort, then they pressed a key. The computer then presented the instruction 'RELAX', and waited 30 seconds before re-presenting the item. If no discomfort was reported, then after 30 seconds of further relaxation the next item in the hierarchy was presented. Nine college students reporting marked test anxiety completed the program in an average of four sessions lasting about 30 minutes each. Their scores on the test anxiety scale demonstrated significant reduction from pre- to post-treatment as well as increased comfort in various aspects of the academic examination process.

Computerized graded exposure: individualized hierarchies

Expanding on this early work two groups of researchers[14–16] developed generic computer programmes for systematic desensitization that permitted both individual behavioural treatment goals and individualized sensitization hierarchies. Both programmes also expanded the locus of the therapeutic setting, incorporating both computer-guided 'thought-experiment' exposure techniques with computer-guided in vivo (live) exposure homework practice, supported by printed information summaries and diary sheets.

Chandler et al[14] presented a case report of a 35-year-old male diagnosed with agoraphobia and obsessive-compulsive ruminations. The subject reported being unable to leave his apartment alone unless he was going directly to his parents' house or other safe place. The computer program presented graded exposure in four stages. The first stage, delivered in the initial session, taught the patient the learning theory perspective on the aetiology of phobias, offered hope, presented the structure of the program and emphasized the patient's responsibility for, and importance of, completing the homework. This stage also included relaxation training delivered by audiotape. The patient was then instructed to practise the relaxation techniques daily before the next computer session, and this practice was supported by printed instructions. The second stage involved the construction of a personalized phobic hierarchy. In later sessions, the presentation of items from the hierarchy and 'thought-experiment' exposure commenced, following a deep relaxation exercise and in vivo exposure, formed between-session homework. During 13 sessions working with the computer program, the patient improved dramatically, achieving therapeutic targets and life goals which were retained, indeed improved, at 8 months follow-up. From not being able to leave his apartment he was able to set up in business as a tradesman working on external jobs, and able to go where he wanted to by himself. Equally dramatic improvements were seen in a case series of five patients suffering from a range of phobias published later by the group.[17]

Ghosh and Marks[15] reported a randomized controlled study of 40 agoraphobics investigating the effectiveness of their graded exposure therapy, comparing computerized instruction with psychiatrist-led therapy and a self-help book. Following a 90-minute assessment with a psychiatrist, patients either met the psychiatrist weekly for exposure instructions, received the book 'Living With Fear',[18] or planned their exposure treatment by interacting with the computer program. All three groups of agoraphobics improved substantially up to 6 months follow-up, with no significant differences between them. As a group, the patients dropped from being 'habitual avoiders with regular phobic panic pre-treatment, to becoming non-avoiders with no phobic panic and only residual slight anxiety at follow-up'.

Concurring with other studies,[19–21] the authors concluded that graded exposure is effective in the treatment of agoraphobia, and on the basis of these research findings, Bloom[1] argued that graded exposure 'does not appear to require interpersonal interaction with a therapist in order to be successful'.

Marks and colleague's treatment package has recently been updated to include screen voice-overs, and to permit web-delivery. Research evidence also suggests that the revised programme FEARFIGHTER (Fig. 20.1) is clinically and cost effective in the self-treatment of specific fears and agoraphobia.[22,23]

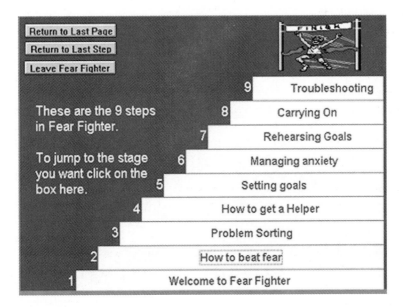

Fig. 20.1. Screenshot from FEARFIGHTER. (Image courtesy of ST Solutions.)

Computerized graded exposure: virtual reality

The use of virtual therapeutic environments has enjoyed some success in the treatment of spider phobia,[24] claustrophobia,[25] acrophobia,[26] social phobia,[27,28] agoraphobia,[29] fear of flying[30,31] and post-traumatic stress disorder (PTSD).[32]

Virtual reality offers an interactive therapeutic paradigm in which users are no longer simply onlookers of images on a computer screen but become active participants within a computer-generated three-dimensional virtual world (Figs 20.2, 20.3). In virtual reality real-time computer graphics, body tracking devices, visual displays and other sensory input and feedback devices are integrated to give the user a sense of immersion or presence in the virtual environment (see Chapter 22).[33] Participants usually wear a head-mounted display presenting a virtual environment display that moves, naturally, in response to head and body motion. Sensor gloves and other features can be used to facilitate and enhance environmental interactions appropriate to the exposure encounter.

In the case of acrophobia, Rothbaum's group has developed virtual reality hardware and software to recreate the experience of a variety of elevation scenes. For example, footbridges above water, outdoor balconies, and a glass elevator simulating the one at the Atlanta Marriot Marquis convention hotel, rising 49 floors or 147 metres. Desensitization conducted during immersion in these environments resulted in substantial incremental improvement over a waitlist control group (i.e. randomized to a delayed treatment group). Following treatment, patients reported significantly reduced fear and avoidance of heights and improved attitudes towards heights. There were similar benefits in a controlled trial where 49 patients with fear of flying were randomly

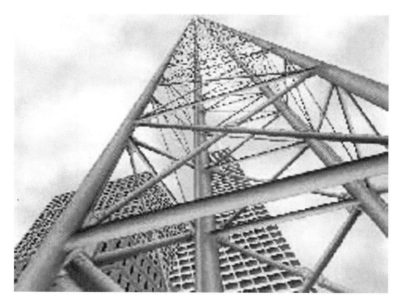

Fig. 20.2. Virtual reality fear of heights simulation. (Image courtesy of the Virtual Reality Medical Centre.)

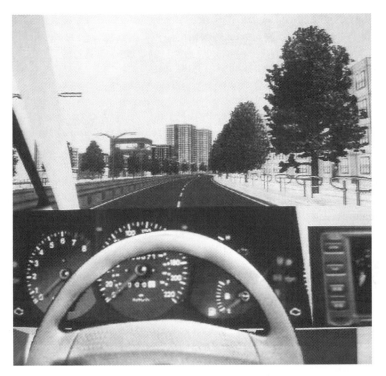

Fig. 20.3. Virtual reality fear of driving simulation. (Image courtesy of the Virtual Reality Medical Centre.)

assigned to virtual reality exposure and desensitization to a flight fear hierarchy, standard therapist-guided exposure, or a waitlist control. Rothbaum et al[31] found that both virtual and standard exposure were superior to waitlist control in reducing fear of flying and in achieving behavioural flight goals, and that these improvements were retained to 12 months follow-up. In the year after the study 92% of the virtual exposure group, and 91% of the standard, in vivo exposure, group took a flight.

The computer generation of virtual reality environments may be more acceptable to anxious clients than in vivo exposure,[34] and also permits much more control over the exposure episodes than is usually possible.[35] In addition it can dramatically reduce the cost of therapist-guided exposure to stimuli which typically require leaving the therapist's office (heights, driving, shopping centres) and exposure episodes, which can be costly and complex in themselves (social performance situations, flights, snakes, tarantulas).

In the case of social and performance anxiety, future virtual therapeutic environments may be augmented with avatars (virtual people) to create the illusion of an interactive audience. Petraub et al[36] recreated a performance anxiety situation by creating a virtual audience of eight male avatars sitting in a semicircle. In order to foster the illusion of life, the avatars exhibited small twitching movements, blinking and shifting about in their chairs. Audience behaviour was presented in two conditions by manipulating facial animations, direction of gaze, posture and physical animation displaying classic non-verbal communications of friendly receptivity and hostility. Petraub et al found that participants, particularly in a high immersion group who interacted with the audience via a head-mounted display (rather than simply a desktop screen), responded to virtual audiences much as they would respond to real audiences. The authors suggested that this indicates that virtual reality scenarios with computer-generated characters could be useful in treating and investigating a range of social performance situations.

Virtual environments can also be used to construct and explore feared or desired spaces which cannot be encountered in real life. Using these techniques, it is possible to transcend the limits of the real world, permitting the shared construction and exploration of memorial, 'thought-experiment' or anticipated events.[37] For example, virtual reality exposure and desensitization has been effectively used to reduce the symptom severity associated with specific traumatic experience in Vietnam veterans using immersion into virtual environments like flying in a Huey helicopter over Vietnam and walking in a jungle clearing – situations that could not be explored easily in real life.[32]

The third wave: computerized cognitive therapy

Cognitive therapy accounts for the symptoms of anxiety and depression in terms of unhelpful thought patterns. The treatment aims to enable clients to identify, challenge and modify negative thinking styles. A substantial body of research evidence supports the value of this approach in the treatment of depression, where its short-term effects match those of pharmacotherapy. An increasing body of evidence strongly suggests that the benefits of cognitive therapy for depression continue after the end of treatment.[10,38] The third wave of computerized therapy systems was characterized by the translation of cognitive therapeutic techniques from human to computer therapists. Here the computer therapist typically adopts a role as instructor and advisor, functions more easily embodied in the computerized therapy paradigm than those of a dynamic analyst.[7]

Cognitive therapy: dilemma counselling system

Wagman's PLATO DCS (DILEMMA COUNSELLING SYSTEM)[7,39] is a good example of the early computerized cognitive psychotherapy approach. Where Weizenbaum[5] and Colby et al[4] had attempted to mimic the most complex and sophisticated forms of psychotherapy, Wagman championed a simpler approach. Wagman developed a psychotherapeutic computer program which he demonstrated was beneficial to its target audience. The systematic dilemma counselling paradigm assumes that discomfort arises from the patient's necessity to choose between what are thought of as two undesirable alternatives, or avoidance-avoidance problems. For example, in the case of career choice for university students, Wagman[7] showcased the dilemma that choosing to be a financier is lucrative but intellectually unstimulating, whereas choosing to be a scientist is intellectually stimulating but not lucrative. The PLATO DCS (DILEMMA COUNSELLING SYSTEM) presents an overview of the rationale for the dilemma counselling method and then offers five stages in resolving each dilemma:

1. it aids the user in formulating the problem as a psychological dilemma

2. it helps the user to develop an extrication route for each dilemma

3. it helps the user to identify a line of enquiry which will help negotiate each extrication route

4. it helps the user to generate solutions for each line of enquiry

5. it guides the patient to rate and evaluate the various proposed solutions.

Early evaluation of the DCS method indicated that it could be valuable for people with a troublesome but clearly articulated dilemma. In a randomized controlled trial, students using the DCS reported greater problem improvement 1 week and 1 month after using the system than co-contact controls. Ninety per cent of those using the system found it at least slightly helpful. Moreover, the majority of participants felt that the system was not too impersonal, and that it was stimulating and interesting, and many participants felt more at ease using the computerized system than seeing a human counsellor.

Cognitive therapies: anxiety

Colby et al[40] have described a method of short-term computer-assisted psychotherapy for anxiety problems, which functions adjunctively to group therapy sessions. THE THERAPEUTIC LEARNING PROGRAMME (TLP) requires 10 hours of group work, in which 6–10 people each work independently on computerized psychotherapy systems and then discuss their individualized printout with the group. The sessions involve eight stages, characterized by Colby et al as:

1. Identify the demand inherent to the patient's interpersonal problem situation that is not being addressed effectively.

2. Identify new proactive behaviour (action steps) that might effectively address the dissatisfied state.

3. Clarify the suitability of the new proactive behaviour and identify the inhibited function that results from the patient's prediction of feared adverse consequences.

4. Identify the incorrect beliefs (thinking errors) that link catastrophic predictions to an action intention.

5. Help the patient to understand the historical origin of thinking errors in childhood adaptations and to sort out present realities from past realities.

6. Help the patient understand that childhood-thinking is no longer appropriate for adult decision-making in interpersonal problem situations.

7.   When the predicted adverse consequences are accepted as incorrect, the patient's fear of transgressing rigid command rules diminish and the patient is more likely to carry out the required proactive behaviour.

8.   The recovery of an inhibited function becomes part of the patient's self-concept as a functioning adult.

Impressive initial outcomes using this technique[41] led to a later study including almost 300 participants. Over 95% reported improvement in their ability to handle the problem situation that brought them to the therapy, 78% reported a drop in general distress and 78% reported a high level of satisfaction with the procedure.[42]

Another approach to offering computerized cognitive (and behavioural) advice for problems of anxiety in primary care is reported in Parkin et al.[43] The prototype programme WORRYTEL was designed to guide users to develop their own self-treatment programme, permitting them to view case vignettes, identify personal symptoms and print out useful screens from the program. A small open pilot study of the program suggested that anxious patients found the system easy to use, acceptable and empathetic, but wanting more specific guidance in how to overcome their current problems.

Cognitive therapies: panic

In a small randomized controlled trial Newman et al[44] demonstrated that a palmtop therapeutic aid could increase the cost effectiveness of cognitive therapy for panic. The traditional therapy group received 12 sessions of individual cognitive therapy, whilst the palmtop group received just four individual therapy sessions and completed the remainder of the course guided by their palmtop panic program. Both groups benefited from the trial and improvements were retained at a 6-month follow-up. The authors estimated that the palmtop treatment saved $540 per panic treatment, which in the face of equivalent clinical outcomes represents a considerable potential health care cost saving.

Cognitive therapies: depression

Selmi et al[45] developed a computerized psychotherapy program based on the work of Beck[46,47] to simulate therapist-delivered cognitive interventions for depression. Selmi et al[48] reported evidence for the efficacy of computerized cognitive therapy for depression. Thirty-six patients meeting clinical criteria for depression were randomly assigned to therapist-led psychotherapy, computerized psychotherapy or waitlist control. Both active treatments were found superior to the waitlist control group.

Colby[49] described a computerized treatment package called OVERCOMING DEPRESSION which was designed to provide cognitive therapy for mild to moderate depression. OVERCOMING DEPRESSION consisted of two sections. One section provided information about depression and possible cognitive strategies for alleviating the disorder and preventing relapses. The second section offered a dialogue mode which allowed the user to engage in therapeutically directed conversations with the program, which was designed to interpret and respond appropriately to everyday language.

The fourth wave: multimedia interactive cognitive behavioural therapy for anxiety and depression

In recent years cognitive behavioural therapies that integrate the principles and treatment methods in cognitive and behavioural strategies have enjoyed their position as the psychotherapeutic techniques best supported by research evidence.[10,11] A primary strategy in this approach is to analyse the interaction of thinking styles and behaviour patterns so that clients can identify antecedents to distressing emotional states and modify them.

As cognitive behavioural techniques are routinely manualized in order to standardize how they are delivered, they are excellent candidates for translation to alternative delivery formats. A review of research designed to test empirically the clinical benefits of earlier waves of computerized psychotherapy systems suggests that these systems can work, can work as well as human therapists and may be especially effective where cognitive and behavioural techniques are employed.

The newest computerized therapy systems combine cognitive and behavioural approaches delivered via multimedia interactive formats (Fig. 20.4). They are designed to embody both the specific active techniques of this therapeutic approach and the non-specific features of the therapeutic relationship known to influence clinical outcomes (e.g. alliance or engagement, empathy, motivation and trust). The multimedia format integrates video, graphics and animations, voice-over and many interactive episodes, including multiple choice responding, distress/success ratings,

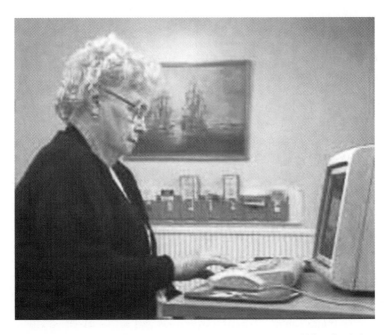

Fig. 20.4. Computerized psychotherapy in progress. (Image courtesy of Ultrasis plc.)

on-screen problem-solving and diary completion. This provides a stimulating and engaging interface.

Two empirically supported interactive multimedia systems are currently available: MIND STREET[50] and BEATING THE BLUES.[51] The former is designed to be used with face-to-face treatment, thus offering a package of 'computer-assisted psychotherapy'. The latter has been designed primarily as a stand-alone tool.

MIND STREET

MIND STREET comprises six modules (Introduction, Basic Principles, Changing Automatic Thoughts, Taking Action, Changing Schemas, and Continuing Your Progress), lasting approximately 3 hours 45 minutes in total and typically completed in 4–8 sessions over 4 weeks. The computer program is designed to socialize the patient to cognitive and behavioural treatment methods, offer psychoeducation, reinforce the utility of self-help exercises, and help free the clinician for interventions that require the sensitivity and expertise of a human therapist.

In an uncontrolled, preliminary trial, 96 inpatients and outpatients, most diagnosed with major depression, were permitted to use the package at their own pace in conjunction with any available treatment as usual (typically a mixture of pharmacotherapy and psychotherapy). Users indicated a high rate of acceptance of this form of computer-assisted therapy, with 78% of patients completing the entire program. Mean scores on a measure of cognitive therapy knowledge were significantly improved.[50]

Patients' scores on the Beck (Anxiety and Depression) scales and Automatic Thoughts Questionnaire were dramatically reduced immediately following the programme. However, the open-nature of the trial and conjuctive administration of the treatment programme (with both client–computer and client–therapist work forming the whole treatment) makes it impossible to attribute this improvement solely to the multimedia package.

A randomized, controlled study has also supported the clinical efficacy of this programme. Drug-free subjects with major depression were randomly assigned to computer-assisted cognitive therapy (CCT), standard cognitive therapy (CT) or a waitlist control group (WL). Treatment consisted of up to nine sessions over 8 weeks. CCT involved abbreviated consultations with a clinician (25 minutes instead of 50 minutes in CT) plus use of the computer package (about 25-minute sessions). Results showed that CCT was equal to CT and both were superior to the WL. The response rate (50% drop in Beck Depression Inventory (BDI) scores) was identical in CCT and CT (70%), and was only 7% in WL subjects. No follow-up data are available yet.

BEATING THE BLUES

BEATING THE BLUES offers cognitive behavioural therapy for anxiety and depression in the form of a stand-alone computer-controlled, interactive multimedia package which can be delivered on a PC located in the primary or psychotherapy care practice or community resource centre. Clinical supervision and responsibility continue to rest with the primary care physician or other appropriately qualified personnel (nurse or clinical psychologist), to whom reports (including warnings of suicide or other risk) are automatically delivered by the program.

BEATING THE BLUES is an eight-session program (each session lasting about 1 hour), plus 'homework' assignments between sessions. The therapy program is readily usable by patients with no previous computer experience. Like other versions of cognitive behavioural therapy, BEATING THE BLUES can be given alone or in combination with pharmacotherapy.

BEATING THE BLUES utilizes a range of multimedia capabilities. It features a series of filmed case studies of fictional patients who are used to model both the symptoms of anxiety and depression and their treatment by cognitive behavioural therapy, as well as animations, voice-over and interactive modules (Figs 20.5, 20.6).

In a recent study,[51] researchers used BEATING THE BLUES with a sample of 170 patients suffering from anxiety, depression or mixed anxiety and depression (CITE). The randomized, controlled trial demonstrated the clinical benefits of BEATING THE BLUES. Patients were first of all prescribed treatment as usual (TAU) by their primary care physician – whatever the physician regarded as appropriate for that patient. They were then randomized separately within two categories, Drug or No Drug, depending upon the physician's prescribed treatment, to TAU alone or TAU plus BEATING THE BLUES. Any other prescribed psychological treatment was removed for those patients randomized to BEATING THE BLUES. All patients completed a number of questionnaires (including the Beck Anxiety and Depression Inventories) at entry to the trial, 2 months later (when patients randomized to BEATING THE BLUES had completed the programme) and at 1, 3 and 6 months follow-up.

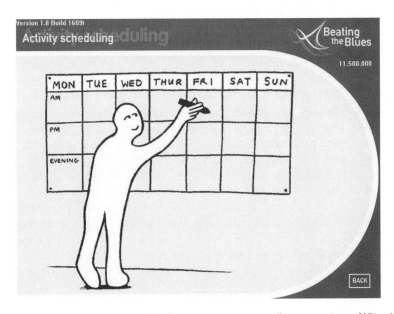

Fig. 20.5. Activity scheduling screen shot from BEATING THE BLUES. (Image courtesy of Ultrasis plc.)

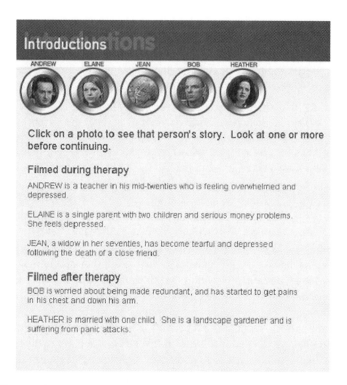

Fig. 20.6. Case study screen shot from BEATING THE BLUES. (Image courtesy of Ultrasis plc.)

At entry, levels of anxiety and depression were in the high–moderate to severe range and comparable to those observed in other studies of general practice. As expected, patients allocated by the physician to drug treatment were more severely ill. The prescribed pharmacotherapy was effective on all measures. Also as expected, patients who, at entry to the trial, had been ill for 6 months or more were more anxious and depressed than those with shorter periods of pre-existing illness.

The most important finding was that computer therapy reduced anxiety and depression significantly and substantially: average scores at the end of treatment in patients allocated to BEATING THE BLUES were barely above the non-clinical range. These effects remained equally pronounced right through follow-up to the final 6-month measurement. Moreover, they did not interact with drug treatment: the beneficial effects of drugs and of BEATING THE BLUES were additive. Nor did the effects of BEATING THE BLUES interact with either the severity or duration of pre-existing illness. Notably, patients more than 6 months ill at the start of treatment responded as well to computer therapy as did those with shorter periods of illness.

In summary, research findings indicate that computer-delivered cognitive behavioural therapy can be a valuable tool for the treatment of anxiety and depression across almost the entire range of patients seen with these conditions in general practice[51] as well as for inpatients and outpatients within the context of psychiatric practices.[50]

What works for whom?

The landscape of mental health service provision varies from country to country, state to state, and indeed, town to town. One shared feature is that national health services, health maintenance organizations (HMOs), employee assistance providers, individual clinicians, community mental health centres and other mental health care providers are all seeking opportunities to increase access to more acceptable, more beneficial and more cost-effective early interventions for mental health problems.

A review of the research literature regarding computerized psychotherapies indicates that where proven techniques are translated for computer delivery clinical outcomes are comparable to traditional face-to-face services and may be indicated for both anxiety and depression. The best supported programs meet recognized standards of proof for psychotherapeutic interventions,[11] as well as independent acknowledgement for the benefits of disseminating these programs within health care systems (E. Kaltenthaler, personal communication).

Little is known about which patient characteristics predict most engagement or benefit from computerized psychotherapy. Research is currently under way to identify predictors of continuation and of outcome.

The future

This chapter offers a snapshot of a very young set of technologies: a brief review of a few dozen papers which largely constitute the published empirical literature regarding computerized psychotherapies. True computerized psychotherapies have just begun. The published literature reviewed here is not wholly representative of the state of the field, as empirical psychotherapy research often follows in the footsteps of clinical pioneers. However, the majority of published research suggests that computerized psychotherapies:

- offer an acceptable format for care
- increase access to effective psychotherapies for people suffering from anxiety and depression
- reduce symptoms and problem severity
- improve functioning and well-being
- reduce the costs of delivering proven techniques in mental health care.

We believe that computerized psychotherapies have an exciting future. They will not replace face-to-face therapies, but will supplement them. It is unlikely that there will ever be enough skilled therapists to meet the needs of all those suffering from the common mental health problems. Computerized therapies will help fill this gap, by engaging patients in self-changing behaviours grounded in many of the psychological principles underlying face-to-face therapy. We envisage a future in which only those patients who cannot be helped by self-help books or computer therapy programmes will need to call upon 'live' therapists. Computerized therapies will also find a place as adjuncts to face-to-face therapy, giving additional opportunities for patients to learn and to overcome their problems. This will reduce the time that the therapist needs to spend with each patient. Therapists will be freed up to focus their efforts on those for whom the need for human contact, or the complexity or rarity of their problems, requires face-to-face work. Philosophically, computerized therapy passes power and control to patients, by providing a resource for them to use as they wish. Computerized therapy therefore has the potential to bring psychological principles to the aid of vast numbers of people with common mental health problems.

References

1   Bloom BL. Computer-assisted psychological intervention: review and commentary. *Clinical Psychology Review* 1992;**12**:169–197.
2   Cavanagh K, Shapiro DA, Zack JS. Computer plays therapist. In:Goss S, Anthony K, eds. *Technology in Counselling and Psychotherapy Practice: a practitioners' guide.* Palgrave, 2003. In press.
3   Marks I, Shaw S, Parkin R. Computer-aided treatments of mental health problems. *Clinical Psychology:Science and Practice* 1998;**5**:151–170.
4   Colby KM, Watt JB, Gilbert JP. A computer method of psychotherapy: preliminary communication. *Journal of Nervous and Mental Disease* 1966;**142**:148–152.
5   Weizenbaum J. ELIZA – a computer program for the study of natural language communication between man and machine. *Communications of the ACM* 1966;**9**:36–45.
6   Weizenbaum J. *Computer Power and Human Reason, from Judgment to Calculation.* San Francisco:WH Freeman, 1976.
7   Wagman M. PLATO DCS: an interactive computer system for personal counselling. *Journal of Counseling Psychology* 1980;**27**:171–178.
8   Wright JH, Wright AS. Computer-assisted psychotherapy. *Journal of Psychotherapy Practice and Research* 1997;**6**:315–329.
9   Servan-Schreiber D. Artificial intelligence and psychiatry. *Journal of Nervous and Mental Disease* 1986;**174**:191–202.
10 Roth A, Fonagy P. *What works for whom: a critical review of psychotherapy research.* London: Guilford Press, 1996.
11 Department of Health. *Treatment Choice in Psychological Therapies and Counselling: evidence based clinical practice guidelines.* London: Department of Health, 2001. Available at http://www.doh.gov.uk/mentalhealth/treatmentguideline/leaflet.pdf [last checked 17 September 2002].
12 Lang PJ, Melamed BG, Hart J. A psychophysiological analysis of fear modification using an automated desensitization procedure. *Journal of Abnormal Psychology* 1970;**76**:220–234.
13 Biglan A, Villwock C, Wick S. The feasibility of a computer controlled program for treatment of test anxiety. *Journal of Behavior Therapy and Experimental Psychiatry* 1979;**10**:47–49.
14 Chandler GM, Burck HD, Sampson JR-JP. A generic computer program for systematic desensitization: description, construction and case study. *Journal of Behavior Therapy and Experimental Psychiatry* 1986;**17**:171–174.
15 Ghosh A, Marks IM. Self-treatment of agoraphobia by exposure. *Behaviour Therapy* 1987;**18**:3–16.
16 Ghosh A, Marks IM, Carr AC. Controlled study of self-exposure treatment for phobics: preliminary communication. *Journal of the Royal Society of Medicine* 1984;**77**:483–487.
17 Chandler GM, Burck H, Sampson, JP, Wray R. Effectiveness of a generic computer program for systematic desensitization. *Computers in Human Behavior* 1988;**4**:339–346.
18 Marks IM. *Living with Fear: understanding and coping with anxiety.* New York: McGraw-Hill, 1978.
19 Jannoun L, Munby M, Catalan J, Gelder M. A home-based treatment program for agoraphobia: replication and controlled evaluation. *Behavior Therapy* 1980;**11**:294–305.
20 Mathews A. Recent developments in the treatment of agoraphobia. *Behavioural Analysis and Modification* 1977;**2**:64–75.
21 McDonald R, et al. The effects of self-exposure instructions on agoraphobic outpatients. *Behaviour Research and Therapy* 1979;**17**:83–85.

22   Kenwright M, Liness S, Marks I. Reducing demands on clinicians' time by offering computer-aided self-help for phobia/panic: feasibility study. *British Journal of Psychiatry* 2001;**179**:456–459.

23   Shaw S, Marks IM. (1996) Computer-aided self-care for agoraphobia/panic. Paper to Annual Meeting of Royal College of Psychiatrists, London, July.

24   Carlin AS, Hoffman HG, Weghorst S. Virtual reality and tactile augmentation in the treatment of spider phobia: a case report. *Behaviour Research and Therapy* 1997;**35**:153–158.

25   Botella C, Villa H, Banos R, Perpina C, Garcia-Palacios A. The treatment of claustrophobia with virtual reality: changes in other phobic behaviors not specifically treated. *CyberPsychology and Behavior* 1999;**2**:135–141.

26   Rothbaum BO, Hodges LF, Kooper R, et al. Effectiveness of computer-generated (virtual reality) graded exposure in the treatment of acrophobia. *American Journal of Psychiatry* 1995;**152**:626–628.

27   North MM, North SM, Coble JR. Virtual reality therapy: an effective treatment for phobias. In: Riva G, Wiederhold BK, Molinari EE, eds. *Virtual Environments in Clinical Psychology and Neuroscience: methods and techniques in advanced patient–therapist interaction.* Amsterdam: IOS Press, 1998:112–119.

28   Petraub DP, Slater M, Barker C. An experiment on fear of public speaking in virtual reality. In: Westwood JD, ed. *Medicine Meets Virtual Reality.* Ohmsha: IOS Press, 2001:372–378.

29   Wiederhold BK, Wiederhold MD. Lessons learned from 600 virtual reality sessions. *CyberPsychology and Behavior* 2000;**3**:393–400.

30   Muehlberger A, Herrmann MJ, Wiedemann G, Ellgring H, Pauli P. Repeated exposure of flight phobics to flights in virtual reality. *Behaviour Research and Therapy* 2001;**39**:1033–1050.

31   Rothbaum BO, Hodges L, Anderson PL, Price L, Smith S. Twelve-month follow-up of virtual reality and standard exposure therapies for the fear of flying. *Journal of Consulting and Clinical Psychology* 2002;**70**:428–432.

32   Rothbaum BO, Hodges LF, Ready D, Graap K, Alarcon RD. Virtual reality exposure therapy for Vietnam veterans with posttraumatic stress disorder. *Journal of Clinical Psychiatry* 2001;**62**:617–622.

33   Kalawsky RS. VRUSE – a computerised diagnostic tool: for usability evaluation of virtual/synthetic environment systems. *Applied Ergonomics* 1993;**30**:11–25.

34   Garcia-Palacios A, Hoffman HG, See SK, Tsai A, Botella C. Redefining therapeutic success with virtual reality exposure therapy. *CyberPsychology and Behavior* 2001;**4**:341–348.

35   North MM, North SM, Coble JR. Virtual reality therapy: an effective treatment for psychological disorders. In: Stanney KM, ed. *Handbook of Virtual Environments:design, implementation, and applications. Human factors and ergonomics.* Mahwah, NJ:Lawrence Erlbaum, 2002:1065–1078.

36   Petraub DP, Slater M, Barker C. An experiment on fear of public speaking in virtual reality. In:Westwood JD, ed. *Medicine Meets Virtual Reality.* Ohmsha: IOS Press, 2001:372–378.

37   Riva G, Molinari E, Vincelli F. Virtual reality as communicative medium between patient and therapist. In: Riva G, Davide F, eds. *Communications Through Virtual Technologies: identity, community and technology in the communication age. Studies in new technologies and practices in communication.* Amsterdam: IOS Press, 2001:87–100.

38   Roth A, Fonagy P. *What Works for Whom:a critical review of psychotherapy research.* London:Guilford Press, 1996.

39   Wagman M, Kerber KW. PLATO DCS, an interactive computer system for personal counseling:further development and evaluation. *Journal of Counseling and Clinical Psychology* 1980;**27**:31–39.

40   Colby KM, Gould RL, Aronson G. Some pros and cons of computer-assisted psychotherapy. *Journal of Nervous and Mental Disease* 1989;**177**:105–108.

41   Talley J, ed. *Family Practitioner's Guide to Treating Depressive Illness.* Chicago: Precept Press, 1987.

42   Dolezal-Wood S, Belar CD, Snibbe J. A comparison of computer-assisted psychotherapy and cognitive-behavioral therapy in groups. *Journal of Clinical Psychology in Medical Settings* 1996;**5**:103–115.

43   Parkin R, Marks I, Higgs R. Development of a computerized aid for the management of anxiety in primary care. *Primary Care Psychiatry* 1995;**1**:115–117.

44   Newman MG, Consoli AJ, Taylor CB. A palmtop computer program for the treatment of generalized anxiety disorder. *Behaviour Modification* 1999;**23**:597–619.

45   Selmi PM. An investigation of computer-assisted cognitive-behavior therapy in the treatment of depression. *Behavior Research Methods and Instrumentation* 1982;**14**:181–185.

46   Beck AT. *Cognitive Therapy and the Emotional Disorders.* New York: International Universities Press, 1976.

47   Beck AT, Rush AJ, Shaw BF, Emery G. *Cognitive Therapy for Depression.* Chichester: Wiley, 1980.

48   Selmi PM, Klein MH, Greist JH, Sorrell SP, Erdman HP. Computer-administered cognitive-behavioral therapy for depression. *American Journal of Psychiatry* 1990;**147**:51–56.

49   Colby KM. A computer program using cognitive therapy to treat depressed patients. *Psychiatric Services* 1995;**46**:1223–1225.

50   Wright JH, Wright AS, Salmon P, et al. Development and initial testing of a multimedia program for computer assisted cognitive therapy. *American Journal of Psychotherapy* 2002;**56**:76–86.
51   Proudfoot J, Goldberg D, Mann A, Everitt B, Marks I, Gray J. Computerised, interactive, multimedia cognitive behavioural therapy reduces anxiety and depression in general practice: a randomised controlled trial. *Psychological Medicine.* In press.

Section 4: The Future

21

Guidelines for Telepsychiatry and E-mental Health

Richard Wootton and Ilse Blignault

Introduction

The term 'guidelines' is used loosely in the literature, often being used interchangeably with 'standards'. However, the two terms have distinct meanings. The dictionary definitions of *standard* include:

- a degree or level of requirement, excellence or attainment
- an acknowledged measure of comparison for quantitative or qualitative value; a criterion.

while the dictionary definitions of *guidelines* include:

- a statement or other indication of policy or procedure by which to determine a course of action
- guidance relative to setting standards or determining a course of action
- a rule or principle that provides guidance to appropriate behaviour.

Standards therefore imply technical compliance with rigid and defined criteria; guidelines imply the following of recommended, and to some extent flexible, practices. Standards are quantitative and are largely prescriptive; guidelines are to some extent qualitative and voluntary.

The aim of guidelines in health care is to promote best practice and to improve the consistency and efficiency of health care delivery, based on scientific and clinical research.[1] That is, guidelines are systematically developed statements to assist practitioners and patients make decisions about appropriate health care for specific clinical circumstances.[2,3] By definition, this implies that guidelines are a tool to aid decision-making, and have undergone extensive evaluation prior to implementation. Guidelines may be employed by several different classes of user, including:

- the general practitioner
- the specialist
- the health service planner.

The ultimate goal of health care guidelines is to improve patient health outcomes, and this has led to the development of databases providing evidence-based guidelines for clinical practice.[4,5] However there is little reference in the literature to guidelines for telemedicine and, in particular, for telepsychiatry and e-mental health.

As the interest in telemedicine techniques for delivering health care increases, guidelines describing best practice are likely to become essential in order to provide appropriate and effective health care. Yet do guidelines exist for telepsychiatry and e-mental health? A formal search of the National Library of Medicine PubMed database was conducted to identify articles containing the terms 'telepsychiatry guidelines', 'telemedicine mental health guidelines' or 'ehealth psychiatry guidelines'. The search was repeated using the search engine of the Telemedicine Information Exchange (TIE) database. The PubMed search produced 37 articles and the TIE search identified seven articles. Table 21.1 lists the guidelines identified in the present review. Although every attempt was made to include the major published guidelines on each topic, some medical and professional societies have published guidelines that are available only to their own members. In addition, hospitals and health services may produce in-house guidelines in the form of policies and procedures, but these are rarely published.

The guidelines that were identified were categorized as:

▶ clinical, i.e. relating to a medical subspecialty practised by telemedicine

▶ operational, i.e. relating to the way that telemedicine techniques are used

▶ technical, i.e. relating to the equipment or telecommunication used in telemedicine.

Clinical guidelines

A number of professional bodies and organizations have drawn up guidelines for clinical practice.[6-13] The guidelines proposed by the American Psychiatric Association (APA), the Royal Australian and New Zealand College of Psychiatrists (RANZCP) and the Queensland Telemedicine Network (QTN) focus on videoconferencing techniques (real-time telepsychiatry). The guidelines issued by the International Society for Mental Health Online (ISMHO) and the Psychiatric Society for Informatics (PSI), the Australian Psychological Society (APS), the American Counseling Association (ACA) and the American Medical Informatics Association (AMIA) refer to online services (i.e. using pre-recorded or store and forward techniques).

The telepsychiatry guidelines recommend gaining informed consent from the patient prior to participating in teleconsultations and ensuring that the patient is made aware of the limitations of the techniques for delivering care, as well as the potential benefits. The guidelines concentrate on the *process* of delivering mental health services remotely, rather than on technical requirements. A general rule of thumb, endorsed by the available telepsychiatry guidelines, is that procedures should be followed in the same way as in face-to-face consultations. The responsibilities and roles of the health care staff should be carefully defined prior to the teleconsultations. There should be appropriate contingency plans in the event of equipment failure. The

Table 21.1. Telemedicine guidelines and standards

(a) Predominantly clinical guidelines

Subject	Author	URL	Status
Real-time telepsychiatry	American Psychiatric Association (APA)[6]	http://www.psych.org/pract_of_psych/tp_paper.cfm	Approved by APA Board of Trustees in 1998
Real-time telepsychiatry	Royal Australian and New Zealand College of Psychiatrists (RANZCP)[7]	http://www.ranzcp.org/statements/ps/ps44.htm#fa1	Appendix to Telepsychiatry Position Statement 1999
Real-time telepsychiatry	Queensland Telemedicine Network (QTN)[8]	http://www.health.qld.gov.au/qtn/pdf/mhg4.pdf	Designed for use in Australia, but more generally applicable 1999
Online mental health services	International Society for Mental Health Society Online (ISMHO) and Psychiatric for Informatics (PSI)[9]	http://www.ismho.org/suggestions.html	Officially endorsed by both ISMHO and PSI in 2000
Psychological services on the Internet	Australian Psychological Society (APS)[10]	http://aps.psychsociety.com.au/about/internet.pdf	1999
Internet online counselling	American Counseling Association (ACA)[11]	http://www.counseling.org/gc/cybertx.htm	Approved by ACA Governing Council in 1999
Clinical use of email	American Medical Informatics Association (AMIA)[12]	http://www.amia.org/pubs/other/email_guidelines.html	Endorsed by Board of Directors 1997, currently being updated for 2002

(b) Predominantly operational guidelines

Subject	Author	URL	Status
Doctor–patient communication by email	American Medical Informatics Association (AMIA)[12]	http://www.amia.org/pubs/other/email_guidelines.html	Endorsed by Board of Directors 1997, currently being updated for 2002
Security issues surrounding patient information systems	British Medical Association[14]		Interim guidelines 1996
Code of Conduct for medical and health websites	Health On the Net Foundation[15]	http://www.hon.ch/HONcode/Conduct.html	Published 1997
Principles to guide the development of website health content, online advertising and sponsorship	American Medical Association (AMA)[16]		Published journal article

Table 21.1. – *continued*

(b) Predominantly operational guidelines – *continued*

Subject	Author	URL	Status
Guidelines for online doctor–patient communication and consultation	US medical malpractice insurers and medical societies[17]	http://www.medem.com/corporate/corporate_erisk_guidelines.cfm	Published 2001
Guidelines for disclosure, patient privacy and quality of content issues of websites	Internet Healthcare Coalition (IHC)[18]	http://www.ihealthcoalition.org/ethics/code0524.pdf	Published 2000
Guidelines for the patient	Yellowlees[19]		Informal guidance
Guidelines for health care delivery via video-conferencing	Queensland Telemedicine Network[20]	http://www.health.qld.gov.au/qtn/guidelines.htm	Designed for use in Australia, but more generally applicable. Updated in 1999

(c) Predominantly technical guidelines and standards

Subject	Author	URL	Status
Guidelines and specifications for videoconferencing equipment, cameras and other technology used in real-time telepsychiatry	Office for the Advancement of Telehealth (OAT) the Health Resources and Services Administration (HRSA), and the Department of Defense[23]	http://telehealth.hrsa.gov/pubs/tech/mental.htm	Developed for use in US Federal telemedicine programs, updated in 2001
Technology and performance requirements for real-time telepsychiatry	Royal Australian and New Zealand College of Psychiatrists (RANZCP)[7]	http://ranzcp.org/statements/ps/ps44.htm#a2	Appendix to Telepsychiatry Position Statement 1999
H.320 standard for video-conferencing using ISDN, and the more recent H.323 standard for video-conferencing using IP networks	International Telecommunication Union (ITU)[24]	http://www.itu.int/itudoc/itu-t/rec/h/h320.html	Mature
Industry standard for Digital Imaging and Communications in Medicine (DICOM)	Radiological Society of North America (RSNA) and others[26]	http://www.rsna.org/practice/dicom/index.html	Mature

remote care of serious cases, such as the suicidal or seriously demented patients, is not generally recommended unless no other alternative is available.

Operational guidelines

There are two distinct classes of telemedicine interaction – those that are pre-recorded (sometimes referred to as store and forward or asynchronous) and those that occur in real time (i.e. interactive or synchronous). Pre-recorded telemedicine often depends on the use of email or Internet access to online care. Real-time techniques often employ videoconferencing, although more basic telephone consulting may be employed where appropriate. Both techniques have their own operational guidelines.

Email communication

The American Medical Informatics Association has issued guidelines for the use of doctor–patient email communication.[12] These guidelines apply to situations where the health care provider has assumed responsibility for patient care – that is, a contractual agreement exists between the two parties. The aim of the guidelines is to enhance the interaction between the doctor and patient. The guidelines cover privacy issues, purpose of consultation, acceptable response time and maintenance of appropriate documentation records. Medical emergencies and sensitive health issues are not suitable for email correspondence. The guidelines recommend the use of computer password-protected screen savers and encryption methods to ensure patient privacy.

Many of the guidelines on the use of email advocate a 'prevention is better than cure' philosophy, since establishing clear procedures and policies prior to any online communication will reduce the risks involved. The US Ophthalmic Mutual Insurance Company (OMIC) has developed such protocols for ophthalmologists as well as providing general examples of disclaimer notices.[13] The British Medical Association has also published guidelines on the security issues relating to patient information systems.[14] These are not restricted solely to computerized systems but also include telephone enquiries where personal health information may be disclosed inadvertently.

Internet access

The Health On the Net Foundation (HON) has issued a Code of Conduct for medical and health websites.[15] Any health or medical advice must be provided by appropriately qualified health professionals unless otherwise stated. The website information is intended to support and enhance the existing relationship between the health care provider and patient, rather than replace it. Owners of a website must provide contact information for those seeking further information and must also respect patient confidentiality, as shown in Figure 21.1.

The American Medical Association (AMA) has also developed principles to guide the development of website health content, govern online advertising and sponsorship, and ensure patients' and consumers' rights to privacy and confidentiality.[16]

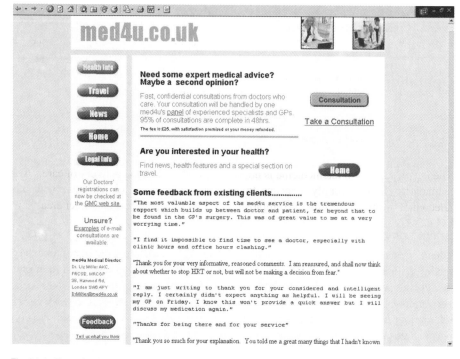

Fig. 21.1. Example of appropriate web page (http://www.med4u.co.uk/).

In the USA, leading medical malpractice insurers and medical societies have developed a comprehensive set of guidelines for online doctor–patient communication.[17] These guidelines recommend that health care providers establish staff policies and procedures regarding online patient interaction and that patient consent must be obtained. Privacy and confidentiality issues are addressed as well as the problems of using third party websites. Disclosure, patient privacy and quality of content issues have also been defined in guidelines formulated by the Internet Healthcare Coalition (IHC).[18]

Informal guidelines for the patient have been suggested by Yellowlees.[19] These include:

► establishing the qualifications, credentials and experience of a potential online health care practitioner

► finding out what clinical and administrative guidelines they follow

► confirming the procedures for consent and confidentiality.

Videoconferencing

Comprehensive guidelines for health care delivery via videoconferencing have been set out by the Queensland Telemedicine Network.[20] Although designed for an

Australian audience, the protocols address issues that are relevant to any user, regardless of country of origin. These range from questioning the need for videoconferencing to the planning and implementation stages. Minimum equipment specifications, proper videoconferencing etiquette and the ideal room set-up are defined. Operational issues such as installation of digital lines, bookings, appropriate documentation and the training needs of users are also addressed.

Technical guidelines

The key to successful telemedicine is not the technology, it is the delivery of care.[21] The technology itself is simply a means to an end. Indeed most of the equipment and telecommunication infrastructure employed in telemedicine are used in other areas such as business and education, and are not unique to health care delivery. Equipment such as personal computers and videoconferencing units have their own technical standards, which are not altered by the fact that they are used to deliver health care. Peripheral equipment such as an electronic stethoscope or a remote blood-pressure-monitoring device in telemedicine should already comply with standards defined for use in conventional health care delivery. The American Telemedicine Association (ATA) Technology Special Interest Group recommends the development of a standard list of specifications and a standard format for reporting the information in sales literature.[22]

The key issue concerning technical telemedicine guidelines is that the technology does not operate in isolation, but as part of a system. Thus guidelines are essential for the entire system rather than for component parts only. A summary of technical guidelines has been formulated in the USA by the Office for the Advancement of Telehealth (OAT), the Health Resources and Services Administration (HRSA) and the Department of Defense. The guidelines, which are intended to ensure the compatibility, interoperability, scalability and reliability of telehealth equipment and systems for use in US Federal telemedicine programs, include a detailed section on mental health.[23]

ITU standards

The main technical standards applicable to telemedicine are those defined by the International Telecommunication Union (ITU) for videoconferencing. The most well known are the H.320 standard for videoconferencing using the ISDN, and the more recent H.323 standard for videoconferencing using IP networks.[24] The Australian Health Minister's Advisory Council (AHMAC) recommended that guidelines are needed for definite categories of technology, such as videoconferencing, telephone advisory services, store and forward data and image transmission, rather than for specific products or vendors.[25]

DICOM standard

The Digital Imaging and Communications in Medicine (DICOM) standard is a widely recognized standard for medical imaging communication. It was originally developed to facilitate transmission and storage of X-ray images, but was subsequently generalized to deal with a wide variety of medical image types. It defines a standard network interface and data model for imaging devices that can facilitate information systems integration. Essentially the DICOM standard enables image acquisition, display of images for reporting and diagnosis, interchange transmission, and an archive medium for long-term storage and compatibility. The key advantage of the DICOM standard is that it allows interoperability between equipment from different manufacturers.[26]

Benefits of implementing telemedicine guidelines

If guidelines in telemedicine are implemented, then a number of benefits can be expected.

Reduced risk of litigation

In general, the purpose of any medical guidelines is to improve the effectiveness and efficiency of clinical practice, provide better clinical outcomes and enhance the reliability of medical services. The introduction of telemedicine techniques does not alter these objectives. From a legal standpoint, adhering to telemedicine guidelines offers a form of immunity to the health care professional, provided that he or she has acted in accordance with a practice accepted as proper by a responsible body of professionals and that reasonable skill and care have been followed.[27] Professional bodies have begun to issue telemedicine guidelines as a result of increasing demands from members. For instance, the College of Physicians and Surgeons of Nova Scotia issued a directive stating that physicians who provide telemedicine services must have the same standards of practice as a physician who sees patients in person.[28]

Standardization of current work practices

Telemedicine affects work practices.[29,30] The use of guidelines in telemedicine encourages standardization of work practices as well as providing evidence of quality assurance. Quality assurance is an area of telemedicine which has been almost entirely neglected to date, and the literature contains few reports.[31] As telemedicine enters the 'mainstream' of routine health care delivery, quality assurance will become essential.

The provision of a minimum acceptable level of care serves to maximize patient outcomes.[25] As with any new clinical intervention, telemedicine interventions should undergo rigorous evaluations before being integrated into mainstream care. Most clinical telemedicine guidelines emphasize the need for periodical review of the existing standards, which ultimately acts as a process for refining the procedures and protocols for health care delivery. Clinical trials and evaluations are needed to assess the most appropriate method of delivering health care remotely and hence provide evidence of best practice and standardization which is essential for clinicians.

Guideline implementation

The fact that relatively few telepsychiatry and e-mental health guidelines exist suggests that there are certain barriers to their development.

Who should formulate telemedicine guidelines?

At present there is no consensus as to who should take the responsibility of formulating telemedicine guidelines. It is accepted that health care professionals should be responsible for clinical standards, and generally the professional bodies such as the appropriate Colleges are responsible for formulating medical standards for each speciality. However the development of telemedicine guidelines does not readily lend itself to this model as telemedicine tends to be multidisciplinary and to involve many areas of expertise. The alternative therefore may be to encourage specific telemedicine organizations such as the ATA or the UK's Telemedicine Forum to assume responsibility for defining telemedicine guidelines. Indeed the World Medical Association (WMA) recommended that national medical associations should develop and implement telemedicine practice guidelines in conjunction with appropriate specialized organizations such as national departments of health.[32]

When should guidelines be updated?

Assuming that telemedicine guidelines have been drawn up, there is a requirement to keep them up to date. As Shekelle et al[33] have pointed out, there are a variety of reasons why a set of guidelines will become outdated. These include:

- changes in evidence on the existing benefits and harms of interventions
- changes in outcomes considered important
- changes in available interventions
- changes in evidence that current practice is optimal
- changes in values placed on outcomes
- changes in resources available for health care.

The most practicable way of assessing whether telemedicine guidelines need updating is to establish a review committee – probably an international expert committee – to review the guidelines regularly, perhaps annually.

Conclusion

Many articles and reports have emphasized the need for developing telepsychiatry and e-mental health guidelines, but few actually exist in practice. This recognized need and the gradual evolution of guidelines reflect the first signs of maturity in this emerging field. Perhaps the dearth of guidelines to date is due to the fact that individual medical and professional groups do not always have the technical expertise or resources to formulate guidelines specific to telemedicine applications. It may be that a collaborative approach is required, involving telemedicine specialists and clinicians from all disciplines involved in the provision of mental health care and from several jurisdictions. Moreover the formulation and implementation of guidelines does not necessarily guarantee improved patient outcomes, and continual monitoring of the effect of guidelines will be required. The process of developing, implementing and evaluating telemedicine guidelines takes time but is essential. The future development of telepsychiatry and e-mental health, including their integration into routine mental health service delivery around the world, will depend on this important work.

References

1 Field MJ, Lohr KN, eds. *Clinical Practice Guidelines: directions for a new program.* Washington DC: National Academy Press, 1990.
2 Woolf SH, Grol R, Hutchinson A, Eccles M, Grimshaw J. Clinical guidelines: potential benefits, limitations, and harms of clinical guidelines. *British Medical Journal* 1999;**318**:527–530.
3 Reed H. Creating a guidelines database. *Health Information on the Internet* 2001;(April):4–5.
4 National Guideline Clearinghouse. Available at http://www.guideline.gov/FRAMESETS/static_ fs.asp?view=about [last checked 20 June 2002].
5 Guidelines in professions allied to medicine (Cochrane Review). Available at http://www.cochrane.org/ cochrane/revabstr/ab000349.htm [last checked 20 June 2002].
6 APA resource document on telepsychiatry via videoconferencing. Available at http://www.psych.org/ pract_of_psych/tp_paper.cfm [last checked 20 June 2002].
7 RANZCP position statement on telepsychiatry. Available at http://www.ranzcp.org/statements/ps/ ps44.htm [last checked 20 June 2002].
8 QTN clinical practice guidelines for using videoconferencing technology in Queensland Mental Health Services. Available at http://www.health.qld.gov.au/qtn/pdf/mhg4.pdf [last checked 20 June 2002].
9 Hsiung RC. Suggested principles of professional ethics for the online provision of mental health services. *Telemedicine Journal and E-health* 2001;**7**:39–45.
10 APS considerations for psychologists providing services on the Internet. Available at http://aps.psychsociety.com.au/about/internet.pdf [last checked 20 June 2002].
11 ACA ethical standards for Internet online counselling. Available at http://www.counseling.org/gc/ cybertx.htm [last checked 20 June 2002].
12 Kane B, Sands DZ. Guidelines for the clinical use of electronic mail with patients. The AMIA Internet Working Group, Task Force on Guidelines for the Use of Clinic–Patient Electronic Mail. *Journal of the American Medical Informatics Association* 1998;**5**:104–111. Reproduced on http://www.amia.org/pubs/ other/email_guidelines.html [last checked 20 June 2002].
13 Protocols for email in the ophthalmic practice. Available at http://www.omic.com/new/digest/10_2/ surfers.cfm [last checked 20 June 2002].
14 Anderson R. Clinical system security: interim guidelines. *British Medical Journal* 1996;**312**:109–111.
15 HON Code of Conduct (HONcode) for medical and health web sites. Available at http://www.hon.ch/ HONcode/Conduct.html [last checked 20 June 2002].
16 Winker MA, Flanagin A, Chi-Lum B, et al. Guidelines for medical and health information sites on the internet: principles governing AMA web sites. *Journal of the American Medical Association* 2000;**283**:1600–1606.
17 Guidelines for online communications and consultations. Available at http://www.medem.com/corporate/ corporate_erisk_guidelines.cfm [last checked 20 June 2002].
18 eHealth Code of Ethics. Available at http://www.ihealthcoalition.org/ethics/code0524.pdf [last checked 20 June 2002].
19 Yellowlees P. *Your Guide to E-Health: third millennium medicine on the Internet.* St Lucia, Qld: University of Queensland Press, 2001.
20 Queensland Telemedicine Network. Implementation of telehealth: guidelines for telehealth development. Available at http://www.health.qld.gov.au/qtn/guidelines.htm [last checked 20 June 2002].
21 Yellowlees P. Successfully developing a telemedicine system. In: Wootton R, Craig J, eds. *Introduction to Telemedicine.* London: Royal Society of Medicine Press, 1999:93–103.

22   ATA Technology Special Interest Group white paper. Available at http://www.americantelemed.org/ICOT/ TechnologySIGRec.htm [last checked 20 June 2002].

23   Telehealth technology guidelines, section on mental health. Available at http://www.hrsa.gov/pubs/ tech/mental.htm [last checked 20 June 2002].

24   International Telecommunication Union: recommendation H.320. Available at http://www.itu.int/itudoc/itu-t/rec/h/h320.html [last checked 25 June 2002].

25   Australian New Zealand Telehealth Committee: report to the Australian Health Ministers' Advisory Council (AHMAC). Available at http://www.telehealth.org.au [last checked 20 June 2002].

26   DICOM: the value and importance of an imaging standard. Available at http://www.rsna.org/practice/ dicom/index.html [last checked 20 June 2002].

27   Stanberry B. Medicolegal aspects of telemedicine. In: Wootton R, Craig J, eds. *Introduction to Telemedicine*. London: Royal Society of Medicine Press, 1999:159–175.

28   Guidelines for the provision of telemedicine services. Available at http://www.cpsns.ns.ca/telemedicine_ guidelines.htm [last checked 20 June 2002].

29   Aas IHM. A qualitative study of the organizational consequences of telemedicine. *Journal of Telemedicine and Telecare* 2001;**7**:18–26.

30   Aas IHM. Changes in the job situation due to telemedicine. *Journal of Telemedicine and Telecare* 2002;**8**:41–47.

31   Wootton R, McNichol B, Byrnes T, et al. Quality assurance in minor injuries telemedicine. *Journal of Telemedicine and Telecare* 2000;**6**(suppl 1):212.

32   World Medical Association statement on accountability, responsibilities and ethical guidelines in the practice of telemedicine. Available at http://www.wma.net/e/policy/17-36_e.html [last checked 20 June 2002].

33   Shekelle P, Eccles MP, Grimshaw JM, Woolf SH. When should clinical guidelines be updated? *British Medical Journal* 2001;**323**:155–157.

22

E-mental Health in the Future

Peter Yellowlees

Introduction

Mental health care will undoubtedly change over the next 20 or 30 years.[1] How will it be delivered in future? It is dangerous to predict technological innovation since it is well known that past e-health or telemedicine systems have suffered from a wide range of difficulties and have not fulfilled the promise that has so often been suggested. The reasons for this[2,3] fall into three main categories:

1. *Human issues*, which include clinicians' concerns about privacy, their own technophobia and lack of training, a lack of leadership in pilot projects, and the inability to diffuse knowledge learnt into the general health care system.

2. *Technological issues*, which include the lack of user-friendly information systems and interfaces, a lack of standards, the inability to move clinical systems close to where doctors work (and especially to their desktops) and the lack of satisfactory bandwidth.

3. *Business issues*, which include the high expense of hardware and software, an inability to remunerate physicians for online work and a general lack of a viable business model supporting e-health activity.

Whatever the future holds, it is clear that mental health care will be an important part of e-health generally.

E-health models of care

At a global level the health care system is moving away from episodic care to concentrating on continuity of care, especially for patients with chronic disease[4,5] who will cause the greatest disease burden in the future. There is a gradual move in many countries away from a focus on the service provider to a focus on the informed patient, and from an individual approach to treatment to a team approach. Increasingly there is emphasis less on the treatment of illness, and more on the need for wellness promotion and illness prevention. This, of course, parallels the shift from traditional care to community care. This is the model of the 'information age care' described by Ferguson.[6]

To move to this future model of health care requires a strengthening of the availability and use of information to facilitate changes in mental health service delivery. The requisite technologies should have four main objectives:

1. to empower consumers and clinicians in day-to-day health care delivery by improving access to evidence-based information at the point of care

2. to facilitate the delivery of a wider range of services to primary and community care

3. to provide accurate data to support research, and clinical policy and governance arrangements

4. to ensure that there is a sustainable, secure, reliable electronic environment, which of course must be underpinned by strong, policy-driven privacy protection.

A 1997 symposium that discussed the future of health care systems concluded that 'no health care system is stable. Changes being driven by growth of the middle-class, the globalization of economies, information technology and consumerism will transform health care worldwide.'[7] There are seven major driving factors that will allow rapid maturation of e-health delivery nationally and internationally in the mental health field:

1. *Economic* – E-health should reduce the fragmentation of our present health system which blocks reform and investment.

2. *Safety and quality* – Improved information access should reduce risk factors and lead to an increased demand for evidence-based information.

3. *Demographics* – The ability to manage chronic illnesses, combined with the increased morbidity towards the end of life, will generate a need not only for the better integration of health services but also for greater health care provision.

4. *Service delivery* – The increasing emphasis on prevention will require more screening processes, registers, monitoring and early intervention programmes for what are preventable illnesses.

5. *Consumer expectations* – As populations become better educated and have more available health information so they will demand more involvement in their health care, and become less tolerant of inequities in health outcomes.

6. *Technology* – New health technologies are often introduced with relatively little monitoring, tracking or quality assurance and IT should assist in these areas.

7. *Information needs* – The predicted changes in service delivery will increase the need for better information particularly in terms of patients' histories, decision support, service options and scheduling, all at the point of care and in any clinical setting.

All of these barriers to e-health adoption are gradually being overcome. Prices continue to fall, technology has become more user friendly, especially software, and doctors themselves have gradually started to become convinced of the usefulness of e-health programmes. The single most important change, however, is the increasing availability of broadband telecommunications which allows the development of new applications, particularly at the doctor's desk. This allows videoconferencing to be combined with distributed electronic health records, allowing psychiatric consultations anywhere, anytime (Fig. 22.1).

When we consider, in addition to broadband access, other expected technological developments, then it is obvious that there will be major changes in future health environments. Futurists such as Satava and Jones[8] suggest that extraordinary health scenarios may result, including complete body scans leading to the immediate creation of whole-body 3D radiological and biochemical records as one walks through a scanning device at the door of a hospital emergency department. Other seemingly bizarre predictions include the ability to continuously monitor individual health indices with the assistance of nanotechnology – microinstrumentation which records from inside the body. All of these scenarios are being examined, some of them by NASA as byproducts of the space programme.[9–11]

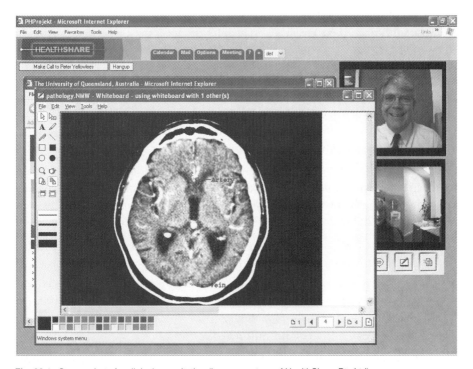

Fig. 22.1. Screen shot of a clinical consultation (image courtesy of HealthShare Pty Ltd).

Networks of the future

Whatever technological changes occur, the major challenge will be to make them available at the point of care, with the patient. Here is where the use of broadband networks is crucial. Perhaps the easiest way of describing the importance of these future health networks is to use the metaphor of the car and the road transport system.

The car is the patient

The car, when purchased, is in perfect condition. It is well known that with regular preventative maintenance, appropriate insurance policies and good documentation the car will last longer, have better resale value, breakdown less often and need fewer replacement parts. This is an accepted fact. Humans should be the same, but are not treated in the same way under our 'health system' that mainly exists to provide care when people have already become sick. In other words it is an 'illness system', rather than a 'health system'. Perhaps humans would be fitter, live longer, have fewer medical crises, complications and hospitalizations if they took the same approach as we do for cars. This involves us in having regular health checks and screening examinations for illnesses such as breast or bowel cancer. It also involves us in having longitudinal records, which we own ourselves, which document our health indices. The latter include everything from our height and weight at various different times, our immunizations and the records of other screening tests and the treatment we have had for our illnesses. Equally these records should be able to receive health monitoring information; further, if we are being treated, for instance, for diabetes, we should be able to keep a regular record of all our blood sugar data, and receive automatic reminders of when the next tests or examinations are due. There is substantial public health evidence that preventative mental health programmes such as this deliver major long-term benefits to humans in the same way that cars receive benefits through preventative car maintenance.

The roads of the health information highway

There are only really two types of roads, major highways and side roads, which deliver people to their homes and cars to their garages. In the IT environment, the Internet, or virtual health network, will be the highway of the future. This superhighway will be extremely fast and will be owned, as are our roads, not only by the government, but also by major corporations or even community organizations, perhaps with a series of different building and leasing arrangements. Undoubtedly the traditional telecommunications providers will be the primary owners, but there will be significant work for those who build and maintain such networks – the equivalent of the road maintenance gangs of today.

International connectivity and cultural exchange

Roads of course exist in all countries of the world. Cars need to vary depending on whether they require left- or right-hand drive and in accordance with different petrol combustion rules, although the underlying model remains fairly similar. Like cars, people are similar, yet have different cultural, religious and philosophical differences, and consequently need their health care delivered in different ways, perhaps through different languages in different countries and environments. The global health superhighway needs to take account of these human differences. Ultimately, however, the move to the global health superhighway should lead to better human communication and understanding, and more acceptance that differences between humans, as in car models, is appropriate and reasonable. This can only have a positive effect on the mental health of the nations of the world.

What, then, will be the technologies that might be used to provide mental health care in future and what will exist on these health superhighways?

Virtual reality and 3D modelling

Virtual reality allows individuals to interact in a different way from what was possible in the past with computers.[12] There have been many definitions but in essence virtual reality is a set of computer technologies which, when combined, provide an interface to a world that in itself is computer generated. The interface has to be convincing enough that the user believes that he or she is actually in such a computer-generated world, and allows users to navigate and interact within that environment in real time. Virtual reality has been used since the early 1990s in a number of centres around the world.[13,14]

Patients have been introduced to virtual reality environments for assessment, therapy and rehabilitation, and their introduction raises important ethical and safety issues. As these environments will be used increasingly in future, these ethical and safety issues will become increasingly important. Special precautions will need to be undertaken to ensure the safety and effectiveness of virtual reality applications, especially when used with patients with, for example, post-traumatic stress disorders or psychoses, who may well be quite vulnerable to developing adverse consequences as a result of a virtual reality exposure. The most successful areas of virtual reality application in mental health at present have been for the treatment of specific phobias, such as fear of flying, a fear of heights, a fear of driving, a fear of public speaking or of spiders, as well as for neuropsychological evaluation and testing.[15] There are at least 15 academic centres around the world addressing these main areas and several hundred publications have emerged. It has been noted[11] that 'earlier results seem to indicate that virtual environments are not only effective but have multiple advantages over conventional therapies in the treatment of specific phobias'. Before a wider acceptance of this new technology occurs however it is crucial that clinical trials and comparisons of outcomes are published and evaluated. It has even been suggested that there are advantages in performing neuropsychological evaluation and testing tasks in virtual environments.

A wide range of 3-D modelling technology is available, ranging from relatively inexpensive helmets, worn by the individual user and which display 3D video, up to room-sized systems for groups. These latter systems are now available in about a hundred sites around the world. Figure 22.2. shows two research workers standing beside a 3D representation of the virtual human in the Visualization Centre at the University of Queensland.

In psychiatry the headset systems are typically used for treating patients with phobias, such as fear of heights, spiders or flying, or for assisting people to cope with anxiety disorders such as post-traumatic stress disorder.[16-20] In these settings patients can be exposed to their fearful situation and treated with cognitive behavioural programmes so that their anxiety reduces. In the future these types of treatment programmes may be available at their primary care practitioner's office by looking at a computer screen, or perhaps by putting on a headset.

A recent project in the larger visualization environment at the University of Queensland, has started to model in 3D the experience of psychosis.[21] Psychosis is a mental disorder affecting 1–2% of the population at some point in their lives and symptoms of psychosis include delusions, hallucinations and thought disorder. Most people with psychotic systems 'hear' voices and a large proportion also 'see' visual illusions. At present patients have to describe their symptoms to their therapists – there is no way for the therapist to share the experiences or to evaluate them objectively. As

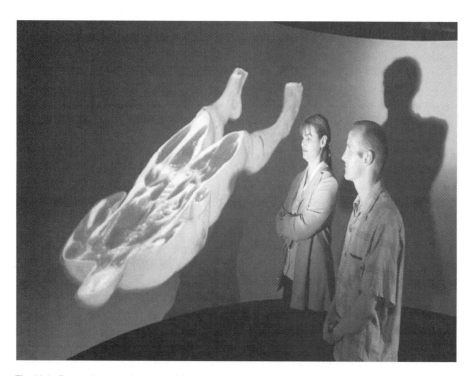

Fig. 22.2. Researchers and the virtual human at the University of Queensland Visualization Centre.

a consequence patients often feel that their therapists cannot really understand them, and the therapists themselves find it hard to understand the exact nature of psychosis as they have no personal experience of it. The project at the University of Queensland aims to model the experience of psychosis in a 3D laboratory. Patients are interviewed by investigators and the interviews are recorded. The transcribed descriptions of auditory and visual hallucinations are then modelled so that the experiences identified by the patients can be artificially re-created. The modelling is an iterative process because it depends on the ability of the patient to describe their symptoms in detail, and for these descriptions to be accurately understood and represented by the clinicians and IT developers. Early experience suggests that re-creation of these environments is possible, although difficult, and the group is looking at improving its methodology and attempting to develop software that will allow rapid production of the simulated psychosis environments.

Apart from the obvious potential teaching value of these environments, and the possible development of what will be effectively a perceptual symptom library, it is hoped that these environments will be useful for diagnostic purposes, and may even be ultimately used as repeatable 'trigger' allowing for neurophysiological examinations of the central nervous system, using, for instance PET scans.

Another interesting use of virtual reality involves NASA.[9-11] The NASA group has always seen telemedicine as important in ensuring that astronauts in space have medical support on their missions. Much work has been done on 'high bandwidth virtual collaboratories' that can assist health care delivery through what is essentially a virtual clinic. The goals of this clinic are to bring the clinic to the patient, no matter how remote the patient is, to provide administrative support for special care or surgery when necessary using virtual environment technology, and to advise about the transport of the patient to an appropriate health service if local treatment cannot be delivered. The NASA approach, although focused on space, has significant earth-based implications. These types of approaches are likely to be used in future, not just in extreme situations such as in space, but linking multidisciplinary teams of experts from different geographical regions so as to provide expert advice on individual patients. Of course this happens already with multidisciplinary clinics for the management of problems such as pain, but virtual clinics will be much easier to organize in future.

Person tracking

A global positioning system (GPS) is a navigation device that provides a very accurate position; miniaturization means that GPS chips can now be embedded in certain makes of watch. There are other location methods based on the use of mobile phones. One can imagine a time when patients with dementia or other forms of cognitive impairment, or those who are deemed to be dangerous to society, are tracked using such technologies. Much more likely though is the use of tracking systems as a routine security device for health professionals who have to make home visits, particularly in dangerous areas or isolated places. For some health workers this may be an unwelcome prospect, because their supervisors will be able to see exactly where they are at any moment. Getting lost, or found, will never be the same again, but these particular mental health workers should certainly be safer.

Wireless computing

The biggest Internet service provider in Japan is the DoCoMo Wireless Company, which has achieved this position in a few months, as a whole generation of youth have taken to the mobile Internet. Wireless access is likely to have a massive influence in the health arena. There are three types of wireless systems:

The mobile Internet using mobile phone networks

The ability to access the Internet without wires permits the provision of information to anyone, anywhere. Doctors will be able to download patient data while they carry out home visits, free of the need to keep paper records, and with the facility for constantly updating themselves about new results. At the same time they will be able to access information to improve their decision-making, as well as to use decision support tools directly from their mobile phones. Video mobile phones are already being trialled and video consultations, by mobile hand-held devices, are not far away. In India 'simputers', effectively wireless versions of hand-held personal digital assistants (PDAs), are becoming popular. These simputers are loaded with translation data to voice systems so that English text downloaded wirelessly to the simputers can be listened to in Hindi by the one third of the Indian population who are illiterate. This suddenly gives access to the Internet to people who are illiterate. Such developments represent an extraordinary potential force to reduce the adverse effects of the digital divide and to provide information about mental health and general wellness to populations that could not previously receive such information.

Wireless local area network

In a wireless LAN your computer is connected to a radio base station, in the same way that a cordless telephone is connected to its base station. Confidential data can be downloaded, fully encrypted, or such systems can be used for audio or video transmissions between professionals. This is effectively a wireless virtual private network. For mental health professionals, who make frequent home visits to patients, this will be an important step forward, as it will allow them continuous access to patient files and other data, and at the same time increase their personal security in what can sometimes be potentially dangerous situations.

Personal area wireless connections

These types of systems use technologies such as Blue Tooth devices to exchange information. The principal uses will be in physiological monitoring. There are major technological challenges in this area, where, although the chips can be made very small, this is much harder to do with batteries. Such devices will ultimately be miniaturized and attached to people's bodies to record ECG, continuous blood pressures and a variety of other monitoring data, and then send all this data automatically to a base station as people go about their daily activities. Undoubtedly in the future high dependency units in hospitals will have most of their monitoring of the patients performed wirelessly, and the same will happen in the area of home care, particularly for the chronically ill and disabled, who will be able to wear cardiac monitors that transmit wirelessly and faultlessly in the comfort of their own homes. This will be important in mental health as many patients who have serious psychiatric disorders also suffer from medical conditions, and it will be of particular value in managing the frail elderly who will increasingly be maintained in their own homes, rather than in nursing homes.

Grid computing

The grid is a network of computers which is accessible from a single originating computer.[22] Grid technologies can therefore be used for solving compute- and data-intensive tasks such as molecular modelling for drug design.[23] Grid computing will allow a doctor to search for data on a single patient across many hundreds of computers or data systems simultaneously, and then to combine all of the data found on that individual in one place. This is the era of what is termed 'distributed computing' where super computers can be linked to increase their power and data accessibility. In the field of health, this will allow us to create individual electronic health records almost instantaneously. Another advantage of distributed computing is that one needs very little computing power to access the grid, and this means that, in third world countries, it should be possible to access extraordinary levels of computing power with a simple PDA. This will allow mental health staff access to parts of the world where there are at present few, if any, effective treatments available.

Biometrics

Security and privacy issues are major problems in any form of e-mental health care. Biometrics will radically change the security issues surrounding health data. This will be particularly important in forensic psychiatry. It is already possible to buy highly accurate retinal scanning cameras, which will of course be increasingly developed to work in combination with ordinary video cameras. This will mean that when you sit at your computer in the future, you will have a retinal scan, and be properly authenticated, every time you commence such a session, thereby guaranteeing the security of your access to patient data. There are many other possible identifiers in biometrics including your whole face, your fingerprints, your handwriting and your voice; some systems are combinations of several of the above. Alternatives, of course, are to have fingerprints scanned digitally on to smart cards which will be read by readers linked to the Internet. Such readers are already very cheap, and one hardware manufacturer has already built a smart card slot and fingerprint reader into one of its laptop computers.

The ability for accurate authentication of individuals on the Internet will substantially increase its business use. For instance it is known that 80% of Internet users browse commercial Internet websites where there are products for sale, yet only 4% are prepared to actually buy on the Internet. This will change significantly when authenticated security systems are available, and should lead to particularly significant changes in the health care area where, as health is already acknowledged as the largest industry in the world, there is huge potential for commercial transactions to occur online. The ability to revolutionize ordering systems and essentially start managing large-scale e-health programmes, integrated into normal face-to-face care, with the assistance of accurate authentication should lead to much greater, and more confident, take-up of these systems.

Digital facial analysis

A number of attempts have been made to automate the clinical skill involved in identifying depression, a disorder characterized by a slowing and paucity of movements. In recent times I have worked with the Australian Commonwealth Scientific and Industrial Research Organization to use signal-processing technologies to assist in identifying image and facial recognition patterns. This work has led to a possible computerized screening test for depression with initial results comparing video images from depressed and non-depressed subjects demonstrating that the technology has excellent potential to be an effective tool. It may be possible to develop a product as a screening tool that would consist of software on a computer analysing images from a digital video camera. Patients would then sit down in front of a video camera and computer which would read a series of questions to them to which they would respond. Analyses would be made of the responses to the structured depression screening questions, and also of their facial movements, and the end result would be an assessment as to whether the patients were definitely depressed, possibly depressed or not depressed. This type of technology would be able to monitor a patient's progression under drug therapy. It is hoped to develop a commercially viable product, which would ultimately be available on doctors' desktops, or even perhaps accessed simply through the Internet by patients themselves.

Autonomic computing

Autonomic computing is the area of artificial intelligence combined with neurophysiological monitoring, where computers may eventually perform many of the skills that doctors nowadays acquire through years of training and experience. Early research in a number of centres, mainly in the USA, has tried to demonstrate that moods can be monitored electrically. It is hoped that this type of work will eventually lead to the development of 'mood clothes' where one might have one's level of, for instance, depression, measured via a monitoring shirt worn over a period of time. At the moment this work is at a very early stage but it is an example of the possible diagnostic tools that may be available in future.

Global clinicians of the future

It seems inevitable that we will move to global health care systems with clinicians and patients interacting in electronically distributed environments around the world, supported by broadband technologies, either wired or wireless. These global delivery environments, on the doctor's desktop, or in the patient's home, will incorporate a variety of features including video technology, to allow video consultations in real time or video email for store and forward interactions, as well as electronic consumer-owned, or provider-shared, voice-driven health records. On the clinician's desktop there will be appropriate practice management and communications software to allow him or her to link seamlessly, in a peer-to-peer relationship, with colleagues. This same desktop will have a very strong educational focus so that health care professionals will be able to receive their continuing health education, for professional credits and re-accreditation needs, via their desktop. They will get this either by taking part in interactive videoconferences given by experts in their field, and relayed to potentially many thousands of different sites, as well as in a large number of flexible, work-based teaching environments, which will allow interactive quizzes to be performed, and marked, as well as recorded for long-term monitoring, simultaneously.

The roles of psychiatrists will change, and specialists will increasingly focus on the teaching and supervision of other health professionals and of groups of consumers. Some specialists, who are particularly good teachers, will probably migrate into the role of 'world authority' in certain areas. This is already happening in commercial university programmes where some individual professors, mainly in areas such as business and economics, and from universities like Yale and Harvard, have already become educational 'superstars'. Students will now enrol as much to hear their lectures, as to take a particular course, and teachers will increasingly be employed to headline particular teaching programmes, which will draw in students, in the same way that sports teams buy particular individuals with special talents. Mental health teaching and learning programmes will as a consequence become more flexible, and will be available ubiquitously.

A future mental health system has to meet the challenges contained in the recent report from the Committee of Quality Health Care in America published by the Institute of Medicine.[11] This influential report notes that 'information technology must play a central role in the redesign of the health care system' and suggests that the USA needs a renewed national commitment to build an information infrastructure to support health care delivery, which 'should lead to the elimination of most hand written clinical data by the end of the decade'.

With the introduction of clinical information and communication systems there is the opportunity to implement this recommendation at a global level, over time. There are a number of exciting technologies that are either becoming available now, or are on the fairly near horizon, and they will without doubt radically change the way that we provide mental health services during the next century.

References

1   Yellowlees P. *Your Guide to E-Health – third millennium medicine on the Internet.* Brisbane: University of Queensland Press, 2001.
2   Treister NW. Marketing and the medical specialist in the managed care environment. *Physician Executive* 1997;**23**:14–19.
3   Yellowlees P. Successful development of telemedicine systems – seven core principles. *Journal of Telemedicine and Telecare* 1997;**3**:215–222.
4   Yack D. Chronic disease and disability of the underprivileged: tackling challenges. *Business Briefing: Global Health Care* 2000;(October):45–49.
5   Murray CJ, Lopez A. On the comparable quantification of health risks: lessons from the Global Burden of Disease Study. *Epidemiology* 1999;**10**:594–605.
6   Ferguson T. From industrial-age medicine to information-age health care. In: Rheingold H, ed. *The Millennium Whole Earth Catalog.* San Francisco, CA: Harper, 1994:170.
7   Smith R. The future of healthcare systems. *British Medical Journal* 1997;**314**:1495–1496.
8   Satava RM, Jones SB. Virtual reality and telemedicine: exploring advanced concepts. *Telemedicine Journal* 1996;**2**:195–200.
9   Ross MD. Medicine in long duration space exploration: the role of virtual reality and broad bandwidth telecommunications networks. *Acta Astronautica* 2001;**49**:441–445.
10 Ross MD, Twombly IA, Bruyns C, Cheng R, Senger S. Telecommunications for health care over distance: the Virtual Collaborative Clinic. *Studies in Health Technology and Informatics* 2000;**70**:286–291.
11 Ross MD, Twombly IA, Bruyns C, Cheng R, Sengers S. *The Institute of Medicine. 2001. Crossing the quality chasm. A new health system for the twentyfirst century.* Albuquerque: University of New Mexico Health Sciences Center, 2002.
12 Renaud P, Singer G, Proulx R. Head-tracking fractal dynamics in visually pursuing virtual objects. In: Sulis W, Trofimova I, eds. *Nonlinear Dynamics in Life and Social Sciences.* Moscow: Advanced Studies Institute of the North Atlantic Treaty Organization, 2000:333–346.
13 Riva G, Wiederhold BK, Molinari E (eds). *Virtual Environments in Clinical Psychology and Neuroscience.* Amsterdam: IOS Press, 1998.
14 Weiss AE. *Virtual Reality: a door to cyberspace.* New York: Twenty-First Century Books, 1996.
15 Westwood JD, Hoffman HM, Mogel GT, Robb RA, Stredney D. *Medicine Meets Virtual Reality 2000.* Amsterdam: IOS Press, 2000.
16 Vince J. *Virtual Reality Systems.* Wokingham, UK: Addison-Wesley, 1995.
17 Bornas X, Fullana MA, Tortella-Feliu M, Llabrés J, García de la Banda G. Computer-assisted therapy in the treatment of flight phobia: a case report. *Cognitive and Behavioral Practice* 2001;**8**:234–240.
18 Rothbaum BO, Hodges L, Anderson PL, Price L, Smith S. Twelve-month follow-up of virtual reality and standard exposure therapies for the fear of flying. *Journal of Consulting and Clinical Psychology* 2002;**70**:428–432.
19 Heading K, Kirkby KC, Martin F, Daniels BA, Gilroy LJ. Controlled comparison of single-session treatments for spider phobia: live graded exposure alone versus computer-aided vicarious exposure. *Behaviour Change* 2001;**18**:103–113.
20 Rothbaum BO, Hodges LF, Ready D, Graap K, Alarcon RD. Virtual reality exposure therapy for Vietnam veterans with posttraumatic stress disorder. *Journal of Clinical Psychiatry* 2001;**62**:617–622.
21 Centre of Online Health, University of Queensland. Available at http://www.coh.uq.edu.au [last checked 6 September 2002].
22 Grid Computing Info Centre. Available at http://www.gridcomputing.com/ [last checked 9 September 2002].
23 Buyya R. The virtual laboratory project. *IEEE Distributed Systems Online* 2001;**2**:(5).

23

The Internet, Social Isolation and Mental Health – future perspectives

Deede Gammon, Gunnvald B. Svendsen, Martin A. Jenssen and Svein Bergvik

Introduction

Once upon a time, physical isolation was tantamount to social isolation. However, technology, such as the postal service, the telephone system or the Internet, has changed that. A prima facie, but perhaps naïve, assumption would be that all new communication technologies reduce social isolation.

In this chapter, we attempt to predict the effects of the Internet on social isolation and mental health. Our approach shares McKenna and Bargh's[1] well-argued view: that the Internet does not, by itself, have the ability to determine isolation/sadness, or inclusion/happiness. Certainly some people will use the Internet to isolate themselves, to nurture subversive environments online and to become crazier. However, some people will use the Internet to promote physical and mental health both for themselves and others. Like earlier technologies, the Internet will be what people make of it.

We have chosen to focus on future opportunities for exploiting technology to reduce social isolation and improve mental health. We present two stories that show these opportunities from two angles: (i) the Internet as a tool in mental health care; and (ii) the Internet as a medium for socializing in daily life. By speculating about the future, perhaps we can gain a better idea of what we can do today in order to maximize the potentials – and limit the pitfalls – of the future.

Social isolation and mental health

Social isolation may be conceptualized along different dimensions:[2] being alone (i.e. the amount of time spent alone), living alone, level of contact with other people and loneliness (i.e. subjective feelings about the level of interaction with others). Social isolation can also be defined as the opposite of social support, which is the availability of significant others to whom one interrelates with, trusts and can turn to in times of crisis,[2] as well as the presence of social nurturing, alliance, guidance and feelings of worth and intimacy.[3]

It is generally agreed that relationships characterized by social support are beneficial to physical and mental health. Such relationships have been found to moderate the effect of stress and burnout,[4,5] reduce grieving periods,[6] increase exercise behaviour,[7] increase health-related quality of life[8] and reduce depression and anxiety.[9,10] While subjects from a normal population have 20–30 persons in their social network, the corresponding numbers for non-psychotic psychiatric patients are 10–12 and four to five for psychotic patients.[11]

However, we must be cautious in assuming that more social support, and larger social networks, are always better. The number of persons in a social network may be of less importance than having at least one person with whom one can share one's innermost intimate feelings and thoughts. Along this line, Schwarzer and Leppin[12] found in their meta-analysis little relation ($\bar{r} = -0.10$) between objective measures social networks (e.g. size) and depression, although the relation between perceived social support and depression was stronger ($\bar{r} = -0.30$). Furthermore, intensely intimate or protective behaviour may in some cases be perceived as a threat to the need for control and freedom, and thus lead to negative outcomes, including psychiatric symptoms.[13,14] A dense family-centred network can have an inhibitory effect on varied social involvement, and some individuals can benefit from having several social arenas which are not closely connected to each other.[15]

The subjective dimension of social isolation underlines the difficulty of measuring the concept because different people may have different needs for support and social networks.

The Internet and social isolation

Concerns about social isolation arose long before the Internet. Increased mobility, urbanization, entertainment media and decomposition of family ties all contribute to our unease about what our social lives will look like in the future. The emergence of the Internet into the social scene has given a new boost to old concerns. For example, Kraut's[16] highly publicized study which resulted in international media headlines such as 'Internet causes loneliness and depression', in fact showed an average (although not significant) reduction in reported depression and an increase in size of distant social networks among the ($n = 169$) subjects. The study found a small positive correlation ($r = 0.15$) between the amount of time online and depression, but a 3-year follow-up study also revealed that the negative effects on depression in the high-frequency Internet users had dissipated[17] (although more so for extraverts than introverts). While the first study has been dismissed by some[1] due to serious weaknesses (e.g. lack of randomization and a control group), it demonstrates the challenges that the Internet poses to traditional conceptions of, and research on, social networks and isolation.

In contrast to concerns about the isolating effects of the Internet, an increasing number of studies demonstrate how it can enhance social inclusion. McKenna and Bargh[1] reviewed many of these and offered a nice summary analysis of the characteristics of the Internet and their implications for self and identity, social interaction and relationships: one's option of being anonymous, the greatly reduced importance of physical appearance and physical distance as 'gating features' to relationship building, and one's greater control over the time and pace of interactions.

These unique characteristics of the Internet are used to explain why 75% of those who responded to a questionnaire about their use of online mental health discussion groups in Norway ($n = 492$) find it easier to discuss personal problems online than face to face.[18] Here, anonymous access to information and peer support was reported to be crucial for many. Similar findings have been reported for persons with serious mental disorders, all with social anxiety, and whose lives were characterized by extreme social isolation along with periodic hospitalization.[19] In this small study ($n = 8$), the five people who used the Internet socially found that it represented a lifeline into normal (non-psychiatric) society and the experience that other 'normal' people found them to be interesting, valuable friends despite their 'craziness'. They reported that access to this type of support helped them to dissipate crises and in some cases prevented hospitalization. The reduction in social cues relative to face-to-face interaction allows access to social environments with less social anxiety, and relieves one from having to think about one's non-verbal behaviour (e.g. blushing, shaking, sweating). Similarly, the Internet also facilitates communication between people by overriding differences that might alienate them in traditional face-to-face settings (e.g. race, social status and gender).

These perspectives show how the social use of the Internet by isolated persons may compensate for the lack of off-line support. This coincides with what Kraut et al[17] have called a 'social compensation' model, which opposes 'the rich get richer' model supported by their own studies. Further research should look into the potential of the Internet for enhancing mental health interventions which aim to develop social skills and self-confidence among those who suffer from social anxiety. The integration of Internet-based methods and activities in treatment and rehabilitation will of course need to build on scientific evidence and accepted standards for clinical treatment. As the field of human–computer interaction research has long taught us, different media are suited for different needs. We see exciting potentials as knowledge from this field merges with and enhances the knowledge and future research in mental health.

Future story 1

The 40 to 60 year olds represent a group underserved by health care despite the risk for suicide and psychosomatic disorders. Adolescents resemble this group in the sense that they often find it difficult to acknowledge and address psychosocial issues before they become serious problems.[20] Even if people do go to the doctor, they may not be able to 'cut to the core', either because they are not at ease putting feelings into words face to face, or they don't feel that their doctor understands them, see the story in Box 23.1. As indicated earlier, electronic-based interaction can lower the threshold for discussing personal problems, and we also know that the public welcomes the opportunity to send email to doctors.[21]

Bill would never have had access to a peer support group without the Internet – whether it was for grief, alcoholism or whatever else. Had there been enough divorcees for a group in his local community, they'd either be related, earlier classmates, neighbours, colleagues or 'someone who knows someone'. Anonymity can be a crucial

---

Box 23.1. Future story 1: The psychosocial prescription

Bill knew he was losing it, but doctors are for wimps. Besides, the new general practitioner (GP) in his north Norwegian village was young and pretty. What could he say? That he cries himself to sleep at night because his wife left him, that his heart races when he meets strangers and that he hates his life? Forget it!

'You look like sh**' remarks Jim, another fisherman. Jim points at the wharf's 'Firstaid tele-kit', indicating that Bill should hook up. But Bill had already done that and it had confirmed what he already knew; that nothing was wrong with him physically. Jim grabs Bill's personal digital assistant (PDA) for a minute, and as he gives it back says, 'Get a grip'. On the screen was a site called 'Your GPs waiting room' and Jim had highlighted a link called 'Let's figure it out'. That evening, Bill started thinking that maybe it would be easier to interact with his GP without her staring at his ugly, miserable self. He ended up asking the system to generate his password for the encrypted service and then interacted with a series of psychosocial instruments (Fig. 23.1). These provided profiles of Bill's needs and resources. 'Maybe it's not so stupid to discuss some of this stuff, after all', thought Bill, and with a 'What-the-hell', pressed SEND.

The next day, he found that Mary, his GP, had booked him an online appointment. 'Thank God I didn't invest in the video mode for my PDA', he thought. Mary opened by praising Bill for not waiting longer to get in touch, and showed him how the system-generated prescription list worked. Bill was relieved that she didn't see the need for pills and therapy 'yet', but was embarrassed when Mary asked why the system would recommend the 'Tropical birds for nerds' site. Birds had been an interest in his youth, but some of his schoolmates had made fun of him, and his wife couldn't tolerate the noise and mess. Mary said she wanted him to try all the sites at least once, as well as complete the site-related 'prescription evaluation diary' (PED). The PED would help him reflect on why he did or didn't like the suggested sites, and provide a better basis for their next consultation.

After several evenings lurking on the various sites, Bill wondered why he hadn't checked them out earlier. 'Divorcees help divorcees' had always been available, but he doubted he would have had the nerve had Mary not given him the push. He slowly but surely started interacting with people who knew just what he was going through, and who gave him invaluable advice and support. One even stayed all night with him during his worse crisis. He now daily visits three to five close friends, among them a fisherman from Alaska who is *proud* of his interest in tropical birds.

Like the majority of those who meet others on the net, Bill was making plans to meet his new friends in real life. Mary is now helping him apply for the special travel rates called 'A friend a day keeps the doctor away', which are offered by his health insurance company.

---

access criterion. As far as finding friends who share common experiences and interests (e.g. fishermen in arctic regions who love tropical birds), the Internet is ingenious.

Mary's role as *general* practitioner may be the most remarkable in this story. She perceives her role as Bill's consultant in finding and using his own resources, and to connect him to the resources of others. Here, the field of medicine converges with the mass of knowledge within the fields of community and health psychology into Mary's role as 'gatekeeper' to specialized health services and insurance coverage. Bill didn't need pills or psychotherapy – yet. He needed a life, and Mary had the tools (thanks to technology) and the legitimacy to help him help himself. We believe consumer pressure will contribute to this type of role among doctors, more or less independently of technology.[22]

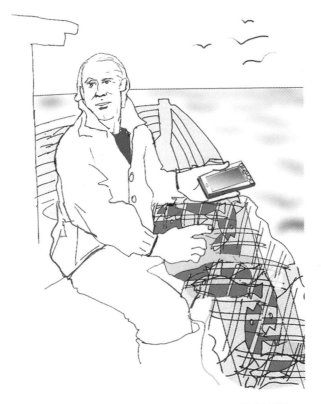

Fig. 23.1. Bill, consulting his primary physician. (Copyright 2002 Molly van Weij, NST.)

Obviously, many things need to happen to make this story come true. We need evidence to quality assure the psychosocial diagnostic and treatment tools Mary used (which also included prescriptions for virtual reality therapy, psycho-educational classes, etc.). Continued testing and deployment of public key encryption and trusted third party (TTP) mechanisms for data security, as well as legal and ethical issues, are essential. Finally, we need continued debate concerning our prevailing tendency to medicalize unhappiness, as well as acknowledgement by insurance companies that prevention pays.

Future story 2

The story in Box 23.2. – possibly a nightmare for some (e.g. son and daughter-in-laws) – shows how technology can enable daily life socializing for physically isolated individuals (and kids who love their grandparents). Up to now, the developments in 'smart house' and home care technology have focused upon physical monitoring devices and access to health care providers. In our efforts to enable the elderly to live at home as long as they wish, attention to their psychosocial needs to prevent

---

Box 23.2. Visiting grandma

'Wake up, grandma! You've got to see this, and besides, you're snoring too loud!' Grandma rolls over and tries to find her glasses. Her wall screen has erupted with repeat after repeat of Johnny's goal from the soccer match at school. 'Wow! That's my boy' she mutters as she tries to gain consciousness. 'What time is it?' she asks as she fumbles for her watch. '1 p.m. our time and 4 a.m. your time, grandma. You can never get it right' chides Johnny. Grandma groans as she recalls her late night bridge game. While receiving the soccer details, Grandma sees from the colour of her lampshade that there's action in Johnny's kitchen. 'Your Mom must be making lunch.' 'Yeah, but please don't tell her I'm here. She saw that you were up late, and I promised I wouldn't visit you until evening. I just *couldn't* wait.'

---

depression and loneliness and ensure quality of life, are as crucial. We believe that the feelings of inclusion, worth and intimacy can be maintained by non-intrusive, socially aware, 'just being there' technology (which does not necessarily involve interactive video). New social norms will be generated and rituals for regulating interaction. It will change our perceptions of privacy, and challenge our norms for including others, for example the elderly, in modern-day family life.

The future of the Internet as an arena for socializing

The above stories raise many issues (e.g. quality assurance, privacy, legal, ethical, and philosophical). We chose to focus on the technological enhancements needed to support opportunities for social inclusion in the next decade, and to what degree such enhancements are likely. We will argue that the development of the Internet into a carrier of high-quality speech and the creation of socially aware everyday things connected to the Internet should be given high priority. Further we argue that both these developments are within reach, although high-quality speech will probably have to rely on the traditional telephone networks.

Theories of communication mediation tend to arrange the mediating technologies along a 'richness' dimension, from the richest, i.e. face-to-face communication, via video and audio down to text chat and email, which is considered the poorest.[23,24] In line with this, video has often been touted as an important communication development. However, after 30 years of research into the effect of video on interpersonal interaction, positive results are few and far between. One comprehensive review[25] found little effect of video over speech on interpersonal interaction, and another study indicated that video might be detrimental if it takes resources from the audio channel.[26] Thus, the support of video does not appear to be crucial when seeking ways to enhance the Internet for social purposes.

Speech, on the other hand, has consistently proved essential in a wide range of tasks,[26] recently also in developing trust between strangers, where it is demonstrated both that trust can develop online and that speech plays a significant part in that development.[27,28] Trust, defined as: 'willingness to be vulnerable, based on positive expectations about actions of others' [27] and trust development, is related to social isolation and supported both directly and through increased willingness and ability to disclose aspects of one's self.[29]

Speech is dependent on timing, and the introduction of small time delays between sender and receiver are detrimental. Thus, a communication network that supports high-quality speech must minimize delay and variations in delay, between sender and receiver. Delay and variations in delay, called lag and jitter, are notoriously hard to handle in the Internet. At present, there are no universally accepted schemes for implementing mechanisms that guarantee that these parameters are within acceptable bounds. Actually the current version of the Internet protocol (IP) is not suited to support these kinds of mechanisms (usually called quality of service mechanisms). Thus, the Internet will probably have to do without them at least until the next version of the IP protocol is implemented. This upgrade will probably not be completed within the next 10 years. Thus, the Internet cannot be expected to deliver high-quality end-to-end telephony services inside the next 10 years. For this we have to rely on conventional telephony (PSTN) and ISDN for the foreseeable future. For the socially isolated, of course, it is probably inconsequential which network technology carries his or her conversation.

On the face of it, integrating high-quality speech into the Internet signifies only another telephony network. However, coupled with advances in terminal technology, it could develop our living quarters into media spaces akin to those envisaged for the office in the early 1990s.[30,31] Developments along these lines are already under way. The Casablanca project is a relevant example.[32] Here a number of social communication devices for the home were designed and evaluated. Consumer preference studies concluded that lightweight communication devices, such as a 'presence lamp', are desirable and that high-quality audio spaces will be well received. The purpose of the TSUNAGARI project[33] was to establish a feeling of social presence by signalling through everyday objects. The project used the Internet to connect the households of family members who were living apart. An artificial flower, fitted with optical fibres, signalled different types of activity between the connected families. In a similar study,[34] picture frames were used to signal the activity between the homes of elderly parents and their children's homes. The Casablanca project concluded that the 'project has demonstrated that the space of new domestic communication technologies is enormous'[32].

By doing away with the traditional input and output mechanisms, and integrating the communication devices into everyday objects, these studies achieved two goals. First, and highly important, the communication technology is made accessible to a wider audience. Keyboards, mice and computer screens may be second nature to some of us, but they represent barriers to others. Second, by signalling through everyday objects, the presence and activity of others can be made continually available, but without any need for conscious attention. This development is akin to the 'coming age of calm computing' conjectured by Weiser.[35]

The availability of these types of technologies depends on developments in sensor, processor and miniaturization technologies, as well as in the way devices are connected to the Internet. To connect the devices to the Internet without difficulty, two conditions must fall into place. One is the advent of so-called always-on connections to the Internet. Another is the availability of inexpensive and small, short range wireless communication devices. Always-on connections are modelled after the local area networks (LAN), where data flows freely between the terminal and the Internet as long as the terminal is on. Both xDSL, cable and wireless connections to the Internet have this 'always-on' characteristic, and they will probably be the most commonly used type of connection in 10 years time. A wireless connection makes it feasible to connect a large number of devices to the Internet without turning a home into a tangle of wires. Currently the 2.4-GHz band has seen a huge increase in popularity, mainly because of agreement on two standards, the IEEE 802.11 and Bluetooth. The 802.11 currently specifies LANs (range of a few hundred metres) with around 10 Mbit/s capacity, while Bluetooth specifies a short-range (few metres) Pico network with 1 Mbit/s capacity. Thus, it is reasonable to assume that everyday objects can be connected continually to the Internet, inside a 10-year timeframe.

The Internet has a potential to bring together social communication devices, buddy-lists, information sources and awareness indicators, with the telephony system's high-quality speech transmission. It can thus create a new type of 'media space' that will be used both by those in need of nurturing and support, and by those who just want to hang out together, probably creating a richer social life for both.

Conclusion

In this chapter we have looked at future opportunities for reducing social isolation and enhancing mental health from two angles: (i) the Internet as a tool in mental health care – 'the psychosocial prescription'; and (ii) the Internet as a medium for daily life socializing – 'visiting grandma'. The opportunities outlined in the first are largely dependent on non-technical factors (e.g. evidence on prevention, new roles for doctors, insurance coverage) which need to be addressed in parallel with developing the technology. The second will, we believe, find a market as soon as the technology is available. We have argued that advances in terminal equipment, especially development of socially aware gadgets and the integration of the Internet with the high-quality telephone systems, are prerequisites for this development.

Interesting episodes will flourish with these new media, and generate new social norms and rituals for regulating interaction. It will change our perceptions of privacy, and challenge our norms for including others, for example elderly people in modern-day family life. Insights from human–computer interaction research will hopefully merge with and enhance future research in mental health.

Social life through the Internet may evolve as an important option for many, not just those who are physically or psychologically disabled. Factors like an ever more global job market, and anxieties fuelled by crime, terrorism and pollution, will play their role. Questions of identity, reality, truth and how we define a healthy life will continue to flourish as availability and variations of social interaction evolve through the Internet.

References

1 McKenna KYA, Bargh JA. Plan 9 from cyberspace: the implications of the Internet for personality and social psychology. *Personality and Social Psychology Review* 2000;**4**:57–74.

2 Hawthorne G, Griffith P. *The Friendship Scale: development and properties*. (Working paper no 114.) Melbourne: Centre for Health Program Evaluation, 2000. Reproduced at http://chpe.buseco.monash.edu. au/pubs/wp114.pdf [last checked 19 September 2002].

3 Weiss R. The provisions of social relationships. In: Rubin Z, ed. *Doing Unto Others*. Englewood Cliffs: Prentice Hall, 1974:17–26.

4 Monroe SM, Steiner SC. Social support and psychopathology: interrelations with preexisting disorder, stress, and personality. *Journal of Abnormal Psychology* 1986;**95**:29–39.

5 Constable JF, Russel DW. The effect of social support and the work environment upon burnout among nurses. *Journal of Human Stress* 1986;**12**:20–26.

6 Stroebe MS, Stroebe W. Who suffers more? Sex differences in health risks of the widowed. *Psychology Bulletin* 1983;**93**:279–301.

7 Resnick B, Orwig D, Magaziner J, Wynne C. The effect of social support on exercise behavior in older adults. *Clinical Nursing Research* 2002;**11**:52–70.

8 Bennett SJ, Perkins SM, Lane KA, Deer M, Brater DC, Murray MD. Social support and health related quality of life in chronic heart failure patients. *Quality of Life Research* 2001;**10**:671–682.

9 Elmore SK. The moderating effect of social support upon depression. *Western Journal of Nursing Research* 1984;**6**:17–22.

10 Dalgard OS. *Bomiljø og psykisk helse*. [Living-environment and mental health.] Oslo: Universitetsforlaget, 1980.

11 Henderson S, Duncan-Jones P, Mcauley H, Ritchie K. The patients primary group. *British Journal of Psychiatry* 1978;**132**:74–86.

12 Schwarzer R, Leppin A. Social support and mental health: a conceptual and empirical overview. In: Montada L, Filipp SH, Lerner MJ, eds. *Life Crises and Experiences of Loss in Adulthood*. Hillsdale, NJ: L Erlbaum Associates, 1992:435–458.

13 Hernes T. Sosiale nettverk, sosial støtte og psykisk helse. [Social networks, social support and mental health.] In: Dalgard OS, Sørensen T, eds. *Sosialt nettverk og psykisk helse*. [*Social Network and Mental Health*.] Otta: Tano, 1988;19–39.

14 Wing JK. Social influences on the source of schizophrenia. In: Wynne LC, Cromwell RL, Matthysse S, eds. *The Nature of Schizophrenia: new approaches to research and treatment*. New York: John Wiley, 1978;599–616.

15 Phillips SL. Network characteristics related to the well-being of normals: a comparative base. *Schizophrenia Bulletin* 1981;**7**:117–124.

16 Kraut R, Patterson M, Lundmark V, Keisler S, Mukopadhyay T, Scherlis W. Internet paradox: a social technology that reduces social involvement and psychological well-being? *American Psychologist* 1998;**53**:1017–1031.

17 Kraut R, Kiesler S, Boneva B, et al. Internet paradox revisited. *Journal of Social Issues* 2002;**58**:49–74.

18 Kummervold PE, Gammon D, Bergvik S, Johnsen JA, Hasvold T, Rosenvinge JH. Social support in a wired world: use of mental health forums in Norway. *Nordic Journal of Psychiatry* 2002;**56**:59–65.

19 Gammon D, Rosenvinge J. Is the Internet of any help for persons with serious mental disorders? *Journal of the Norwegian Medical Association* 2000;**120**:1890–1892.

20 Norwegian Medical Association. *Forskning og fagutvikling i forebyggende helsearbeid blant barn og unge*. [Research and strategy in health promotion among children and adolescents.] Oslo: Norwegian Medical Association.

21 Andreassen H, Sandaune AG, Gammon D, Hjortdahl P. Use of Internet health services in Norway. *Journal of The Norwegian Medical Association* 2002;**17**:1640–1644. Reproduced at http://www.tidsskriftet.no/ pls/lts/PA_LTS.Vis_Seksjon?vp_SEKS_ID=565067 [last checked 19 September 2002.]

22 Hjortdahl P, Nylenna M, Aasland OG. Internett og lege-pasient-forholdet – fra 'takk' til 'hvorfor'? [The Internet and the doctor–patient relationship. From 'Thank you' to 'Why?'] *Journal of The Norwegian Medical Association* 1999;**29**:4439–4441.

23 Daft R, Lengel RH. Information richness: a new approach to managerial behaviour and organizational design. In: Staw B, Cummings LL, eds. *Research in Organizational Behaviour*. Greenwich, CN: JAI Press, 1984:199–233.

24 Short J, Williams E, Christie B, eds. *The Social Psychology of Telecommunications*. London: Wiley, 1976.

25 Whittaker S, O'Conaill B. The role of vision in face to face and mediated communication. In: Finn KE,

Sellen AJ, Wilbur SB, eds. *Video-mediated Communication.* Mahwah, NJ: Lawrence Erlbaum Associates, 1997:23–49.

26   O'Conaill B, Whittaker S. Characterizing, predicting and measuring VMC. In: Finn KE, Sellen AJ, Wilbur SB, eds. *Video-mediated Communication.* Mahwah, NJ: Lawrence Erlbaum Associates, 1997:107–131.

27   Bos N, Olson J, Gergle D, Olson G, Wright Z. Effects of four computer-mediated communication channels on trust development. In: *Conference on Human Factors in Computing Systems.* CHI 2002 Conference Proceedings. New York: ACM Press, 2002:135–140.

28   Jensen C, Farnham SD, Drucker SM, Kollock P. The effect of communication modality on cooperation in online environments. In: *Conference on Human Factors in Computing Systems.* CHI 2000 Conference Proceedings from The Hague, Netherlands. New York: ACM Press, 2000:470–477.

29   Turkle S, ed. *Life on the Screen. Identity in the age of the Internet.* New York: Simon and Schuster 1995.

30   Fish RS, Kraut RE, Root RW, Rice RE. Evaluating video as a technology for informal communication. *Computer–Human Interaction (CHI)* 1992;37–48. Reproduced at http://pages.cpsc.ucalgary.ca/~saul/601.13/readings/evaluating_video.pdf [last checked 19 September 2002].

31   Bly S, Harrison S, Irwin S. Media spaces: bringing people together in a video, audio and computing environment. *Communication of the Association for Computing Machinery* 1993;**36**:28–47.

32   Hindus D, Mainwaring SD, Leduc N, Hagstrøm AE, Bayley O. Casablanca: designing social communication devices for the home. In: *Conference on Human Factors in Computing Systems.* CHI 2001 Conference Proceedings. New York: ACM Press, 2001:325–332.

33   Itoh Y, Miyajima A, Watanabe T. 'TSUNAGARI' communication: fostering a feeling of connection between family members. In: *Conference on Human Factors in Computing Systems.* CHI 2002 Conference Proceedings. New York: ACM Press, 2002:810–811.

34   Mynatt ED, Rowan J, Jacobs A, Craighill S. Digital family portraits: supporting peace of mind for extended family members. In: *Conference on Human Factors in Computing Systems.* CHI 2001 Conference Proceedings. New York: ACM Press, 2001:333–340.

35   Weiser M, Brown JS. The coming age of calm computing. In: Denning PJ, Metcalfe RM, eds. *Beyond Calculation: the next fifty years of computing.* New York: Copernicus, 1997:75–85.

24

Unique Aspects of Internet Relationships

Esther Gwinnell

Introduction

Psychotherapy has developed from an interaction between two people face to face to include more complex interactions such as group therapy and therapy conducted via satellite on video screens. Psychotherapists are now exploring therapy over the Internet, by email, by instant messages and even group therapy in a chatroom setting.

The process of conducting therapy by email or other Internet options brings up new questions for the therapist. How does email affect transference? Are there aspects of Internet therapy that increase some symptoms? What are the danger zones in e-therapy versus face-to-face therapy?

There are new psychiatric complaints related to Internet use. Some individuals have become 'addicted' to the Internet, to email relationships, to chatrooms and to Internet pornography. Obsession and Internet stalking have become more common; preoccupation with fantasy games have led some users to lose contact with reality, to neglect their families and jobs as they pursue their virtual reality adventures.

In my work researching Internet romance, I interviewed dozens of individuals and couples who had fallen in love with someone they met on the Internet. They met in chatrooms, discussion groups and bulletin boards. In answering the question 'how do you fall in love with someone on the Internet?' I was presented repeatedly with special aspects of communication on the Internet that echoed phenomena found most commonly in the psychotherapeutic relationship.

In my psychiatric practice, I have used email as a therapeutic tool, bringing up entirely new questions about the effects of faceless, bodiless communication in a clinical setting. Although this chapter addresses these questions, these are early explorations of a rapidly changing technology.

Internet romance

Human beings learn from birth to relate to each other through all the senses. Infants respond to the sound of their mother's voice, her familiar smell, even before vision becomes important. Throughout our lives, we develop ways of understanding the people in our lives that include even such tiny cues as the enlarging or shrinking of the pupils of the eyes. Although we are not consciously aware of these many cues, we respond according to our learning.

Equally important in our development is the sense of who we are, what we are like and how we are perceived by the people around us. The Internet provides an anonymous forum for exploration of the self, and can allow people to develop entirely new personas which have little or no relationship to day-to-day life. Writing to strangers from the safety of home can allow individuals to pretend to be anything or anyone they can imagine. One of the primary attractions of chatrooms and fantasy games appears to be the opportunity to interact with many strangers and to create new selves unfettered by the perceptions of others.[1] On the screen, we are not subject to the instantaneous assessment we face in daily life.

Transference

In the early work of psychoanalysis, the ordinary social cues were minimized as much as possible to allow for the presentation of a blank slate upon which a patient might project his/her internal world. The analyst was taught to avoid emotional inflection of the voice, minimize facial expression and even to avoid allowing the patient to see his/her face. Patients were encouraged to bring their life experience with relationships into the analytical session by the analyst avoiding bringing his actual self into the session – as much as possible. But even in that setting, with the therapist sitting out of sight of the patient, speaking little, providing as few individual cues as possible, there was a wealth of information about the therapist available to the analysand.

Entering Sigmund Freud's office, a patient would smell the cigar smoke, see innumerable objects relating to him, would hear his voice, see how he walked and talked, and would be able to form valid conclusions about what kind of a person he was in the room with, even without seeing Freud throughout the course of a session. Although the decrease in visual and auditory cues would allow for the development of transference, the real man was still available as a reference point.

In this setting, transference was quite powerful, even to the point of developing transference psychosis. With the Internet, there are so few social cues that the development of transference can be powerful, rapid, and take place without the intrusion of the 'real person' into the experience. Information may be completely fictitious; statements about gender, age, physical appearance and social class may be entirely absent or unreliable.

Since this information is, in essence, necessary to human beings, much of what is unavailable is supplied from previous experience and fantasy. In effect, the development of transference is not only easy and rapid on the Internet, it is required in order to have a relationship with another person.

R.J. met a man in a chatroom. He used the name 'Zorro' online. He initially attracted her attention because of his somewhat morbid sense of humour, and she began to correspond with him. She reported that immediately upon reading his first communication 'a picture of him came into my head. He was tall and thin, with dark hair and high cheekbones. I could picture his cynical smile, and even the way he would move his shoulders when he gestured. It was so vivid that I could have picked him out of a crowd. I fell in love with that picture.' (Quotations in this chapter, for the most part, come from email communication with individuals either interviewed for my book[2] or who have subsequently sent email to me after reading my book or visiting my website.[3])

When she explored this image, R.J. found it was composed of characters she had seen in movies who demonstrated cynical humour, combined with an old boyfriend whose black wit had initially attracted her but then repelled her. The online name of Zorro contributed to her internal image; and added an appealing sense of dangerousness to her emotional drawing of him. She experienced intense feelings and fantasies about Zorro, which hearkened back to feelings she had about her old boyfriend, but also to feelings she later related to childhood emotions. R.J. exchanged email messages with Zorro for some months. When he sent her a photograph, her feelings for Zorro vanished – he didn't look or feel anything like her image of him.

Obsession or addiction?

The Internet is available 24 hours a day and is constantly open for business. Email can arrive at any moment of the day or night. Some individuals in my research exchanged email as frequently as 50 times per day, or spent hours chatting live online long into the night.

Constant checking for new email becomes a part of any Internet relationship. The cycle of anticipation, fantasy, anxiety, relief from anxiety and new anticipation seems to produce obsessive-compulsive behaviour patterns in most participants.

E.M. used the name 'Natasha' on the Internet. She met a man, 'Hitchcock', in a discussion group devoted to old movies. They exchanged email about a particular film they both liked, and over the course of several days they had exchanged approximately 25 email messages. E.M. started checking her email every half an hour while working, and stayed online continuously at home to monitor her email. She began to check her email at night whenever she awoke, and would go to her computer immediately in the morning when she arose. She described having very strong feelings of disappointment if there was no email from Hitchcock and then pleasure each time she saw his name on her email list.

E.M. began to think about Hitchcock continuously, intruding into her thoughts about any topic. She composed email messages in her head and had fantasies about conversations that she would have with him. On vacation, she went to considerable trouble to find an Internet access site that would allow her to check her email, and found herself anxious and preoccupied when she could not. She described herself as 'in love' with Hitchcock.

Dr Kimberly Young described a group of individuals that appeared to be addicted to the Internet, meeting the basic criteria for the diagnosis of 'addiction' according to the DSM-IV.[4] People with previous addiction problems or eating disorders were more prone to this problem than others, but people who were house-bound or disabled were also more likely to develop significant emotional dependence on Internet-related activities. Especially concerning were role-playing games or virtual reality sites where people construct a fantasy life, complete with buying homes, furnishing apartments, starting businesses and essentially creating entire alternate lives for themselves.

Although there is no evidence for physical addiction per se, some individuals engaging in Internet pornography or participating in sexual chatrooms clearly become profoundly preoccupied. There does appear to be an emotional withdrawal syndrome, with anxiety, restlessness, depression and even some physical symptoms such as shakiness, tremor and sleep disturbance associated with attempting to discontinue Internet use.

Shapira et al[5] evaluated 20 people whose use of the Internet was clearly pathological in scope. He found that 80% of these individuals fulfilled the criteria for major mental illness. It appeared from his research that the illness predisposed them to various types of Internet activities, from virtual reality sites to fantasy games and Internet pornography.

C.B. was undergoing long-term treatment for obsessive-compulsive personality disorder and bipolar affective disorder. She had a long history of compulsive shopping, severe depressive episodes and periods of hypomania.

C.B. was unemployed when she first began participating in chatrooms. She began to have private chats with men, with whom she would exchange sexual fantasies. She spent time in explicit sexual chatgroups, and spent increasing amounts of time on the Internet while her husband was at work. She reported that she was masturbating dozens of times a day while engaged in these sexual chats; she reported that most of her other responsibilities were ignored while she obsessively sought sexual 'partners' on the Internet.

Her attempts to disengage from these Internet activities made her feel depressed and anxious. She could not resist checking her email at night after her husband had gone to bed, and could not leave her house for more than a few hours during the day because she could not tolerate being away from the computer. She felt empty and irritable when her husband was present and she could not use the computer.

In C.B.'s case, her previous history of psychiatric illness to some extent predicted the kind of Internet problem she developed. The hypersexual behaviour and obsessive-compulsive style of chatroom usage were consistent with her prior difficulties with compulsive shopping and subclinical manic symptoms. Her style of Internet use is also consistent with an addictive-type process, and she could be viewed as fulfilling the criteria for Internet addiction.

The Internet is like a dream

The unreal quality of email and chatroom interactions, empty of ordinary human information, feels very like a dream to some people. Fantasies are readily exchanged and created, and the development of an internal fantasy image of other people on the Internet reduces the intensity of ordinary defence mechanisms. For example, in the course of exchanging email with a stranger, G.R. felt free to discuss daydreams and then sexual fantasies – things that were too uncomfortable or anxiety provoking to share with her spouse. She told her Internet friend things about herself that she would have been ashamed to tell someone in a face-to-face setting. As a result, she experienced herself as being very intimate with someone she had never actually met. One man in a chatroom said 'I find myself saying things in email that I would never say in a telephone conversation. Even with years of experience in dealing with email, it still surprises me how much of my inner self I reveal. When I sit down at the computer, it feels always like I am communing with myself, even though I plan to send the email to someone.'

This sense of intimacy springs from the absence or breakdown of social boundaries. The lack of significance of the relationship initially allows for social experimentation. The anxiety present in our first meeting with a stranger is absent. Safe at home or in a perceived safe place, without personal contact, hidden behind a false name, many people are willing to be intimate almost immediately. 'There are no safety belts here – the things you learn not to talk about from childhood on seem reasonable on the net.'

My exploration of Internet romance has found repeated examples of men and women who were not intending to become involved with someone on the Internet, but started their relationships with the idea that 'It doesn't count. It isn't real. I'll never even meet this person.' The sense of make-believe in these relationships can have devastating consequences as people continue to experience a stronger sense of intimacy with a pretend person than they do with a spouse.

The masquerade ball

One of the more prominent aspects of Internet communication is that people feel free to be anyone they want. Male newspaper writers have pretended to be women in chatrooms to see how long it would take for someone to discover their pretence. One writer observed that he was shocked that no one found out that he was not a woman until he confessed. There are dozens of tales of Internet relationships where one party was not what they purported to be – from men pretending to be women, to men and women pretending to be much older or much younger than they were in real life.

This is not, in most cases, a deliberate attempt to deceive people for malicious reasons. Rather, the anonymity and unreality associated with chatrooms and email brings out a playful side to people. As one cartoon put it, 'on the Internet, no one knows you're a dog'. Much of the alarm and suspicion that people have about Internet relationships comes from this awareness: not only are other people not necessarily what they seem to be, but I may also be playing a role or inventing a character.

D.A. invented several characters for his Internet activities. He had separate names and email addresses for all of them, pretending at times to be a young woman in pornographic chatrooms and pretending at others to be gay or lesbian or a very old man. He had multiple romantic and erotic relationships based on these characters and spent hours each day creating email responses that would be 'in character' for each of his conquests. He did eventually reveal the truth of his identity, and was shocked at the angry responses. One woman threatened suicide at the loss of her fantasy lover. D.A. wrote, 'I didn't think it was serious. I thought everyone was just playing around – but I guess I was the only one playing around.'

The masquerade aspect is encouraged by several aspects of email and chatroom conventions. Choosing a false name is similar to choosing a costume. The anonymity is also similar to wearing a mask. Finally, a sense that it would be better to hide one's real self – for self-protection or out of a desire to remain anonymous – powerfully encourages participants to choose some other screen identity.

In responses to Internet questionnaires, people have admitted to choosing 'handles' on the Internet that have special meaning to them. Some handles are intended to attract certain people; others are simply intended to provide a façade to maintain anonymity. Participating in a political discussion group or religious discussion group online can make one a target for angry responses; the fear of some kind of retaliation is widespread.

Disinhibition

The fear of retaliation is a valid one. Without the face-to-face social structure, many participants in Internet interactions do not demonstrate ordinary levels of politeness, reserve, or, indeed, ordinary levels of restraint in any area. Similar to road rage, people on the Internet may lose control of angry impulses. The lack of facial expression or voice modulation can make interpreting some interactions very difficult, and some individuals can respond with rage or 'flaming', safe in the knowledge that they are hidden from view.

A sense of anonymity can also allow participants to be more overtly sexual, or to explore more unusual sexual activities. The belief that Internet activity is not real, has no consequences and is completely safe can decrease an individual's inhibitions about sexual exploration. As with C.B., this exploration can become obsessive or addictive in nature.

'Angelina' had been in many flame wars on the Internet. She sought out discussion groups or chatrooms, and deliberately made provocative or insulting remarks for the effect they would cause. She especially enjoyed baiting individuals she thought were pompous or prissy, based on the limited information available in their email messages or Internet names. It was not accidental that she chose the Internet name Angelina; she saw herself as the opposite of an angel and took great pleasure in her ability to stir up a chatroom. She could not imagine any repercussions from this. She could not envisage any consequences because she wasn't really there: 'after all, no one could hit me'.

In her daily life, she had never raised her voice in anger in any public setting. She was polite and neatly attired, respectful of her superiors and pleasant to shop assistants. On the Internet, she felt free to surrender to all her angry impulses and was actually rather proud of being able to do so. She saw this as 'a kind of catharsis, a kind of letting my hair down after a lifetime of never being able to be angry. I've always been a good little girl, but sometimes I'm boiling with anger and the Internet is a place I can have a good fight and work off some steam.'

Exacerbation of some psychiatric processes

Paranoia

Since Internet interaction increases the speed and intensity of the development of transference, some psychiatric illnesses may be aggravated by increased Internet activity. The fantasy image is not necessarily a pleasant one. As B.T. participated in a chatroom, he noticed that some of his comments would be carried through in other people's discussions. He began to wonder if they were deliberately quoting his words back to him in different contexts as a way of testing him or mocking him.

As B.T. spent more time surfing the Internet, he noticed that things he would say to people around him in daily life would be repeated in websites or in chatrooms. His ideas of reference were rapidly expanding as he began obsessively to monitor chatrooms from a 'lurker' position. He read extensively about Internet spying and the various methods of tracking people from Internet sites, and became convinced that people from his chatroom were watching or knew about his every activity. He was certain that his chatroom acquaintances were attempting to harm him.

Although an individual with paranoid ideas can find evidence of being malevolently pursued anywhere, the Internet offers many more opportunities for projection and ideas of reference without the added information about the event that face-to-face contact normally provides. The opportunity to engage in obsessive searching for evidence allows individuals to gather in more and more information that supports a paranoid idea.

In fact, as the Internet expands to include more and more previously isolated individuals, it is possible to build up a social network of people who believe the same kind of paranoid ideas. Then, within that group, ideas that would be met with disbelief or derision outside are instead supported and strengthened. B.T. discovered a website dedicated to the uncovering of cults and conspiracies. His social network rapidly constricted itself to only others from this website and every interaction confirmed his belief that his former chatroom was actually a recruiting site for a satanic cult.

Obsession and stalking

An unfortunate consequence of being able to make contact with so many strangers who are essentially fantasy figures is the increased potential for pathological obsession and stalking. Combining the elements discussed above, the required development of a fantasy image, the opportunity for obsessive behaviour, and the decrease in ordinary social restraint allows for the development of the psychotic transference or pathological obsession that leads to stalking.

Movie stars are frequently subject to this kind of psychotic transference, but in the usual course of daily life, few people are exposed to stalking by strangers. In chatrooms and discussion groups, however, a man or woman can be exposed to hundreds of individuals who all form a fantasy image of that person. If the fantasy is powerful enough, or the audience is ill enough, anyone can be a victim of a pathological obsession.

The scope for stalking on the Internet is substantial. It is possible to track down an individual's home address, even download maps to that address. Alternate screen names can be found, as can references to participation in discussion groups or newsgroups. Everything ever written for general consumption can be accessed. More private information can frequently be found by searching for financial and credit histories.

Lack of social cues

A prominent concern is the lack of social and interpersonal information between the patient and the therapist. Much of therapy depends on the assessment of body language, facial expression, voice tone and speech patterns, the spontaneous introduction of new material and the ability to respond to that information. Thus email must be seen as a very limited setting. Diagnosis in psychiatry can rely on latency of response, depressed affect, speech pattern abnormalities and behavioural assessment. By contrast, everything is based on the patient's self-report by email or in a chatroom or support group type setting on the Internet.

It may be that this communication is substantially more honest and introspective than face-to-face conversation. As noted above, the experience of communicating via email may be free enough from anxiety to allow some individuals to reveal themselves in ways not available to them in therapy.

H.W. has been receiving treatment for some years. An exquisitely shy man, he talks in a voice so quiet that I frequently need to ask him to repeat himself during sessions. He also has little ability to be introspective in my office; his anxiety causes him to have tremendous problems with thought-blocking and dissociation. His interpersonal sensitivity is extreme – he watches for any possible sign of impending rejection and abandonment. Many sessions end with a question about whether I am going to stop seeing him.

But in sending me email, H.W. is eloquent and expressive. His thoughts about his situation and his fears are clearly and even poignantly developed and, unlike his presentation in my office, he can be assertive and even enthusiastic about new ideas. For H.W. email has offered a different format for his therapy. I would not describe this as truly psychotherapy, however. He and I have come to think about this as a kind of 'interactive diary'. Because he does know me and has come to my office, he does have an image of me that is reasonably reality-based.

But because I am not in the room, he relates in his writings to his fantasy of me; with a sense that he is truly alone and writing in his own journal, which then somehow leads to a response. There is a kind of magical thinking involved in this interchange, which has been commented on by other patients, and by patients involved in Internet therapy with other therapists. His journal writes back to him with ideas about new ways to think about problems or anxieties; which he can then explore in private writings or return to email.

Both transference and countertransference can be altered in an email exchange. My internal image of H.W. is very different when we are exchanging email. This person who writes so eloquently and easily seems like a different person from the painfully shy man who speaks so softly and so little. It is all too easy for me to lose contact with his reality if I don't insist on regular office visits. In my interviews with patients, it is clear that patient and therapist share this loss of the real person.

Several qualities of this interchange have been problematical. Unlike the verbal give-and-take of a session, email sessions must take place over the course of some days. Although he may write to me in the middle of the night, my responses may take a day or two. And rather than the ephemeral quality of conversation, he has the opportunity to obsess for days over every tiny aspect of my response. He will become preoccupied with my specific choice of a word, and will respond to emotions he has interpreted from my writing that would be experienced very differently had they been communicated with my voice and body language. The multiple possible interpretations of various written phrases can be alarming. Humour, irony, sarcasm, witticisms, clever turns of phrase – they can all be distressingly misinterpreted in writing. A delay of a day in responding to an email can be interpreted as lack of interest, even when rules for communicating in this way have been clearly established.

Boundaries

As with other Internet-based relationships, it is difficult to establish appropriate boundaries. If a patient writes email at 02 : 00, and the therapist responds within a few moments because she happens to be online, does that create a new and false expectation of immediate reply? Does this enhance a magical view of the therapist, that she is watching over her patients, constantly checking email and providing a pervasive presence that can either seem intrusive or supportive? If portions of an email are not specifically addressed, does that represent lack of interest? Or perhaps, lack of attention?

Reading email takes time, and composing a reasonable reply takes additional time. If email is considered to be a part of the therapy, discussing and understanding the time limitations is essential. Some patients will write email messages that run to 10 or 15 printed pages. This exemplifies both transference and counter-transference issues – the patient may have fantasies of limitless access to the therapist, and the therapist may in turn be overwhelmed at the quantity that must be read.

Deliberate deception

In pure Internet therapy, where there has never been a personal interaction, these hazards are greater, and are complicated by the unreal quality of the communication. There is a strong opportunity for deliberate deception by the patient, especially in support groups or therapeutic chatrooms.

In one support group for mothers with ill children, a woman participated in the support groups for some time, detailed her child's horrible progressive disease and then related that her child had died. All the women in the group were very sad, and rallied around with their support. However, some time later in a different support group, it was discovered that this woman was engaged in a series of elaborate lies with which she effectively traumatized multiple support groups. While pathological liars are certainly a part of the ordinary world, the therapeutic chatrooms and bulletin boards offer a powerful and even dangerous forum for acting out and victimizing more vulnerable individuals.

Therapy online

Some formats have been suggested for conducting therapy online on a fee-for-service basis. For the past 5 years, the American Psychiatric Association annual meeting has included presentations and seminars relating to conducting therapy over the Internet. Research on the usefulness and safety of these protocols continues, but the results are not yet available. The interactive diary approach is being evaluated, as are much more structured cognitive behavioural programmes that allow the patient to use computerized self-assessment tools and monitor behavioural changes online.

Conclusion

It is increasingly clear that human beings are not emotionally prepared to cope with the faceless and bodiless communication that email and other Internet settings present. The intensity of the relationship is disproportionate to the information available. Learning to relate to other people without the thousands of social cues available in face-to-face conversation may never be adequate to allow therapists to conduct true psychotherapy over the Internet. However, understanding the pitfalls of email and chatroom relationships may make it possible for therapists to help patients deal with the confusion and distress these relationships can generate.

References

1   Turkle S, ed. *Life on the Screen: identity in the age of the Internet*. New York: Simon and Schuster, 1995.
2   Gwinnell E. *Online Seductions: falling in love with strangers on the Internet*. New York: Kodansha International, 1998.
3   Available via e-mail at strangers@nocouch.com. see http://www.nocouch.com [last checked 3 September 2002.]
4   American Psychiatric Association. *Diagnostic and Statistical Manual of Mental Disorders*, 4th edn. Washington, DC: American Psychiatric Association, 1994.
5   Shapira NA, Goldsmith TD, Keck PE Jr, Khosla UM, McElroy SL. Psychiatric features of individuals with problematic internet use. *Journal of Affective Disorders* 2000;**57**:267–272.

25

The Road Online to Empowered Clients and Empowered Providers

John M. Grohol

Introduction

The Internet allows professionals to reach out and offer a wider range of affordable services to more consumers than ever before. The therapist is not only a direct provider of services in this new paradigm of the empowered client, but also the coach and consultant to the patient. This new role allows the professional to help the client be a more educated consumer of the growing set of resources available to them online.

Historically, psychotherapists and psychiatrists have acted as the gatekeepers to mental health services. While this role changes marginally from decade to decade, most therapists act as the expert to guide the client to a successful resolution of their problems. No matter what the specific psychological orientation of the therapist is, whether a Freudian or a cognitive behavioural therapist, the professional nearly always takes the lead in guiding therapy, dispensing information about the specific disorder and acting as a conduit for additional support services in the community.

Therapist as expert

These roles are defined by specific boundaries, which are often explicitly elucidated early on in the therapeutic relationship. 'Here is how I work. These are my expectations of you as the client, and these are the expectations you can have of me as your therapist. Here is what you do in case of an emergency.' The therapist makes it clear that while she is not a friend or advice-giver to the client, she is acting in the role as an expert in human behaviour and experience. This role often translates simplistically to the client as 'Doctor knows best'. If the professional says that a psychiatric consultation is necessary in order to evaluate the client for medications, the client goes along with it. If the professional says that he or she works using cognitive behavioural techniques in order to help effect change in the client's life, the client goes along with it. If the therapist suggests that couples counselling is in order, the client goes along with it. Very rarely do clients express disagreement with choices made about their treatment, and the clients that do are sometimes labelled as 'resistant' or some similar psychotherapeutic mumbo-jumbo.

At this point, many professionals will object to this characterization of the traditional psychotherapeutic relationship, claiming, 'Oh no, I don't act like that. I'm a partner with the client in helping them change'. While that may be many therapists' orientation, their practice is often reduced to making specific recommendations for behavioural or thought changes in order to effect emotional change. Clients who do not follow the recommendations often spend a great deal of time in therapy, and the therapist is left scratching his or her head as to why.

Dissemination of information

Until recently, nearly all the information that clients wanted to know about their disorder or diagnosis was delivered to them by their mental health professional. 'What is depression?' would be answered in session by the 'expert' therapist or doctor. Ten years ago, this was the clients' primary, and often only, source of such information. Many therapists refused (and still refuse) to share even the clients' own diagnosis with them, often with the claim, 'Well, they wouldn't understand what that means'. The idea of explaining the assorted complexities of the diagnosis, and the entire diagnostic system used within mental health, was unthought of.

If the client was prescribed a psychotropic medication by a psychiatrist or a primary care doctor, the client was often left with very little information about the possible side effects or even the insert accompanying the medication. 'What should I expect while taking this medication' was often met with a short reply, and no place for the client to get additional information. Few clients felt brave enough to ask questions. Many clients are intimidated by their doctors and defer questions altogether, preferring to take a 'wait and see' attitude – 'If it doesn't hurt me, I won't bother the doctor with all of these silly questions'.

Stages of care

The average client comes into treatment only after having lived with their problem for a period of time. It may have been a few weeks, a few months, or a few years. The client will have often tried resolving the problem on his or her own, talked to family members or friends about it, and perhaps tried to obtain books on the subject.

Once in the mental health system, whether the client sees a psychiatrist or therapist first, the professional does an intake and makes a diagnosis. Then a course of treatment is defined, often with a specific treatment plan written out on a form. Sometimes the client is a part of defining their treatment, sometimes not. Even if the client does collaborate with the therapist on the treatment plan, how he or she actually obtains the goals defined therein is left to the therapist's training, experience and knowledge.

Treatment ends when the client's symptoms have decreased to the therapist's or client's satisfaction, when the client's insurance coverage is exhausted, or the client is frustrated with the lack of progress. More recently, the onset of managed care in many health care systems around the world means trying to better define outcomes and measure progress in therapy. This can be done with a variety of measures, including treatment plans, symptom checklists or other measures of the client's well-being.

The potential of the Internet

The Internet is turning on end the traditional psychotherapeutic relationship. No longer are clients content to sit back and be told how to change. Instead, they are taking a more proactive role. Clients are learning more about their disorders and diagnoses ahead of time. Many high-quality websites provide comprehensive lists of diagnostic symptoms for various disorders, as well as the usual and standard treatments prescribed.

Some clients are even helping to narrow down possible differential diagnoses by taking interactive, self-help quizzes online. Clients are finding others online with a similar diagnosis and joining self-help support groups that make living with the disorder easier and more understandable. For some people, the convenience and lower cost of the emerging e-therapy modality is attractive.

Psycho-education

A wide variety of websites provide a virtual encyclopaedia of knowledge about mental health disorders that was not readily available to the lay public before 1995. These sites were first begun by a handful of professionals who understood the Internet as an inexpensive transmission medium for disseminating information. By learning a simple language called HyperText Markup Language (HTML), anyone could publish a website on any topic they chose.

Given the paucity of consumer-focused information on mental health issues, these websites quickly gained a following of mental health consumers. Government-funded institutes, such as the National Institute of Mental Health (Fig. 25.1), worked hard to bring their sites online and provide the wealth of consumer information that they had developed over the years in paper format. Before the Internet, even getting a simple list of what constitutes a diagnosis of 'major depression', for instance, was extremely difficult if a person didn't know a cooperative mental health professional. These websites provided valuable resources on mental disorder symptoms, diagnoses and treatment to a much larger audience than before.[1]

This reluctance on the profession's behalf to share this knowledge is less surprising when considered in the context of the evolution of our modern mental disorder diagnostic system. This system, codified within the *Diagnostic and Statistical Manual of Mental Disorders*,[2] really only gained widespread acceptance a decade earlier, and was still making slow inroads in many established therapeutic practices. Before this more scientific model of diagnosis was adopted, most professionals handed out diagnoses in a very personalized, experience-based manner that had little empirical support or reliability between professionals. Given the diagnostic system's overall young age, the lack of information supplied about diagnoses derived from it (and subsequent empirical diagnostic systems) is perhaps more understandable.

In addition to basic information about how mental disorder diagnoses are made, websites offered increasingly detailed information about theoretical orientations practised in psychotherapy and the techniques that accompany them. Not surprisingly,

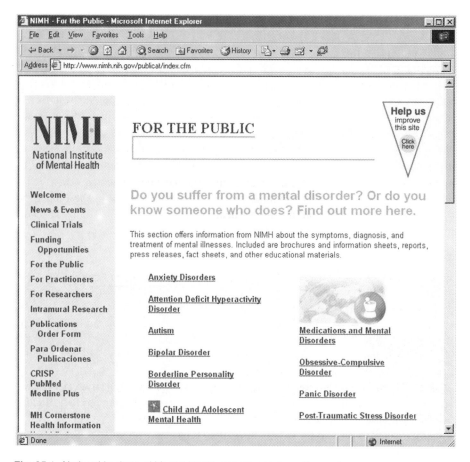

Fig. 25.1. National Institute of Mental Health consumer information web page.

many consumers' impressions of psychotherapy are still rooted in the traditional psychology 101 teachings of Jung and Freud, of clients lying on couches discussing their dreams with a distant, unattached therapist. The Internet put to rest many of these inaccurate characterizations and illuminated the wide range of orientations practised in psychotherapy today. Clients learned that therapy does not have to last for years and cost a substantial sum of money. Instead, therapy can be short-term, goal-oriented and valuable from time to time as life gives a person something unexpected to handle.

Reference information

As managed care has swept through many health care systems in the 1990s, it has led to an emphasis on outcome research and improving client outcomes with definable, clear treatment goals. This emphasis has led to shorter treatment periods and, often, more paperwork. It also means that professionals providing mental health services often have less time to discuss everything that they would like to in a session. In addition to researching symptoms or treatment modalities online, clients can also turn to the Internet for access to medication databases. If the client forgot something told to them, or the psychiatrist failed to mention a specific side effect, the client can easily go online, look up the medication, and read in great detail all about it. This was not easily possible before the Internet and can help to answer common questions about what to expect from a medication including any side effects.

Databases made available through the Internet also help professionals. A psychiatrist can go online and check drug interactions quickly and more easily than looking them up in a large tome that may or may not have been updated with the most recent information. When the National Library of Medicine brought the MEDLINE medical research database online, a great deal of free research information was made available (Fig. 25.2). Now a research citation can quickly be looked up online, rather

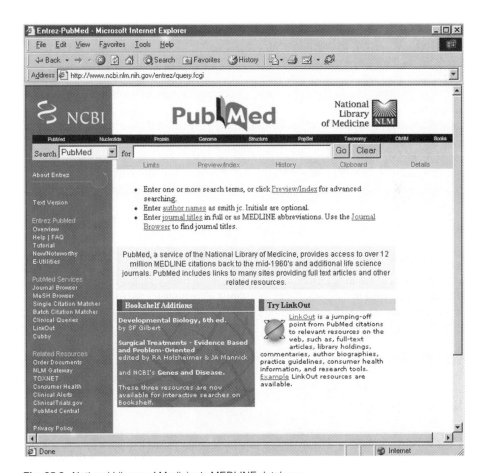

Fig. 25.2. National Library of Medicine's MEDLINE database.

than trudging off to a local university or medical school library. Professionals can stay up to date on the latest advances, and as more and more journals offer the full text of their articles online, professionals have the potential to stay more current than before.

Other databases of information are also made readily available through the Internet. The American Self-Help Clearinghouse's Sourcebook[3] of self-help support organizations around the world makes it much easier to find a support group in one's community, or learn how to start one if none exists. Similar databases of health information, glossaries and medical dictionaries are also available online. Many of these types of resources were not available or not accessible before the Internet.

Interactive quizzes and support groups

Interactive online quizzes have made it possible for someone who suspects that they have a problem in a specific area to get immediate feedback about their symptoms (Fig. 25.3). This immediate feedback provides clients with a valuable resource, even if the results of the quiz are not always as empirical or as accurate as an in-depth intake evaluation by a trained mental health professional or a standard paper-and-pencil measure. The fear of the unknown, of suspecting a problem without knowing whether you have one or not, is often as debilitating as the disorder itself. While some of these quizzes are not as accurate as their paper-and-pencil counterparts, others are empirically based and validated. They also open the door to potential treatment, encouraging the client to seek out professional assistance if the questions answered suggest a possible diagnosis. Since the US Surgeon General's Mental Health Report[4] in 1999 showed that most people who qualify for a mental health diagnosis never seek out professional treatment, any method that may increase the number of people who are encouraged to seek treatment must be examined. Interactive quizzes are one such method.

These quizzes can also be used in another manner. Some measures are available online that allow an individual to monitor and track their scores on the quiz over time (see http://PsychTests.com for examples). Such measures allow clients, whether they are undergoing treatment or not, to track the progress of their moods and symptoms. These measures offer immediate feedback, they are psychometrically validated and are available to the client at any time.

Online support groups offer the Internet-aware client the chance to talk to others who suffer from a similar disorder. The positive, therapeutic effect of peer-run, self-help support groups has been well documented.[5] As available online, they offer a greater range of variety of topics from which to choose, as well as the convenience of participating in them as one's schedule allows. For instance, a client seeking a support group in their local town on dissociation may find it difficult to locate such a group. There are dozens of such online groups, however, available for the choosing. Often a person will turn to an online support group before seeking out professional treatment. The group can advise the client on different treatment modalities, what to expect from a competent and caring therapist, and what possible medications (and their side effects) are available. This information is often offered in a more opinionated and

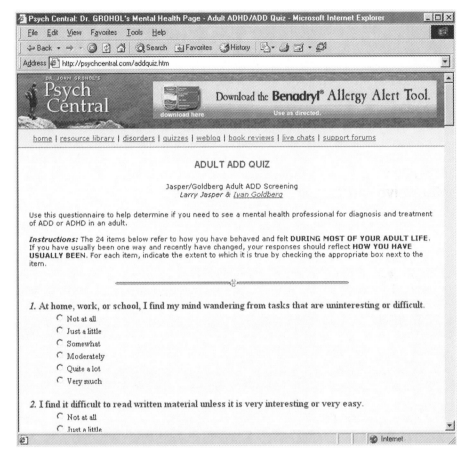

Fig. 25.3. An example of an interactive quiz from PsychCentral.com.

personalized manner than on a website. The social nature of the support group usually makes the information more digestible and easier to understand. The members of the group are speaking in a language that every other member understands (often very unlike the language used when professionals speak to clients). In addition, every member knows that most other members have been there themselves, making it feel like they 'are all in this together'. That group effect usually has a positive, beneficial impact for each of its members.

E-therapy

The most controversial of Internet innovations is e-therapy, a new modality of psychotherapy that takes places in many different forms. In its most common manifestation, e-therapy is performed as a stand-alone treatment via ordinary email.

Each 'session' is composed of an email from the client to the therapist, and the therapist's response back to the client (Fig. 25.4). Some therapists set limits on the length of the email message, while others charge on the basis of the time it takes for them to read and respond to the client's message. Generally these email exchanges cost less than half of a traditional face-to-face psychotherapy session.

Less commonplace are the use of real-time chat applications, instant messaging or videoconferencing modalities for e-therapy. Videoconferencing is generally similar to face-to-face psychotherapy, is covered under telemedicine guidelines and standards (see Chapter 21), and is most often used in rural environments. Chat applications, such as Internet Relay Chat (IRC) and instant messaging (IM), are also similar to face to face as they are real time and require scheduled appointment times; however they still take place in a text-only environment. Because all of these modalities require appointment times and take place in real time, they tend to lose many of the benefits traditionally associated with e-therapy, including anonymity, lower cost and greater convenience.

In addition to using e-therapy as a stand-alone treatment modality, many clients are using it as an adjunct to traditional psychotherapy care. Clients who can no longer

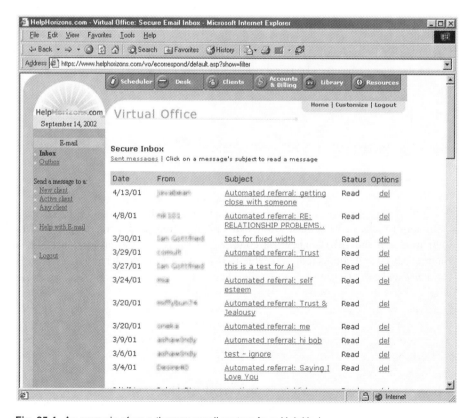

Fig. 25.4. An example of an e-therapy email system from HelpHorizons.com.

afford to see their regular therapist every week for treatment might add e-therapy to their treatment regimen as a way of filling in the gaps of their standard care. For instance, it is often impossible to express a reaction to a dream or other immediate crisis event to the person most able to help you cope or interpret it. E-therapy allows the client to record their thoughts and feelings whenever they have them, and have a much quicker reply than if they had to hold on to the event for a few days or even a week or more before getting some feedback on it. This greater immediacy can often lead to the client obtaining a more intensive treatment, which in turn leads to quicker positive outcomes.

Ferguson[6] differentiates these email modalities as Type 1 and Type 2. Type 1 email is when a client emails a doctor with no prior relationship established; Type 2 email is when the client has a pre-existing relationship with the doctor. Traditional physicians are already using email to help supplement ongoing patient care (Type 2), much as a telephone call, while other doctors are offering direct advice and information to individuals who ask for it online (Type 1). Both modalities fit well into the concept of e-therapy and can be useful for different types of individuals seeking care, under varying circumstances.

Therapists who support the e-therapy modality in their own practice often worry that it will lead to a greater workload, answering emails in their spare time and not getting paid for doing so. While it is currently true that under most conditions, insurance companies do not reimburse for e-therapy, such issues can be dealt with by directly billing the client for the service, or limiting the type or amount of care given via email. For instance, simply using email instead of the telephone to change or cancel an appointment can be more convenient for both parties, because neither is stuck playing an endless game of 'telephone tag'.

New paradigms: empowered clients, empowered providers

These Internet innovations are the tools that are empowering a new generation of clients. Some have called them the Y Generation of patients.[7] No longer limited by a lack of information about disorders or their treatment, this generation of clients is beginning to take more control of their treatment options and demanding more from their treatment providers. They are coming to expect that the professional will be Internet savvy and connected, to be able to reach their provider when it is convenient for them, and even to suggest a modality of care that may fit in better with the client's needs.

A side effect of all this greater information becoming available online is that professionals have to learn how to properly and positively deal with this information being brought into session. Clients become more educated consumers when the therapist goes over the information found online in this context, learning to distinguish accurate, objective information from inaccurate or biased opinion. Another side effect is that the more people put to rest their old stereotypes of psychotherapy and the more that people seek it out, the less stigma is associated with mental health problems in general.

Instead of the professional acting as the paternalistic expert, clients will increasingly look to the therapist or psychiatrist as a filter, a guide to the widening variety of treatment choices available. For instance, a client brings in information found online discussing a new relaxation technique that they would like to try. Some therapists might be offended by the suggestion, or feel embarrassed by their own unfamiliarity of the technique. The empowered provider will recognize the limits of their own knowledge, however, and work with the client, either to learn the technique if they believe it has any value, or to refer the client to another provider for this component of the client's treatment.

The therapist becomes the partner in care with the client, not the hand-holding empathetic expert. How can a professional understand what it is like to feel the symptoms associated with schizophrenia if they have never had it themselves? An online group allows the client to find genuine empathetic support from a group of others who truly know and understand the experience that they are going through. Instead of trying to be all things to all clients, therapists can use their skills and experience to help the client choose the treatments best suited for them. Perhaps face-to-face therapy once a week is simply not possible given the client's lifestyle. E-therapy becomes a viable alternative for the Internet-experienced client, after an initial face-to-face intake evaluation establishes the parameters of the therapeutic relationship.

If providers need convincing, they need look no further than a recent Harris poll.[8] The survey found that patients want more online doctor/patient communication, would pay for it, and it would even influence their choice of providers. Employers are also supportive and encourage employees to conduct more doctor visits by email.[9] They believe, with evidence to support their position, that such visits will increase the quality of health care for their employees. The empowered patient is not just a fad or passing phenomenon, it is the future of health care, and by extension, mental health care.

We can see the effects of this new paradigm already as a whole new field of professional coaching has gained exposure. These professionals view themselves as paid supporters or surrogate, upbeat friends for the client, helping to emphasize the positive aspects and resources in the individual's life, and working with them on ways to improve social skills and resources. Therapists can adopt some of these positive components for their own practices, looking to guide their clients in an active role of discovery, insight and change. Rather than being, as is often the case nowadays, the sole change agent in the client's life, empowered providers will help clients make use of many different possible resources that are available to help them change. In this role, therapists will actually have less work to do because the client is taking on more of the work themselves, or the work is being spread out amongst a wider array of helping resources (such as online support groups, adjunctive e-therapy, and the client's own online reading and journaling).

The professional's paternalistic attitude toward their clients is often characterized by the argument 'My clients are too sick to know what's best for them'. Indeed, when disorders such as major depression or schizophrenia are diagnosed, the client may often be in a state of mind where decisions about their own care cannot be made easily. Therapists do not have to give up all rights to helping guide a client to the choices that they believe will offer the best outcomes for their clients. By adopting a more open, flexible attitude to treatment that incorporates many of the components discussed above, the therapist can help the client discover resources and give them a sense of wonder and empowerment from the experience. All too often, clients feel overwhelmed by their disorder, and feel very alone and misunderstood with their feelings. A simple suggestion for joining an online support group, for instance, can make a significant difference to the client's life.

There are several useful sources of information to professionals who are contemplating the online road. MDNetGuide has an article[10] on this topic and Daniel Sands[11] has compiled an excellent website and written some useful guidelines about doctor–patient email that should be read (Fig. 25.5). Professionals who adapt their practices to this new generation of Internet-savvy patients will find their work often easier and perhaps more gratifying. The key to addressing the empowered client's needs is not to cater unquestioningly to them, but to understand and help guide them through the multitude of choices.

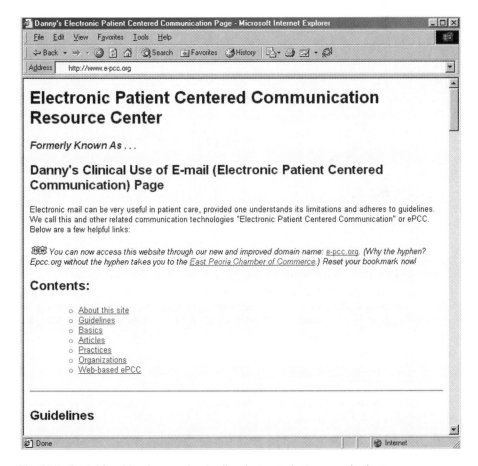

Fig. 25.5. Daniel Sands' web page about online doctor–patient communications.

Conclusion

Internet-savvy practitioners will embrace the empowered patient as an advancement in providing higher-quality care. Rather than adding to the professional's workload, the online client will reduce it, because the clients can better understand the difficulties they are facing and the treatment choices available. With added support from online peer groups, with added information from online websites, and with added opportunities for professional care, the empowered client is likely to be an individual who needs less direct care and less direction in implementing change. The client in the future will be better informed, not only of the possible disorder or dysfunction they are facing, but also of the treatment options available. Some will choose a treatment provider based on their own needs and the efficacy of the treatment after having done their own online MEDLINE research. Others will be content to discover that they are not alone in facing the disorder and to find other like-minded individuals in online support groups. Working online will mean less time spent on explanation and education with the client, and more time on actual change work and progress. The client will feel less helpless, better educated and a more active participant in their own treatment.

References

1   Grohol JM, ed. *The Insider's Guide to Mental Health Resources Online*. New York: Guilford Publications, 2000.
2   American Psychiatric Association. *Diagnostic and Statistical Manual of Mental Disorders*, 4th edn. Washington, DC: American Psychiatric Association, 1994.
3   White BJ, Madara EJ, eds. *The Self-help Sourcebook*. Denville, NJ: American Self-Help Clearinghouse, 1998.
4   US Department of Health and Human Services. *Mental Health: a report of the surgeon general*. Rockville, MD: US Department of Health and Human Services, Substance Abuse and Mental Health Services Administration, Center for Mental Health Services, National Institutes of Health, National Institute of Mental Health, 1999.
5   Kyrouz EM, Humphreys K. Research on self-help/mutual aid groups. Available at http://www.mentalhelp.net/poc/view_doc.php/type/doc/id/993 [last checked 3 September 2002].
6   Ferguson T. From doc-providers to coach-consultants: Type 1 versus Type 2 provider–patient relationships. The Ferguson Report. Available at http://fergusonreport.com/articles/tfr07-01.htm [last checked 3 September 2002].
7   Cascardo DC. Getting ready for the new generation of savvy patients. *Medscape Money and Medicine* 3(1). 2002. Available at http://www.medscape.com/viewarticle/436315 [last checked 14 September 2002].
8   Taylor H, Leitman R, eds. Patient/physician online communication: many patients want it, would pay for it, and it would influence their choice of doctors and health plans. *Harris Interactive Health Care News* 2002;**2**(8):1–3.
9   Carrns A. In effort to boost health-care quality, employers urge doctor visits by e-mail. *Wall Street Journal* 2001;23 March. Reproduced at http://www.genesispartners.co.il/html/news_23032001_wsj.shtm [last checked 15 September 2002].
10 How to make online patient communication work for you. *MD Net Guide Magazine, Primary Care Edition* 2002;**4**(3). Reproduced at http://www.mdnetguide.com/v4n3/pc_march/CoverStory_pc.shtml [last checked 3 September 2002].
11 Sands D. Electronic patient centered communication resource center. Available at http://www.e-pcc.org/ [last checked 3 September 2002].

26

Conclusion

Paul McLaren, Peter Yellowlees and Richard Wootton

Introduction

The experiences of the authors in this book demonstrate that telepsychiatry can be used in a variety of differing ways and for a broad range of purposes. The basic applications are clinical and educational but, in an increasingly patient-centred health environment, many applications particularly the educational and self-help ones, are relevant not only to clinicians, but also to patients. Perhaps the most important message of this book is that e-mental health offers a wide range of choices. The type of clinical or educational approach taken depends on the context in which the e-mental health service operates, and while most of the services to date have been performed in real time, particularly using videoconferencing or telephony, it is likely that in future more store and forward psychiatry will be practised. This is particularly the case for the provision of professional supervision and secondary patient consultations, all of which are likely to be available via email in the future.

Email has major advantages for e-mental health care because it is cheap and convenient for doctors and patients, but there is a need for research in this area in terms of its efficacy. Guidelines for the use of email between patients and doctors exist (see Chapters 5 and 21) and apply to the psychiatric consultation in the same way that they apply to consultations in other medical areas. Even if secondary consultations by email do not ultimately become common, the incorporation of email into the referral process will almost certainly occur because of its obvious cost and clinical advantages over the traditional postal system. Just as mental health services vary enormously in the face-to-face environment, so ultimately will e-mental health services vary and it is probable that a range of differing clinical electronic options will be utilized in differing places at differing times.

The issues in technology adoption have been well described. In the case of e-mental health they are not very different from those originally discussed by Rogers.[1] Rogers demonstrated that about 5–10% of any population were 'early adopters', and at present for most areas of e-mental health, it is these people who drive utilization. Telepsychiatry is on the verge of being adopted into the mainstream in some areas of Australia, where it has strong political support. Rogers hypothesized that 70–80% of providers will adopt technology if there is evidence to support its adoption. Rogers' final group were the last 10–15% of any population who are described as 'laggards'. This is the group who is least likely to change. The evidence base needs to be further strengthened to generate the critical masses of adopters required to make e-mental health and telepsychiatry economical.

Younger mental health professionals are entering the field with much stronger information technology skills and they are much more aware of the power of information and communication technology to enhance efficiency at work. This will lead to further innovation, more rapid adoption and ultimately improve the provision of e-mental health services around the world.

Future challenges

The challenges for e-mental health are of the human, rather than the technological variety. There are still major difficulties with licensure, registration and professional insurance both within countries, and across national, regional or international boundaries. Changes to legislative frameworks tend to be reactive, following changes in practice. Recognition that adequate assessments can be made by videoconferencing for the purposes of compulsory treatment will be important developments. So also will the development and adoption of national and international guidelines to ensure that the increased access offered by e-mental health service does not result in harm.

Many clinicians remain wary of practising e-mental health across national boundaries. This is a novel way of working, and one which requires substantial attitudinal change, with clinicians moving towards a philosophical perspective that puts the patient at the centre of any clinical or information exchange. This cultural change is being driven by the global consumer movement in mental health, where consumers are insisting on being partners in their own care, and in being kept fully informed. The Internet has proved to be a powerful tool for such groups of consumers, many of whom have set up impressive websites for their members, or for anyone interested in the disorders on which they focus.

A third challenge is remuneration for e-mental health activities. Governments have on the whole been slow to remunerate doctors for providing services using videoconferencing, although this does now happen in the USA. Other health systems have only allowed payment for videoconferencing when it is undertaken as part of the clinician's daily work, as in the case of public sector health systems in Australia and Canada. There has not yet, however, been general acceptance by governments of the process involved in videoconferencing in terms of making payments for it in the same manner as for face-to-face services. Payments for email and telephony services are most unusual. There are some health sectors in the USA that will pay for short email consultations, although not usually in psychiatry. In health, time on the telephone has not been paid for, unlike in the practice of law.

Technological developments

There is also the question of technology. E-mental health in future will probably use Internet protocols in a broadband environment, and the speed of their implementation will depend in part on the rate of broadband roll out. This is less of a problem in public sector services, where fibreoptic networks are increasingly being deployed, but will be difficult in terms of covering 'the last mile' to a patient's home, or to the clinics of individual mental health practitioners. The emergence of broadband networks will undoubtedly accelerate the use of e-mental health services. It will be interesting to see whether health practitioners and services can work more closely with telecommunications providers in future.

Further research

The final problem area relates to the need for further research in e-mental health, and a stronger evidence base. Whilst there are now increasing numbers of papers focusing on the reliability of the diagnosis of psychiatric disorders via communications technology, there are very few that look at mental health outcomes following treatment in an online environment, or in a combination of online services and face-to-face consultations. There have been very few long-term randomized controlled trials of e-mental health in any of its forms. Getting funding for trials with sufficient power to demonstrate clinical effectiveness in a range of disorders and settings has proved difficult. There is also a need for larger economic evaluations. Most benefits derived from telepsychiatry services in areas with low population density accrue to service users, who have to travel less and spend less time away from home. The financial benefits for health services are much less certain and need further clarification. An additional complication is the rapid development of the technology. In the 2–3 years that it takes to complete a clinical trial the specification of the equipment tested is likely to become obsolete. It seems probable, however, that e-mental health services will become increasingly cost effective as they migrate to the broadband Internet.

The ultimate proof of success for an e-mental health application is long-term funding and, in particular, the integration of e-mental health services into mainstream budgetary processes. This is still a relatively rare occurrence, and unfortunately around the world many projects continue to be funded only as pilot projects, often reinventing the wheel in terms of research objectives and outcomes, and petering out because they have been too small to create their own cultural change or statistically powerful results. Much more could be gained from telepsychiatry research if smaller projects could be combined to improve statistical power and reduce administrative costs.

Relatively little is known about the significance of image parameters in videoconferencing for clinical processes. In the telepsychiatry research reviewed in this book videoconferencing equipment with a broad range of specification has been used. The experience of communicating over a videophone connected by the telephone network and a rollabout videoconferencing unit connected by a T1 digital line is very different. High specification equipment costs more to buy and costs more to operate. It produces a better quality image but what quality of image is good enough for which task? Basic information on the relationship between image parameters, such as definition, colour scale, frame rate and image size, and clinical outcomes is still lacking.

E-mental health and the future of psychotherapy

The educational and information-gathering components of the cognitive behavioural therapies (CBT) are ideally suited to computerization. The building blocks of the therapeutic relationship, which are central to all therapies, are still poorly understood and still too nebulous to digitize. This may lead to the development of hybrid models of CBT with the information-gathering, self-monitoring and educational components delivered by information technology while the therapist focuses on live sessions. This will allow the total time in therapy for service users to be increased, while the therapist's time is reduced and better focused. The efficiency and effectiveness of the psychotherapies could be improved and if the relationship component is delivered by communications technology then access will be improved and costs to service users reduced.

The delivery of psychotherapy by intelligent information systems should not be seen as a threat to existing service providers. Attempts should be made to integrate the technology into other service delivery models. In the next phase of e-mental health development we are likely to see more people having therapy on the Internet or on computer in their family doctor's surgery. This will be a particular advantage to those living in rural and isolated areas.

E-mental health and service users

Most service users who have been asked have found that e-mental health services were acceptable.[2] They like the increased access and the choice that they have via such services, and it has been suggested that they also like to have the ability, if they so wish, to 'switch off' the practitioner. Some authors have suggested that some service users may prefer being assessed or treated electronically, namely those patients who are paranoid or avoidant.[3] There are also those who live a very long way away from conventional health services and for whom these types of services are much more convenient. The potential of e-mental health to improve access for those with severe and enduring mental illnesses needs particular attention.

E-mental health and professional users

Psychiatrists have been the professional group most often associated with the development of e-mental health services, perhaps because they are in a more clinically powerful position and are more likely to be paid for such services. There are a number of psychiatrists around the world who have amassed considerable clinical experience in providing e-mental health services, mainly by videoconferencing. One of the problems for providing telepsychiatry services is that it is patients and GPs, in rural areas on the whole, who have the main gains from the services. Psychiatrists who provide these services, typically from major cities, have usually done so through a sense of altruism or because of a research interest.

Psychiatrists using videoconferencing have had issues with picture resolution and video frame rate.

GPs, nurses, clinical psychologists and social workers provide the bulk of mental health services. Their role in e-mental health service provision has, on the whole, been one of supporting the patients, of being part of the consultation from the patient end and of being on the receiving end of educational activities. It is reassuring that GPs, in particular, are increasingly taking a more proactive role in e-mental health service provision, and in this book there are good examples of nurses and psychologists taking up similar roles. It is to be hoped that e-mental health practice will become much more widespread in nursing and psychological practice in future.

The future of e-mental health services

E-mental health services are likely to continue to expand as communication technologies become integrated on to an Internet protocol platform and delivered via broadband links. Patients will have access to their own electronic health records, which will be available to their clinicians. During consultations, either face to face or online, clinicians will be able to access health information on the Internet, and share this with patients through the use of distributed systems technology.

Policy makers need more outcome-focused research and economic data on e-mental health to guide investment. It is clear from this book that at present we have the technology to deliver mental health services to more people in more places. We are not far from being able to conduct videoconferencing in people's homes. The entertainment industry will drive the connectivity and technology development for home communication. Health services will have much to gain. While technology races ahead the challenge is its integration to harness the benefits for all.

In respect of community mental health services, e-mental health has still to make a major impact. A key research question to be asked in community mental health care, is 'Which communications medium is most appropriate for which task?'. Most community mental health services use the telephone, the postal system and the face-to-face mode for communication with service users and between professionals. Videoconferencing will soon be widely available and can be added to that repertoire. Face-to-face communication, which in distributed community services requires travelling, is expensive for services and service users. Travel time is wasted time for both parties. The costs of travel will vary with population density. Using communications technology may offer significant savings. More research is required to analyse the costs and benefits of using the telephone, videoconferencing, email, the post and face-to-face communication for core clinical tasks.

There is a need for international standards development in telemedicine and e-health in general, and this may require the involvement of groups. Guidelines and pathways for mental health care will be incorporated into day-to-day practice, and many of these are already being produced in electronic format, and in a manner that will allow them to be integrated with Internet based e-health systems. The IT industry has tended not to focus on product evaluation, and it will be up to clinicians in particular to ensure that any new IT products are properly evaluated, and that evidence in support of them is acceptable to the greater body of health professionals. Without this continuous evaluation and research it will be hard for e-mental health care to move forward as rapidly as it should, and to become sustainable.

There are a range of exciting advance technologies on the horizon, particularly the use of three-dimensional technologies, image processing and data mining (see Chapter 22), and this makes it likely that the psychiatrist's role will change to that of being an expert in data analysis and teaching, with less time spent on individual patient consultations, and more time spent working with groups of other mental health professionals in a supervisory or secondary consultation approach, all facilitated by information and communications technology. A major role is going to be that of guiding the patient through the problems of information overload.

Mental health professionals will have their most important role as face-to-face clinicians for the foreseeable future. E-mental health services will not completely replace face-to-face work, but rather supplement these activities, particularly in areas of low population density or where service users, who because of their particular attitudes or psychopathology, prefer the balance of power, level of intimacy or anonymity offered by a digital consultation.

Communications technology stimulates communication and this book is the result of many new collaborations and friendships which the technology has supported. Authors from five different countries have contributed in a spirit of international collaboration which will grow with the opportunities to communicate.

We hope that you have enjoyed this book.

References

1   Rogers EM. *Diffusion of Innovations*. New York: The Free Press, 1962.
2   Hilty DM, Luo JS, Morache C, Marcelo DA, Nesbitt TS. Telepsychiatry: an overview for psychiatrists. *CNS Drugs* 2002;**16**:527–548.
3   Yellowlees P. *Your Guide to E-Health – third millennium medicine on the Internet*. Brisbane: University of Queensland Press, 2001.

Index

Page numbers in **bold** refer to boxes, figures and tables